Autoimmune Endocrine Disease

Autoimmune Endocrine Disease

Edited by

Terry F. Davies

Associate Professor of Medicine
Division of Endocrinology
Mt. Sinai School of Medicine,
New York, New York

A Wiley-Interscience Publication

JOHN WILEY & SONS

New York • Chichester • Brisbane • Toronto • Singapore

Library of Congress Cataloging in Publication Data:

Main entry under title:

Autoimmune endocrine disease.

    ''A Wiley-Interscience publication.''
    Includes index.
    1. Endocrine glands—Diseases—Immunological aspects.
2. Autoimmune diseases.   I. Davies, Terry F. (Terry
Francis), 1947-   .   [DNLM: 1. Autoimmune diseases—
Physiopathology.   2. Endocrine diseases—Physiopathology.
3. Autoimmune diseases—Immunology.   4. Endocrine diseases—Immunology.   WL 100 A9385]

RC649.A97   1983   616.4′079   82-17318
ISBN 0-471-09778-0

Printed in the United States of America

10   9   8   7   6   5   4   3   2   1

Contributors

Duncan D. Adams
Autoimmunity Research Unit
Medical Research Council of New Zealand
University of Otago Medical School
Dunedin, New Zealand

Nobuyuki Amino
The Central Laboratory for Clinical
    Investigation
Osaka University Hospital
Fukushima-ku, Osaka, Japan

John C. Bear
Division of Community Medicine
Faculty of Medicine
Memorial University of Newfoundland
St. John's, Newfoundland, Canada

Kirk W. Beisel
Department of Immunology and Infectious
    Diseases
Johns Hopkins University School of
    Hygiene and Public Health
Baltimore, Maryland

Terry F. Davies
Division of Endocrinology
Mount Sinai School of Medicine
New York, New York

Erica DeBernardo
Division of Endocrinology
Mount Sinai School of Medicine
New York, New York

George S. Eisenbarth
Joslin Diabetes Center
Brigham Hospital
Harvard Medical School
Boston, Massachusetts

Melissa Elder
Division of Clinical Chemistry

Department of Pathology
University of Florida College of Medicine
J. Hillis Miller Health Center
Gainesville, Florida

Nadir R. Farid
Division of Endocrinology and Metabolism
Department of Medicine and Thyroid
    Research Laboratory
Memorial University of Newfoundland
St. John's, Newfoundland, Canada

Norbert Gleicher
Department of Obstetrics and Gynecology
Mount Sinai Hospital Medical Center of
    Chicago
Chicago, Illinois

Leonard C. Harrison
The Endocrine Laboratory and Department
    of Medicine
The Royal Melbourne Hospital
Victoria, Australia

Gilbert G. Haas, Jr.
Department of Obstetrics and Gynecology
The University of Pennsylvania School of
    Medicine
Philadelphia, Pennsylvania

Paula Heyma
The Endocrine Laboratory and Department
    of Medicine
The Royal Melbourne Hospital
Victoria, Australia

Åke Lernmark
Hagedorn Research Laboratory
Gentofte, Denmark

Noel Maclaren
Division of Clinical Chemistry
Department of Pathology

University of Florida College of Medicine
J. Hillis Miller Health Center
Gainesville, Florida

Sandra McLachlan
Department of Medicine
Royal Victoria Infirmary
Newcastle Upon Tyne, United Kingdom

Kiyoshi Miyai
The Central Laboratory for Clinical
    Investigation
Osaka University Hospital
Fukushima-KU, Osaka, Japan

George K. Papadopoulos
Hagedorn Research Laboratory
Gentofte, Denmark

Nelson Rassi
Universidad Federal beGoias
Goiania, Brazil

Noel R. Rose
Department of Immunology and Infectious
    Diseases
Johns Hopkins University School of
    Hygiene and Public Health
Baltimore, Maryland

Israel Siegel
Department of Obstetrics & Gynecology
Mount Sinai Hospital Medical Center of
    Chicago
Chicago, Illinois

Bernard Rees Smith
Endocrine Immunology Unit
Department of Medicine
Welsh National School of Medicine
Cardiff, United Kingdom

W. M. G. Tunbridge
Newcastle General Hospital
Newcastle Upon Tyne, United Kingdom

Preface

The escalation in our knowledge of immune mechanisms has spilled over into many areas of medicine. In no area has this been greater than in the delineation of a variety of diseases of the endocrine gland which have now been recognized to be secondary to immune dysfunction. Although such diseases may afflict up to 5% of the population, there are few books available which bring them together and allow both physicians and scientists to obtain an overall grasp of the subject and a clear introduction to the important literature. In fact, it is only very recently that immunologists and endocrinologists have begun meeting to discuss their views on these important diseases.

It was not our intention, therefore, to produce a textbook of medicine which would outline the causes, the presentation, and the treatment of the various autoimmune endocrine diseases since this type of information is available in numerous textbooks of medicine. Rather, we have tried to provide a modern update on the principles of autoimmunity as applied to the endocrine system and to bring together some of the rapidly advancing knowledge on endocrine-related immune dysfunction. The book is aimed not just at the clinical investigator, but at scientists in the biological and immunologic fields who wish to gain a grasp of the various entities from a mechanistic point of view. Needless to say, it has not been possible to cover everyone's area of interest adequately. In particular, parathyroid failure and Graves' ophthalmic disease receive little attention in this volume. There are few new immune data to report on these diseases, but this may change in the near future.

Data documented in the following pages provide evidence that many answers appear to be within technological reach; my colleagues have all contributed enlightening chapters, some controversial, to help disseminate this message. I thank them all most sincerely for giving me such a pleasant task in bringing them together.

TERRY F. DAVIES

New York, New York
January 1983

Contents

1

Autoimmune Mechanisms

Duncan D. Adams

Autoimmunity Research Unit
Medical Research Council of New Zealand
University of Otago Medical School
Dunedin, New Zealand

Contents

1. INTRODUCTION

It is a little more than 100 years since Louis Pasteur laid the foundations of immunology by introducing the germ theory of disease (1), in opposition to the prevailing theory that life was generated spontaneously in decaying organic matter. Pasteur obtained experimental evidence against this, discovered that wines could be spoiled by infection with living microorganisms, and went on to demonstrate the existence of diseases of animals and man caused by infection with microbial parasites. The period from 1880 to 1900 was a golden age for medicine, during which the causes of a score of common diseases were revealed. Moreover, the intellectual foundations were laid for aseptic surgery and for the discovery of antibiotics. Meanwhile investigators such as Paul Ehrlich became conscious of the existence of the immunity system, with its antibodies, of myriad specificities, and of a nonspecific executive system (complement) which would lyse bacterial cells selected by antibody. This was the first great epoch of immunology—the discovery of the immunity system as our defense against infectious diseases and the consequent development of a technology which has culminated in today's superb clinical competence in the prophylaxis or therapy of these diseases.

The second great epoch of immunology is the current, unfinished struggle against autoimmune disease. This research was slow to be initiated. Ehrlich and his contemporaries, observing that an erythrocyte could be lysed by antibody and complement, similarly to a bacterium, wondered whether the immune system ever malfunctioned and attacked the host. However, Ehrlich's own attempts to induce goats to make autoantibodies against their own erythrocytes failed, leading him to propound the dictum of "horror autotoxicus," which held that autoimmunity does not normally occur (2). Nevertheless, Ehrlich appreciated that autoimmunity might happen as an abnormality and be responsible for the occurrence of disease (3). Unfortunately, in the confusion of World War I Ehrlich's caveat was forgotten and after the war for several decades young immunologists were taught that Ehrlich had proved that autoimmunity was impossible. Once again, a blocking concept became popular and obstructed progress. In 1938, for example, Dameshek and Schwartz (4) demonstrated the existence of autoantibodies against erythrocytes in cases of hemolytic anemia, but this had little influence, being ascribed to "autoallergy" or "socalled" autoimmunity (5).

Endocrinologists can take satisfaction in knowing that it was workers in their field who broke the intellectual shackles against autoimmunity. In London, Doniach and Roitt looked for and found autoantibodies against a thyroid antigen in cases of Hashimoto's disease (6). In Buffalo, Witebsky's team demonstrated that autoimmune thyroiditis could be induced in rabbits by use of Freund's adjuvants (7). The year was 1957. Since then, progress in autoimmunity has come painfully slowly, so that 25 years later only Graves' disease and myasthenia gravis are understood in detail, the pathogenic clones for a number of probable autoimmune diseases remain to be demonstrated, and no general principle of therapy for autoimmune disease has emerged. The inherent difficulty of the scientific problems involved is obviously the main reason for this failure, but it behooves us to ask two questions. First, have our researches been concentrated in the most likely directions, and second, are we being hindered by any false concepts, as has happened so often in the past?

Chapter 2 considers the genetics of autoimmunity from a viewpoint most properly influenced by the findings and concepts of recent experimental immunology, including the ingenious research on the histocompatibility antigen system. In this chapter, I include some concepts which are different from and, I think, simpler than their counterparts presently fashionable in some circles in immunology. With the major problems of autoimmune disease unsolved, some variety of interpretation is obviously most desirable. Being a clinician, working in comparative isolation remote in the South Pacific, I have been partially insulated from popular research fashions, but have been heavily influenced by (i) the concepts of the two great immunologic thinkers, Macfarlane Burnet and Nils Jerne and (ii) the great wealth of information available from clinical autoimmune disease.

2. AN ENDOCRINOLOGIST'S VIEW OF THE IMMUNITY SYSTEM

2.1. The Fundamentals

The Purpose of the Immunity System

In attempting to understand the immunity system it is helpful to bear in mind its purpose, that is, the reason for its development by the process of evolution. Observations on individuals in whom the immune system is genetically deficient or artificially suppressed by irradiation or drugs show clearly that the system's purpose is the defense of the host against infectious disease and malignant neoplasm. For achievement of this defense, the immunity system has one basic tool, a machine that can stamp out an unlimited variety of polypeptide chains. The variety of these chains is provided by random gene mutation and recombination in both germ cells and somatic cells, together with DNA and RNA rearrangement in somatic cells. The specificity of the chains is governed by Charles Darwin's principle of natural selection of random variants for reproductive advantage. Operating on populations of people and their ancestors, natural selection has provided the necessary components of the immunity system, including granulocytes, macrophages, T cells, B cells, immunoglobulins, complement, and the histocompatibility system. Additionally, in the continuing struggle against constantly mutating pathogenic parasites, natural selection continues to alter the range of specificities in the system, steering a course between the Scylla of infection and the Charybdis of autoimmune disease. For example, when Europeans colonized New Zealand, the indigenous Maori people, although possessing all the organs and cell types of the Europeans, were nearly exterminated by diseases such as measles, whooping cough, and tuberculosis. It is likely that the reason for this was a difference in immune response repertoire (see below) between the two populations, partly genetic (caused by different microbial pathogens acting on ancestors) and partly environmental (caused by exposure to a different spectrum of microbial antigens in childhood). Subsequently, this difference in susceptibility to infection has been largely corrected by natural selection and intermarriage.

Selection

The immunity system has to be able to distinguish an invading pathogenic microor-

ganism from a host component. This is the function of antibodies, including those expressed as receptors on T lymphocytes (see Section 2.2). Originally it was believed that foreign antigens were ingested by immunocytes and used as templates for the construction of a complementary antibody receptor. However, in 1955, Nils Jerne, with extraordinary scientific intuition, put forward the theory that the process was not one of induction, but of *selection* (8). Jerne postulated that antibodies are not built to fit an antigen but are preformed in large variety, awaiting selection by a complementary antigen, like readymade suits in a shop, awaiting the arrival of a customer who fits. Macfarlane Burnet, another powerful scientific thinker, accepted Jerne's selection theory but realized that behind each antibody there must be a cell. An extensive experience in microbiology had given Burnet a deep understanding of the behavior of large populations of living cells. With cultured bacteria, he had seen mutation and natural selection in action. Burnet's famous "*clonal selection theory of acquired immunity*" (9) is now universally accepted. Before consideration of the immunological clone, it is pertinent to note that immunologic selection occurs in two senses. Antibody or the corresponding T cell receptor selects the foreign target for attack by the executive system, but the foreign antigen can also be thought of as selecting its complementary clone from the large number existing, and stimulating it to proliferate.

The Clone

If a potato is divided into pieces and these are put into the ground, the resultant group of genetically identical plants is known in horticulture as a "clone." Burnet (9) introduced this term to immunology to describe a group of immunocytes with identical receptors for antigen. Implicit in the clonal concept are two assumptions, namely, (1) that a single immunocyte produces antibody of only one specificity and (2) that antibody of a single specificity is produced by more than one immunocyte. Both these fundamentally important assumptions now have experimental confirmation.

The need to be able to provide a clone for any possible microbial pathogen, present or future, necessitates provision of a large variety or *repertoire* of clones. These originate as undeveloped or *virgin clones*, devoid of experience of contact with complementary antigen. The great majority of clones probably remain in this state. When, however, a virgin clone does meet a complementary antigen, its cells enlarge (blast transformation) and divide to form a *developed clone* of greatly increased numbers. Every time a cell divides its DNA has to be copied. This process has a finite chance of error. Such copying errors in somatic (nongerm-line) cells are known as *somatic mutations* (see below). During the very large numbers of cell divisions that occur in a clone after antigenic contact, somatic mutations are inevitable. When these involve variable region genes (see below) they alter the antigenic specificity of the cell, creating a new clone.

The forbidden clones of autoimmunity are discussed in Sections 3 and 4.

Somatic Mutation

Whereas the phenomenon of germ-line mutation is at the forefront of every biologist's mind, the equivalent process occurring in dividing somatic cells has been rather overlooked, especially by students of immunology and pathology. Clonal diversification by somatic mutation occurring during the mitotic stimulus of antigenic contact is probably essential for effective immune defense against infection. Similarly, T cells developing in the thymus, subject to a mitogenic stimulus from the thymic hormone, thymosin, must also undergo clonal diversification by somatic mutation. Jerne has described the thymus as a mutant-breeding organ (10).

In medicine, the initiating factors for many diseases are unknown. For many years it was popular to ascribe the onset of Graves' disease to a psychological factor, or "stress," meaning a severe fright or other psychological upset.

However, a controlled study of Graves' disease showed psychic traumata to be no more frequent in the patients than in controls (11). Furthermore, Graves' disease was not more common in soldiers suffering the terror of World War I trench warfare or in Russians or Jews suffering under the Nazis. In reality, the probable initiating factor for Graves' and other autoimmune diseases is the occurrence of a somatic mutation in a V gene in an immunocyte, with the formation of a forbidden clone from what might be described as a pre-forbidden clone.

Most somatic mutations cause death of the cell involved and thus are of little consequence apart from slowly reducing the number of cells in a tissue. The important exceptions are (i) in immunocytes, where a single mutant cell can found a new clone, which may be helpful in overcoming an infection or harmful in initiating autoimmunity, and (ii) when the new cell has neoplastic property, initiating growth of a tumor.

Geneticists, preoccupied with various germ-line genes and their mutations, curiously tend to ignore somatic mutation, ascribing its effects to "environmental factors." This has some truth in it, for most somatic mutations probably occur during the cell divisions occasioned by antigenic stimulus from infecting microorganisms, which are indeed environmental factors. However, the increased precision of thought that would result from recognition of involvement of somatic mutation is obviously desirable.

Figure 1 depicts clonal selection by antigen and clonal diversification through somatic mutation. Weigert et al. (12), after obtaining clear evidence from amino acid sequence studies of lambda light chains from mouse plasmacytomas, have provided a lucid account of the role of somatic mutation and antigenic selection in amplification of clonal diversity. Further evidence has come recently from DNA sequencing by Bernard et al. (13).

The Limitations of Somatic Mutation. It is crucial to realize that the occurrence of

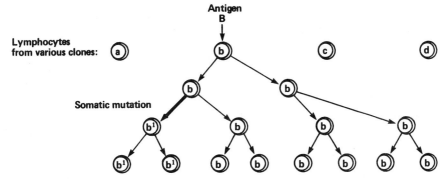

Figure 1.   Clonal selection by antigenic stimulation and clonal diversification by somatic mutation. Concept of Jerne (8) and Burnet (9); biochemical evidence of somatic mutation by Weigert et al. (12) and Bernard et al. (13). *Clone*: a set of lymphocytes with identical receptors for antigen.

somatic mutation does not mean that all clones are interconvertible. Mutation is responsible for the differences between animal species, yet a man cannot mutate to a monkey because an impossibly large number of randomly determined events would be needed. In antibody combining sites (paratopes, see Section 2.2), the six hypervariable regions each involve at least 3 of the 20 available amino acids, allowing 20^{18} or 2.6×10^{23} different amino acid combinations apart from variations in the intervening (framework) portions of the variable (V) region. This means that, as with animals, there are *species* of antibodies, and mutation from one species to another is not possible.

Regulation of the Immunity System

In endocrinology, negative feedback, in which a hormone acts to inhibit its own production, is the mechanism by which secretion of thyroid, adrenal, ovarian, and testicular hormones is regulated, through the mediation of the pituitary gland with its specific trophic hormones. No such mechanism is apparent in the immunity system, which appears to be largely governed by local effects, like a free-enterprise, local market-governed economic system as opposed to a centrally controlled system.

In considering immune regulation it is obviously essential to distinguish between control of cell numbers and control of clonal specificity.

Quantity Control.   This is the defense against occurrence of leukemia or lymphoma. Taussig (14) was quick to recognize that the function of suppressor T cells (see below) is to limit cell division in a clone expanding under antigenic stimulation. Philip et al. (15) have observed that neutrophil granulocytes from some patients with chronic granulocytic leukemia fail to release an inhibitor of granulopoiesis. On the other hand, helper T cells play an essential role in enhancing the cell divisions involved in the mounting of an immune response. Quantity control by helper and suppressor T cells and their soluble factors is discussed in Section 2.3.

Specificity Control.   Failure of this function is the crux of autoimmunity and is considered in detail in Section 2.4 (tolerance), Section 2.5 (immune response repertoire), and Section 3 (genesis of forbidden clones). Mechanisms subserving tolerance to self-antigens appear to be invariably successful for the major histocompatibility antigens and the ABO blood group antigens, but unreliable for certain other self-antigens. Natural selection acting on random specificity variants is probably the main mechanism governing range of specificity (repertoire of clones). Allison (16) observed that people heterozygous for sickle cell anemia have increased resistance to malaria. This explains why sickle cell anemia, which is lethal in the homozygous form, is unusually common in people living in regions where malaria occurs. The lethality of the sickle cell anemia gene in the homozygous state confers a reproductive disadvantage, but this is balanced by the reproductive advantage of resistance to malaria conferred by the gene in the heterozygous state. The phenomenon is described as *balanced genetic polymorphism*. The relatively high incidence of autoimmune diabetes and thyroid disease (both of the order of 1% of the population) may be due to a similar balanced polymorphism; the genes predisposing to these autoimmune diseases, when in different combination, may be advantageous for defense against important infections.

2.2. Basic Anatomy and Physiology

In this section, the bare bones of immunology are sketched, with a view to providing clinicians with the rational framework needed for their work. Where more detail is required an ideal source is Roitt's *Essential Immunology* (17).

Antibodies and Their Genes

Just as the molecular structure of DNA and RNA is entirely comprehensible in the light of knowledge of what these molecules do, so the complexity of antibody molecules and their structural genes becomes elegantly simple when considered in relationship to their function.

Discovery of Antibody Structure. Rodney Porter (18) made a remarkable discovery when he tested the effect of the plant enzyme papain on antibody molecules in the form of gamma globulins from rabbit blood. Instead of splitting the antibody molecules into a large number of haphazard peptide chains, as would be expected, the papain treatment produced only three fragments. One of these was crystallizable (fragment C), which indicated that it was composed of identical or closely similar peptides. The other two fragments were not crystallizable, indicating a heterogeneity consistent with inclusion of the antibody combining sites (fragments Ab). Meanwhile, Edelman had applied reducing agents to gamma globulins (19). These cleaved disulfide bonds, showing that antibody molecules are composed of two types of polypeptide chains —long, or *heavy* chains and short, or *light* chains. Further progress was hindered by the myriad diversity of antibody molecules in gamma globulin preparations. However, pioneers such as Henry Kunkel overcame this problem by obtaining monoclonal antibodies from patients suffering from tumors originating in single antibody-producing cells (multiple myeloma). Such patients secrete monoclonal antibody light chains (Bence-Jones protein) in their urine. Determining the amino acid sequence of such light chains, Hilschmann and Craig (20) found that the 100-odd amino acids at the NH_2 terminal end were different in sequence for each patient tested, but that the remaining 100-odd amino acids at the COOH end of the peptide were virtually identical for all patients. Similarly, heavy chains of myeloma proteins obtained from plasma were found to be variable in the first 100-odd amino acids from the NH_2 end but relatively constant in the sequence of the remainder of the chain comprising about 300 amino acids.

Thus the molecular basis of antibody specificity was discovered to lie in the sequence of amino acids occupying the first 100 positions from the NH_2 terminals of the light and heavy polypeptide chains which form antibody molecules. Subsequent detail has been provided by (i) the discovery of *intrachain disulfide bonds* which contribute to the folding necessary for the three-dimensional configuration of the molecules, (ii) the finding of three or four *hypervariable regions* (21) distributed along the variable regions, comprising a few amino acid positions each and being approximated in the antibody combining site by chain folding, and (iii) the discovery of minor variations in amino acid sequence in the "constant" region of the heavy chain, accounting for the various *classes* of antibody needed for various executive roles.

Definitions.   The chemists coined the term "immunoglobulin" at a time when they were unsure that all the gamma globulins and myeloma proteins with which they were working were in fact antibodies. This is no longer in doubt, but the term "immunoglobulin" has remained and is conveniently abbreviated to describe the various classes and subclasses of antibody. Jerne (22) has provided the terms "epitope" and "paratope" (from the Greek *topos*, a place) to sharpen thinking of antigen–antibody reactions. "Tope" is conveniently changed to "type" to describe an individual specificity.

Epitope   That part of the antigen molecule which actually fits into the complementary combining site of the antibody.

Paratope   The combining site of an antibody molecule, known to be a molecular cleft.
Antibody molecules are themselves antigenic and therefore possess their own epitopes. These are of two types.

Idiotope   An epitope on the variable part of an antibody, formed by the same two polypeptide chains which form the paratope and hence coded for by the same two V genes (see below). This arrangement, which provides each paratope with an antigenic handle in the form of an idiotope, attackable by the paratope of another antibody, may be important for avoidance of autoimmune disease, as discussed below.

Allotope   An epitope formed by the polypeptide chains that constitute the constant region of the molecule and hence are coded for by the heavy or light chain constant region (C) genes (see below).

Allotopes provide genetic markers for immunoglobulin C genes. They are somewhat analogous to the ABO red cell antigens. For example, about 50% of Europeans have the allotype Gm1 and 50% do not. Idiotopes have special significance as clonal markers, markers for V genes.

How Antibodies Function.   Figure 2 depicts an antibody molecule of IgG class (see below, this section). There are two identical paratopes in the form of clefts at the ends of the two arms of the Y-shaped molecule. Selection of the foreign target subserved by the paratopes is linked to executive action through the activation sites for complement, situated in the hinge region at the junction of the stem and the arms of the Y. These sites are nonfunctional until the antibody molecule combines with a complementary epitope, when attachment of the first component of complement occurs, triggering the enzymatic cascade which culminates in lysis of the bacterial or other cell bearing the complementary epitope. This ingenious arrangement allows a powerful, nonspecific, cell-destruction mechanism (complement) to be brought to bear on foreign targets selected with great precision by the antibody molecules (see below).

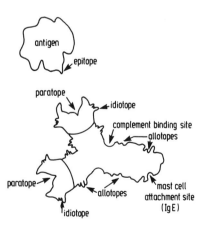

Figure 2.   An antibody molecule of IgG class, showing the two identical *paratopes* (combining sites for antigen) (22) and the complementary *epitope* (22) of the antigen molecule. Also shown are the *idiotopes* (constant region epitopes) and the attachment sites for the C1q molecule of the complement system. Additionally, an attachment site for mast cells, present on IgE molecules, is depicted.

In Figure 2 the epitopes of the molecule, both idiotopes and allotopes, are depicted as protrusions because they are complementary to paratopes, which are clefts.

The basic antibody molecule, as depicted in Figure 2, is composed of four polypeptide chains, two identical heavy chains, and two identical light chains, joined by disulfide bonds. As already mentioned, the first 100-odd amino acids from the NH_2 terminal end of the heavy and the light chain form the variable region of the antibody molecule, with its paratope and idiotope(s), the remainder of the chains forming the constant region. Variations in the amino acid sequences of the polypeptide chains forming the constant region give rise to the various *classes* of antibody.

IgG molecules (Figure 2) with the basic configuration are the most abundant in the blood and afford prophylaxis against infection by any incoming pathogen for which they have a complementary paratope. Some IgG molecules (when their paratopes are occupied by a complementary epitope) activate complement; some do not.

IgM molecules are big pentamers of five IgG-like molecules, with 10 radially disposed paratopes giving powerful agglutinating power, like a bidibid, useful early in infection before high affinity for the microorganism has developed by somatic mutation. IgM molecules, in combination with epitope, are always complement activators.

IgA molecules are dimers of two IgG-like molecules with a protective shield blocking proteolysis of the vulnerable hinge region, so that they can retain activity in the acid secretions of the nose and stomach.

IgE molecules have attachment sites for mast cells, which they cause to release histamine when their paratope is occupied by a complementary epitope. This may be a device for expelling worms from the gut by local inflammation and violent peristaltic movements. Allergy is probably a malfunction of this system, owing to the presence of IgE clones with appropriate paratope specificity.

How Genes for Antibodies Function. Three chromosomes bear the structural genes for antibody molecules (23). The heavy chain genes are on chromosome 14 (24). Light chains, as obtained from the urine of myeloma patients, were found to be of two antigenically different types, designated kappa and lambda, the genes for each type being on separate chromosomes.

The finding that polypeptide chains for antibodies have variable and constant parts was an intriguing challenge to understanding how their genes function. Dreyer and Bennett (25) solved the puzzle, correctly postulating that separate genes code for the variable and constant parts and that any one of a considerable number of V genes can combine with one of the few C genes to produce a single messenger RNA molecule coding for the entire heavy or light chain. After the junction of the heavy and light chains by disulfide bondage, the antibody-producing cell secretes the complete antibody molecule.

Recently it has become possible to determine the nucleotide sequences in the DNA of antibody genes. This has shown that several short J (joining) and D (diversity) genes can combine at random with the major portion of the V genes, a process of somatic recombination which greatly increases the variability of the third hypervariable region (26). The variability of the first two hypervariable regions, however, appears to depend entirely on somatic mutation and selection by antigenic stimulation.

The Complement System

In the words of Manfred Mayer (27), ''A foreign cell in the body is identified by antibody, but the cell is destroyed by other agents. Among them is 'complement,' an intricately linked set of enzymes.''

Now, largely owing to the recent work led by Rodney Porter and Hans Müller-Eberhard, the complement system is understood in impressive detail (28). As well as mediating lysis of foreign cells, the complement system is involved in facilitation of phagocytosis (opsonization), mediation of inflammatory changes, and the attraction and retention of leukocytes. The complement system can be activated in two ways, by the classical and the alternative pathways.

The Classical Pathway. When certain antibodies combine with their antigens a site in the hinge region of the antibody becomes active, affording attachment to a globular head of C1, the first complement component (Fig. 3). C1 has a body from which radiate six collagenous stalks, terminating in six globular heads for attachment to the activated antibody sites. This attachment causes a site on the body of C1 to become an active enzyme which converts C4 and C2 into active forms. The upshot is the formation of a protein complex, *C3 convertase*, with enzymatic activity for native C3, splitting it into small and large components, the latter reacting with C5, C6, C7, C8, and C9 to form the *membrane attack complex*. This is a hollow tube with a flanged head, which can punch a hole in a cell membrane. During complement-mediated cell lysis, hundreds of membrane attack complexes, visible by electron microscopy, act on a cell to cause its disruption by osmotic forces.

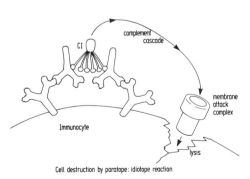

Cell destruction by paratope: idiotope reaction

Figure 3. Immunocyte lysis by paratope-idiotope reaction. The idiotopes on the receptors of the cell being lysed have complementary specificity for the paratopes of antibodies from another clone. After attachment, these antibodies fix complement and so mediate lysis of the cell bearing the particular idiotopes. This reaction, which has been demonstrated experimentally, is the basis of Jerne's concept (22) that a network of clonal deletions occurs after every antigenic stimulus, altering the immune response (clonal) repertoire.

The Alternative Pathway. The complement system can be activated in the absence of antibody by certain bacteria, viruses, or virus-infected cells. Five proteins are involved in this system together with C3 of the classical pathway. Cell lysis is mediated by the same membrane attack complex (made of proteins C5 to C9) used by the classical pathway. The alternative pathway would seem to provide a resistance to bacterial infection, which does not depend on the presence of specific antibody.

The Cells

Polymorphs and Macrophages. The protective role of the polymorphonuclear leukocyte and its big colleague, the macrophage, has long been appreciated. Countless house surgeons have had experiences similar to mine when I was confronted with a lady severely ill with meningitis. A lumbar puncture provided fluid for microscopic examination, whereupon I saw large numbers of polymorphs, with their characteristically lobed nuclei and conspicuous granules, containing lysosomes for digesting phagocytosed material. Among these granules, in many cells, I could see the darkly stained little double disks of meningococci. Here was the cause of the illness! Sulfonamides were administered and within hours complete recovery was underway. Polymorphs form about 70% of the blood leukocytes, they rush to sites of infections, they increase their numbers to cope, their sacrificed bodies form pus—they are our gallant little soldiers, defending us from nasty germs by devouring them.

Lymphocytes. These cells, with barely enough cytoplasm to contain their round nuclei, form about 20% of the blood leukocytes. For many years they were regarded, in the words of the Johns Hopkins pathologist Arnold Rich, as "phlegmatic spectators watching the turbulent activities of the phagocytes." The person who did most to change this and so to found modern cellular immunology was J. L. Gowans (29). In 1962, Gowans et al. (30)

made a monumental contribution by demonstrating that the lymphocyte, far from being an end cell, under the stimulus of an antigen is capable of transforming into a large cell which undergoes rapid division and multiplication. Next McGregor and Gowans (31) showed that animals depleted of lymphocytes by thoracic duct drainage or irradiation cannot make antibody in response to an antigenic challenge, but that this function can be restored by injection of lymphocytes. Thus the role of lymphocytes as precursors of clones of antibody-forming cells was discovered. The reason for their apparent phlegmatism lies, of course, in their clonal nature. For any particular antigen the great majority of lymphocytes have a nonreactive receptor. Similarly understandable is the paucity of their cytoplasm. They need just enough to make a receptor for their antigen and only if they meet it do they need to enlarge in order to multiply or differentiate into the antibody-producing factories that we call plasma cells. The primary feature of a lymphocyte is its specificity for antigen, carried in its nucleus in the base sequences of its chosen heavy and light chain V genes.

T Cells and B Cells. Quite apart from clonal differences, lymphocytes are heterogeneous. J. F. A. P. Miller, a pioneer investigator of the thymus, was one of the discoverers of the two major divisions of lymphocytes, that is, T cells, which have differentiated in the thymus, and B cells, arising directly from the bone marrow. About 85% of lymphocytes in the blood are thought to be T cells and 15% B cells. Morphologically, it can be seen by the electron microscope that B cells, which are covered in antibody molecules and secrete antibody in small quantity, have appreciable rough-surfaced endoplasmic reticulum, needed for protein synthesis. T cells lack this and lack surface antibody but of course do possess surface receptors for their specific antigens. As discussed in Section 2.3, T cells have a special role in defense against intracellular parasites such as viruses and mycobacterium

tuberculosis, whereas B cells are particularly important for defense against bacteria, though the two roles overlap, as discussed in Section 2.3.

Types of T Cells. T cells subserve three very different activities. *Helper T cells* greatly enhance antibody secretion by B cells. In a spectacular experiment, Claman et al. (32) showed that thymus cells and bone marrow cells, put into heavily irradiated mice, enable them to make copious antibodies against injected sheep erythrocytes but that thymus cells or bone marrow cells alone do not. The helper effect on B cells is mediated by soluble *helper factors* (33) (see Section 2.3). Separate *suppressor T cells* inhibit immune responses by secretion of soluble *suppressor factors* (34). Helper and suppressor T cells seem to be very important regulators of immune responsiveness, in the quantitative sense. This is not to be confused with control of the specificity of immune response. *Cytotoxic T cells*, with paratopes of the appropriate specificity, can destroy virus-infected cells, tumor cells, and transplanted foreign cells.

The Histocompatibility System

Recently the reason for the existence of the histocompatibility system has become apparent, as described below, but surprisingly, this great advance is not yet generally appreciated.

For years it has been known that tumors or tissues transplanted from one animal to another are rejected. This does not happen, however, between identical twins, a finding that prompted oncologists to develop strains of genetically identical inbred mice (by brother-sister mating) to facilitate tumor propagation. Naturally, the genetic basis of graft rejection attracted attention. It was found, in all species tested, that a single gene region on one chromosome has a predominant influence. The genetics of graft rejection has been pioneered in the mouse, initially by P. A. Gorer and G. D. Snell, as most interestingly described by Klein (35). In man, the major gene region for graft rejection, the *major histocompatibility complex (MHC)*, is on chromosome 6 (36), where the two main loci, A and B, have approximately 20 and 40 alternative alleles each (37). Since chromosomes are paired, each person has two A locus and two B locus genes, which allows 172,200 different combinations of antigens. These antigens are on most cells in the body, apart from erythrocytes. The cells used for testing are the blood leukocytes, hence the name *human leukocyte antigen (HLA)* for the A and B locus products, for example, HLA-A3 and HLA-B8.

Zinkernagel and Doherty's Discovery.   A long-standing puzzle has been the biological purpose of the histocompatibility system. Why has evolution provided us all with virtually unique sets of antigens on our cells and why can we react particularly strongly against each other's antigens (alloaggression)? Obviously the histocompatibility system does not exist merely to frustrate transplant surgeons. The key to its understanding seems to have come from Gordon Ada's Canberra laboratory, where Zinkernagel and Doherty made the famous discovery that histocompatibility antigens are involved in the immune destruction of virus-infected cells (38, 39). Setting out to test the role of cytotoxic T cells in defense against a virus infection, Zinkernagel and Doherty infected mice with lymphocytic choriomeningitis (LCM) virus. Seven days later spleen cells from the infected mice were added to various cultures of LCM-infected fibroblast cells. The totally unexpected observation was that the spleen cells did not lyse the virus-infected fibroblasts unless they bore the same histocompatibility antigens as the spleen cells themselves. This discovery has provided a very attractive explanation for the existence of the major histocompatibility system, as described in Section 2.3.

Immune Response (Ir) Genes, Ia Antigens, and D Locus Antigens.   Seeking knowledge of genes governing immune response specificity, Benacerraf and McDevitt pioneered lines of research in mice and guinea pigs which revealed an influence of the MHC (40). Since a direct effect of the histocompatibility antigens themselves was incomprehensible before the advent of Jerne's concept (22) that the clonal repertoire is altered by a network of clonal deletions based on paratope-idiotope reaction (Section 2.5), Benacerraf and McDevitt postulated the existence of a new type of gene, the immune response (Ir) gene. A set of these Ir genes appeared to exist in the MHC of the mouse, in between the two loci for histocompatibility antigens (41). However, it now seems more likely that the genes affecting the immune response repertoire are the histocompatibility antigen genes themselves, together with immunoglobulin V genes (42, 43), as discussed in Section 2.5.

There is evidence that the MHC contains genes for surface components on lymphocytes, distinct from the major histocompatibility antigens, but necessary for effective T cell help of B cell function (44). These lymphocyte antigens are called Ia (immune associated) antigens and some biochemical studies support their existence, but the technology is difficult with possibility of deception by experimental artifact. Ia antigens are heterogeneous and appear to include differentiation antigens (45). In man, the Ia antigens include the B cell alloantigens (46), thought to be coded for by genes of the D locus of the MHC, but not yet fully understood. There seems to be a possibility that these are at least partly sets of immunoglobulin idiotopes, in which case they would be multiclonal markers rather than alloantigens. To cap the fascinating complexity of MHC gene function, Taussig and Munro (47) discovered that T cell helper factors (see above) appear to be partly encoded for by MHC genes, as are T cell suppressor factors (48).

2.3.   The Response to Infection

It is easy to understand how an invading bacterium can meet and be phagocytosed by a prowling polymorph or macrophage, but how does a bacterial antigen meet the one lymphocyte in a million which bears its complementary paratope? Gowans (29) and Morris (49) have provided most readable reviews of the clear and simple research findings which answered this fundamental question.

The Function of Lymphatic Vessels

Having penetrated skin or mucosa, bacteria are in the tissue spaces. Here there are lymphatic vessels with valves and with contractile smooth muscle cells, conferring a capacity to suck. Plasma proteins that have passed out from the blood through capillary walls cannot pass back that way, but together with cells that have escaped from the blood and foreign material, such as invading bacteria, are sucked up by the lymphatic vacuum cleaners and carried to lymph nodes. Plasma proteins traverse the lymph nodes and are carried on by efferent lymphatic vessels, eventually returning to the circulation via the lymphatic duct. Foreign material, however, is removed by phagocytic cells which line the lymph sinuses in the medulla of lymph nodes. There is evidence that foreign antigens, phagocytosed in this way, are returned to the surface of the phagocytic cell and presented to T and B lymphocytes in an optimal fashion for triggering an immune response, should a lymphocyte of a complementary clone be present. It was Gowans who discovered how such a meeting is achieved.

Recirculation of Lymphocytes

By removing lymphocytes from the thoracic ducts of rats, tagging them with a radioactive label, returning them to the circulation, and studying their distribution by autoradiography, Gowans and Knight (50) discovered that lymphocytes continually recirculate through the lymph nodes of the body. They arrive at a lymph node in the arterial blood, passing through the capillaries to reach the postcapillary venules, where specialized endothelial cells absorb them and extrude them into the tissue space of the lymph node cortex. From here the lymphocytes pass through the medulla, out into the efferent lymphatic vessel, and back to the circulation by the thoracic duct. One purpose of this recirculation is clear—it enables representatives of every clone to be present in every lymph node and so facilitates the meeting of a foreign antigen with a complementary clone.

Events Following the Arrival of a Foreign Antigen in a Lymph Node

By cannulating the efferent lymphatic vessel of a lymph node in a sheep and injecting an antigen subcutaneously into the region drained by the node, Hall and Morris (49, 51, 52) gained a detailed knowledge of the cellular response to an antigenic stimulus.

Lymphocyte Retention.   Within 4 hours of injection of the antigen, there is a fiftyfold fall in the number of cells leaving the node (51). This lasts for up to 24 hours, when the cell numbers rapidly return to normal. The phenomenon may be due to inhibition of lymphocyte migration from the blood into the node, which may be necessary to protect circulating lymphocytes from exposure to paralyzing concentrations of antigen, and so to ensure an immune response. Alternatively or additionally, there may be a cessation of migration of cells from the node, increasing the time for inductive association of antigen with macrophage and lymphocyte.

Lymphocyte Recruitment.   Following the lymphocyte retention phase, the number of lymphocytes leaving the node increases, up to tenfold above normal. These cells are inactive, mature lymphocytes, apparently recruited from the bloodstream specifically to the node where the foreign antigen is localized. In this way, vast numbers of lymphocytes are brought into association with the antigen, enabling cells of any complementary clone to meet the antigen and be triggered.

Clonal Proliferation and Mutation.   In the next phase, starting about 3 days after the injection of antigen, new types of cell appear in the efferent lymph (52). These are large blast cells, which can rise in number to reach 5% of the cells present. Many of these blast cells can be seen to be in mitosis and almost all incorporate tritiated thymidine, showing that they are doubling their DNA ready for cell division. These cells are the multiplying descendants of lymphocytes of clones bearing paratopes complementary to the foreign antigens. There are also more differentiated, smaller cells, full of polyribosomes, which shows that they are actively engaged in protein synthesis. The rate of multiplication of the responsive clones in the lymph node becomes very rapid, exceeding that of spermatogenesis in the testis (49). Because every cell division requires copying of the DNA base sequence and this process has a finite chance of error, somatic mutations are inevitable. When they involve the V genes, new clones are created. Most are likely to have reduced affinity for the foreign antigens present, but occasionally, especially when the mutation involves the hypervariable region and hence the paratope itself, the new clone has increased affinity for one of the foreign antigens present and so is selectively propagated.

Antibody Synthesis.   In the course of the clonal expansion, two distinct populations of antibody-producing cells develop (49). There are B lymphocytes with only elementary rough-surfaced endoplasmic reticulum, but with copious numbers of polyribosomes, enabling them to form and secrete appreciable amounts of antibody (53). These cells are mobile, migrating into the lymph stream from their origin in the lymph node. The major production of antibody, however, is by plasma cells, probably differentiated from B cells, which remain in the medulla of the lymph node where their vast numbers give the tissue a glandular appearance (49). These cells have much more cytoplasm than lymphocytes, with prominent rough-surfaced endoplasmic reticulum, being veritable antibody factories. They do not migrate from the lymph node. Any antibody detectable in the circulation is likely to be the product of plasma cells resident in the lymph nodes or spleen.

Clonal Dissemination.   At the height of the immune response as many as 1 in 20 of the cells in the efferent lymph can be shown to be a synthesizing antibody (53). If all the cells leaving the stimulated node are drained from the body through a fistula of the efferent lymphatic vessel, no antibody appears in the systemic blood, although the antibody titer of the lymph coming from the stimulated node rises. If, however, the removed cells are reinfused, intravenously, the antibody titer in the systemic circulation does rise.

These observations show that the activated cells leaving the stimulated node in the efferent lymph propagate the immune response throughout the body.

Cell Cooperation

Mention has been made of the discovery by Claman et al. (32) that bone marrow cells transferred to an irradiated host need the help of thymus cells in order to make appreciable antibodies to sheep red blood cells. Mitchison (54) showed that mice primed to a hapten on a protein carrier give a good secondary antibody response to a second immunization but not if the carrier protein is changed. The "helper" cells specific for the carrier protein can be shown to be T cells. T cells and also macrophages may play an important helper role by arranging aggregates of antigen molecules on their surface for effective presentation to B cells, but additionally T cells secrete potent soluble factors.

Helper Factors.   Feldman and Basten (55) showed that T cells primed to the carrier protein keyhole limpet hemocyanin (KLH) would send a KLH-specific helper stimulus to B cells across a millipore filter, thereby starting the study of soluble antigen-specific T cell mediators. T cell helper factors may be shed T cell receptors (47). As well as possessing a receptor for their specific antigen, T cell helper factors possess an MHC-coded region which may have affinity for a B cell surface receptor, also MHC-coded (factor-acceptor hypothesis) which needs to be occupied, as well as the B cell's paratope, to trigger the B cell to divide, secrete, and differentiate to a plasma cell (47). MHC genes coding for helper and suppressor factors are not those for the major transplantation antigens of the human HLA-A and HLA-B loci, or the mouse H-2-K, and H-2-D loci, but separate genes from an adjacent region, known in the mouse as the I region (56). T helper factors have been shown to be involved in the immune response to synthetic polypeptides, bacterial antigens, foreign serum albumin and globulin, foreign red cells, and foreign major histocompatibility antigens (47).

Suppressor Factors.   These are analogous to helper factors, but are made by suppressor T cells and inhibit specific immune responses (47). Suppressor T cells are discussed more fully in Sections 2.4 and 3.3 in relationship to their possible role in preventing autoimmunity.

Viral Infection

Nothing in biology is more fascinating than the nature and activity of viruses. Pieces of genetic information in the form of DNA or RNA are associated with a few proteins, and these constitute an entity which can reproduce itself by entering a living cell and preempting the cell's protein synthesizing machinery for its own reproduction. The surface protein components of viruses, necessary for attachment to cells, enable host defense by specific antibodies which will muffle these proteins and so prevent cell entry. However, viruses change their surface proteins by mutation, and when a neutralizing antibody is not present, cell entry occurs. Fortunately viral antigens remain on the surface of infected cells, affording a target for cytotoxic T cells, if any of the requisite specificities are present. However, an undeveloped, virgin clone of cytotoxic T cells lacks adequate numbers,

and with each lymphocyte cell division requiring nearly a day, numbers build up painfully slowly. This is dangerous, for there is a logistics race between extension of the virus infection by release of newly formed viral particles from infected cells and generation of sufficient cytotoxic T cells to contain the infection. It would be interesting to know whether the great reptiles had histocompatibility systems. If not it may have been virus infection, as discussed in the next section, which caused their extinction.

The Purpose of the Major Histocompatibility System—To Speed Defense against Virus Infection?   Zinkernagel and Doherty's discovery (see Section 2.2) that cytotoxic T cells from virus-infected animals attack cultured cells infected with the virus only if these cells bear major histocompatibility antigens in common with the infected animal can be explained in two ways (57). The viral antigen on the surface of the infected cell may fuse with an adjacent major histocompatibility antigen to form an antigenic compound, the *"altered self"* concept. Alternatively, the *"dual recognition"* concept postulates that cytotoxic T cells have receptors for their own histocompatibility antigens as well as receptors for the foreign, viral antigen, and both receptors must be occupied for the virus-infected cell to be lysed. Decisive evidence between the two theories has been provided by Finberg et al. (58) who immunized BALB/c (H-2^d) mice with syngeneic cells coated with Sendai virus. The resultant cytotoxic T cells lysed Sendai virus-coated BALB/c target cells, as expected, but also lysed, in varying degree, uncoated cells of several different histocompatibility types, viz. H-2^r, H-2^k, H-2^b, H-2^s and H-2^q. This shows that a major histocompatibility antigen, altered by association with a virus antigen, can resemble other major histocompatibility antigens, strongly favoring the "altered-self" hypothesis. Similar evidence from von Boehmer et al. (59). involves the H-Y antigen, supporting the H-gene theory's interpretation of how sex affects the prevalence of certain autoimmune diseases (140) (see section 3.5).

Gordon Ada, the instigator of Zinkernagel and Doherty's famous discovery, interpreted the phenomenon as revealing the fundamental purpose of the major histocompatibility system. Anticipating Finberg et al.'s (58) evidence, Ada (60) saw that the system provides developed clones against potential virus infection of host cells, greatly reducing the time needed to mount an effective immune defense. Additionally, the system prevents the muffling of T cell receptors by free virus particles, a function better reserved for neutralizing antibodies. Today it seems clear that Ada was correct in his perceptive conclusion that the role of the histocompatibility system is to facilitate defense against virus infection.

2.4. Tolerance to Self-Antigens

Definitions of "Tolerance"

Once I spent a year unsuccessfully trying to induce guinea pigs, rats, and mice to make thyroid-stimulating antibodies (TSAb) similar to those present in my scores of thyrotoxic patients. This failure illustrates the existence of a natural, apparently absolute tolerance. This could well depend on a different mechanism from the tolerance that can be induced by excessive antigen dosage. Partial and temporary tolerance may be a "submaximal immune responsiveness," distinct from natural tolerance.

Burnet's Theory and Medawar's Evidence

Whereas natural selection could operate to prevent autoimmunity against antigens common to all members of a species, some other mechanism must be involved in prevention of immune reaction against self-histocompatibility antigens, for parents have the capacity to react to each other's histocompatibility antigens and impart to their offspring all the genes necessary for such reactivity. In 1959 Burnet (9) put forward a brilliant hypothesis which remains viable today. He proposed that nascent immunocytes in the fetus pass through a stage in which contact with complementary antigen causes their deletion. All host antigens present at this stage would thus impose tolerance by clonal deletion. Subsequently, the surviving clones differentiate so that antigenic contact causes not deletion, but stimulation. Burnet's hypothesis received spectacular support from the famous experiments of Medawar's group (62). In one of several similar studies, six fetal mice of CBA strain were injected, in utero, with a mixture of spleen, testis, and kidney cells taken from adult mice of A strain. Five mice were born and 8 weeks later were "challenged" with a skin graft from an adult A strain donor mouse. Two grafts were promptly rejected, but three survived for 75 days, after which one began to be rejected. The remaining two lasted until 77 and 101 days, when their hosts were injected with lymph node cells from CBA mice which had been immunized against A strain skin. Within 14 days of receiving the lymph node cells the two mice rejected their grafts, showing that the observed tolerance was not due to antigenic loss by the grafted skin.

Dependence of Tolerance on Inoculum Cell Survival

With characteristic perspicuity Medawar considered it likely that "at least some of the cells of the fetal inoculum survived as long as the tolerant state which they were reponsible for creating." Subsequently, Billingham and Brent (63) found that varying degrees of tolerance to foreign skin grafts could be induced by injecting *newborn* mice with spleen cells from the donor strain. The results depended strongly on the strains involved. Thus 79% of CBA grafts were accepted by A strain mice, but no A strain grafts were accepted by C57 or AV mice. Moreover, C57 spleen cells and AV spleen cells always killed A strain recipients, but A strain spleen cells never killed C57 mice. One envisages a fight between the foreign spleen cells and the host immunocytes, sometimes won by the inoculum (host death), sometimes won by the host (no tolerance), and sometimes drawn, with inoculum cells and host both surviving in mutual tolerance.

Evidence from Nossal and Pike

In most interesting experiments, Osmond and Nossal studied the multiplication and differentiation of lymphocytes in the bone marrow of adult mice (64). Impending cell division was revealed by uptake of ^{3}H-thymidine given in vivo and presence of immunoglobulin (Ig) on the cell surface was detected by adherence of ^{131}I-labeled antiserum to Ig, added in vitro. It was found that the bigger cells (8–12 μ diameter) were dividing rapidly to produce small lymphocytes (5–8 μ diameter) which lacked surface Ig but acquired it during a nonmitotic maturation period lasting about 2 days. The newly formed lymphocytes were found to be continually leaving the marrow, at random times with respect to their age. When, however, bone marrow was placed in tissue culture, making cell emigration impossible, the proportion of Ig-positive cells rose, as did the antibody-forming capacity of the cultured tissue (65).

Nossal and Pike (66) then set out to test whether the nascent lymphocytes, caught in tissue culture during the nonmitotic phase of progressive Ig display, are susceptible to clonal abortion by contact with specific antigen. Bone marrow cells from adult mice were cultured with and without antigen, in the form of dinitrophenol (DNP) attached to human gamma globulin (HgG) as a carrier. After culture, the cells were injected into irradiated mice which were challenged with the DNP antigen and killed 9 days later so that the number of cells in their spleens which were making antibodies to DNP could be determined by Jerne's plaque-forming cell (PFC) technique (67). Figure 4 shows the findings. The DNP-HgG antigen, at the low concentration of 4 μg/ml, completely prevented the fivefold rise in number of antibody-forming cells developing in the control culture, without antigen present. Tests with a nitrophenylacetic acid derivative (NIP) as an alternative antigen showed the effect to be antigenically specific.

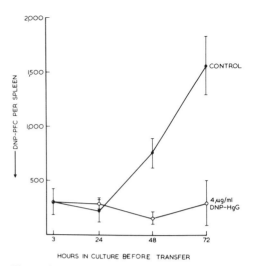

Figure 4. Evidence for clonal abortion by antigenic contact in immature bone marrow lymphocytes from adult mice. These cells differentiate during 72 hours in culture, to acquire antibody-secreting capacity (curve labeled ''control'') as shown by the plaque-forming cell (PFC) technique. If an antigen (in the experiment illustrated, dinitrophenol on human gamma globulin, DNP-HgG) is present in the medium, reactivity to it does not develop (curve labeled 4 μg/ml DNP-HgG). Reproduced with permission from G. J. V. Nossal and B. L. Pike, *J. Exp. Med.* **141**, 904 (1975).

Modification of Burnet's Theory in the Light of Nossal and Pike's Findings. The ingenious and fundamentally important studies of Nossal and his colleagues provide experimental support for Burnet's theory that tolerance to self-antigens is achieved by clonal abortion, but indicate that the process is confined not to a prenatal phase in the life of the whole animal, but instead to an early phase in the life of each maturing lymphocyte. The realization that tolerance by clonal abortion may continue to occur in adult life is of immense significance for the understanding and the future therapy of autoimmune disease, as discussed in Sections 3 and 5.

Suppressor T Cells

When laboratory animals are given excessive dosage of antigen they may fail to make an immune response. Transplanted syngeneic (from genetically identical animals) lymphocytes do not restore responsiveness, unless the host is irradiated. McCullagh (68, 69) obtained evidence that "there is some factor in the tolerant rat inimical to the initiation of an immune response in transfused normal lymphocytes." It is now widely accepted that the inimical factor is the presence of T cells which suppress the specific immune response, and are therefore named suppressor T cells. When washed lymphoid cells from animals, made tolerant to a certain antigen, are mixed with spleen cells of normal responsive syngeneic animals and transferred to a lethally irradiated syngeneic host, the cells from the tolerant animals reduce the immune response of the normal cells to the antigen (70). In beautifully clear experiments, Nachtigal et al. obtained evidence that suppressor T cells arise by differentiation from immature, radiation-sensitive, cortisone-sensitive precursors, in response to a signal transmitted by the antigen (70). These investigators have formulated the following very attractive hypothesis to explain the suppressor T cell phenomenon.

The Hypothesis of Nachtigal et al. (70). It is postulated that, on contact with complementary antigen, immature thymocytes differentiate into suppressor T cells, whereas mature thymocytes differentiate into effector T cells (helper or cytotoxic) (Fig. 5). It is further postulated that the immature T cells are more sensitive to antigen than the mature, thus accounting for the phenomenon of *low zone tolerance*, in which subimmunogenic dosage of antigen causes suppression of response to subsequently administered immunogenic dosage (71). Because the immature thymus cells are mostly concentrated in the thymus itself, any antigen reaching that organ preferentially would tend to induce tolerance rather than response, explaining why aggregate-free proteins, which bypass phagocytic mechanisms, are tolerogenic (72, 73).

This theory provides a most plausible mechanism for the control of clonal expansion. Ordinarily, foreign antigen is presented to mature lymphocytes of a complementary clone in lymph nodes (Section 2.3) inducing clonal

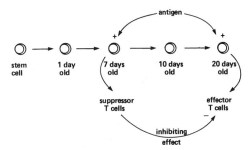

Figure 5. The hypothesis of Nachtigal et al. (70); immature T cells, meeting complementary antigen, differentiate into suppressor T cells, in contrast to mature T cells which become effector cells. Such a mechanism could effectively control the magnitude of an immune response. It could also account for tolerance to self-antigens, but this is much less certain, clonal abortion being the favored alternative.

expansion. However, available immature precursor cells of the clone would be stimulated too, differentiating into suppressor cells which would eventually limit the magnitude of the expanding clone, Without such control a persistent antigen could conceivably induce a leukemic state.

The Remarkable Effect of Total Lymphoid Irradiation

Setting out to improve radiotherapy of Hodgkin's disease, Kaplan (74, 75) used a linear electron accelerator to produce a more penetrating, megavoltage X-ray beam. Aiming at killing all the neoplastic lymphoid cells, he devised a procedure of "total lymphoid irradiation (TLI)," administered in daily doses over several weeks and aimed at all the lymphoid structures in the body. To avoid leukopenia, Kaplan carefully shielded a significant fraction of the bone marrow. This intensive but selective radiotherapy procedure, supplemented with chemotherapy, now gives a 10 year survival of 62% compared with 0.5% for untreated patients with Hodgkin's disease (74). However, this was only the beginning of Kaplan's contribution.

Applying TLI to mice, Kaplan and his colleagues administered dosages of 200 roentgens per day, 5 days a week for a total of 17 days, to the major lymphoid organs, with the hind legs, skull, chest, and tails shielded (76). All T cells and B cells are destroyed by this procedure, but return within 2 months, from progeny of the shielded stem cells in the bone marrow. The remarkable finding was that foreign bone marrow cells, injected immediately after the course of irradiation, survived indefinitely, making the mice chimeras. Furthermore, when foreign skin from the donors of the bone marrow cells was grafted on to the irradiated mice, it survived indefinitely (>120 days) in seven out of eight mice, whereas it was rejected within 20 days in 12 unirradiated mice. In 16 mice similarly receiving TLI and foreign skin grafts, but no bone marrow, all the grafts were rejected within 31 to 70 days. Initially, the foreign grafts were only semi-allogeneic, from F_1 relatives of the graft recipients, but it was found that totally allogeneic grafts were accepted just as well and graft versus host disease did not occur (77). Using rats to facilitate surgery, Kaplan's team showed that their procedure secures indefinite acceptance of transplanted foreign hearts (78).

The Author's Current Opinion

Existing evidence on the mechanism(s) subserving tolerance to self-antigens is not yet conclusive. However, it seems to me that Nossal and Pike's evidence and the spectacular transplantation success of Kaplan's team support clonal deletion of immature immunocytes by antigenic contact as the essential mechanism. Suppressor T cells seem to have to outnumber responding cells to be effective (79) and their effect is only partial (80). This favors the view that the function of suppressor T cells is the control of clonal quantity, of immunocyte numbers, rather than clonal specificity, in accord with Taussig's view (14).

A major question is whether we have suppressor T cells against our own histocompatibility or A and B erythrocyte antigens? If we do not, then clonal deletion would be the likely mechanism subserving tolerance to self-antigens. Perhaps the most favored possibility based on present evidence is that nascent immunocytes go through three chronological stages of differentiation: in the first, antigenic contact may cause deletion; in the second, suppressor T cell development; and in the third, immune response.

2.5.   The Repertoire of Clones

We need at least a million different clones (Section 2.1) of B cells and T cells to be reasonably safe from infection. Our repertoires are determined partly by our *genetic* endowment and partly by *dynamic* influences. The latter include Jerne's network of interclonal deletions and also the somatic mutations occurring in the V genes of cells in clones expanding under antigenic or other mitogenic stimulus (Section 2.3; see also below) (Fig. 1).

Germ-line Genes Involved
Immunoglobulin V Genes.   Because these genes code for the specificity of receptors for antigen on both B and T cells (81, 82) they are major germ-line determinants of the clonal repertoire, as first demonstrated by Dorf et al. (42) and Riblet et al. (43). The number of germ-line V genes is not known but is probably on the order of 1000. However, ingenious nuclear mechanisms bring various subcomponents of V genes together at random to increase the repertoire (83). For example, in the mouse about 600 V genes on the kappa light chain chromosome can combine at random with about five short J (joining) genes to give 3000 variants from 605 genes (84). The major amplification of the repertoire by gene combination is subserved by the cytoplasmic combination of the polypeptide chains coded for by the randomly chosen heavy and light chain V genes used by each clone. Thus 500 heavy chain V genes and 1000 light chain V genes would give 500,000 specificities from 1500 genes.

Histocompatibility Antigen Genes.   By whatever mechanism, all animals appear to succeed in securing lack of reactivity to their

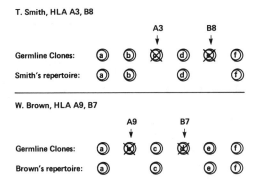

Figure 6. Alteration of the immune response repertoire (set of clones) by the deletions imposed by histocompatibility antigens.

own histocompatibility antigens. Major alloantigens, such as the erythrocyte ABO antigens in man, and minor histocompatibility antigens also appear to be universally successful in imposing blanks in the repertoire. It follows that genes for the major histocompatibility antigens and for other alloantigens are negatively acting genetic determinants for our immune response repertoires (Fig. 6). These are probably the major germ-line genes influencing the occurrence of autoimmune disease (Section 3.5).

Dynamic ("Environmental") Influences

Although our histocompatibility antigen genes and our germ-line V genes give us our initial clonal repertoire, it does not remain static. Apart from alteration by somatic mutation of V genes (Section 2.1; also see below) there is also alteration due to the capacity of certain clones to destroy certain other clones.

Jerne's Network of Interclonal Deletions by Paratope-Idiotope Reaction. As mentioned in Section 2.2, antibodies possess idiotopes, which are epitopes (antigenic determinants) on the variable region (85, 86), adjacent to and possibly sometimes partly incorporating the paratope (combining site) (Fig. 2). Working with antibodies against chemically defined haptens, Cosenza and

Köhler (87) and Hart et al. (88) were able to show that specific immune responses could be inhibited by administration of anti-idiotypic antibodies. The mouse myeloma protein known as T15 was found to bind the hapten phosphorylcholine (87). Immunizing mice with phosphorylcholine, Kluskens and Köhler (89) found the animals produced antibodies against the hapten, as expected, but also produced antibodies reactive with T15. This indicated that the induced antibodies to the hapten had acted as immunogens, inducing secondary antibodies against their idiotopes. T and B cells reactive with the same antigen were found by Binz and Wigzell to share idiotypes (90). Working with antibodies to Group A streptococci, Eichmann discovered that the corresponding anti-idiotypic antibodies had to be of a complement-fixing class (guinea pig IgG_2) in order to suppress the immune response (91).

Marshaling these highly significant discoveries, Jerne (22) proposed that in the immunity system a continuing series of interclonal deletions occurs, forming a "network" of reactions. A complement-fixing clone whose paratope has specificity for the idiotope of another clone (Fig. 2) destroys that clone by complement-mediated cytolysis (Fig. 3). In this way, clones determined by germ-line V genes interact to alter the original repertoire (Fig. 7). Furthermore, new clones emerging by somatic mutation during an immune response may also make deletions. There are additions to the repertoire as well as subtractions, because deletion of an anti-idiotope clone allows survival of its target clone. Thus throughout life the repertoire of clones is constantly altering, by both addition and subtraction of clones. This, together with somatic mutation, is highly relevant to the largely random age of onset of autoimmune diseases as discussed in Section 3.

In imagining paratope-idiotope reaction, it seems important to remember that paratopes appear to be molecular clefts (92) so that complementary idiotopes are probably molecular projections, as depicted in Figures 2

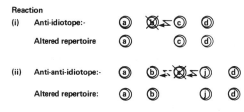

Figure 7. Alteration of the immune response repertoire by interclonal deletions, based on paratope-idiotope complementarity (Jerne's networks).

and 3. Thus it seems unlikely that a paratope can combine with another paratope or an idiotope with another idiotope. This has important logical consequences for envisaging clonal interaction.

It is not yet known whether every idiotope induces a reactive anti-idiotypic clone. This is a point of great significance. If anti-idiotypic reaction occurs only haphazardly, then Jerne's networks provide a medium on which natural selection could act to reduce the prevalence of autoimmune disease by favoring the evolution of V genes with the requisite paratope-idiotope combinations.

Somatic Mutation of V Genes. This has already been discussed as a cause of continual alteration in the repertoire (Section 2.1). Apart from the mitogenic effect of antigenic stimulus, it seems inevitable that *thymosin*, causing massive lymphocyte cell division in the thymus, will also cause somatic mutations and so increase the repertoire of emerging T cell clones. Additionally, T cells activated by antigenic contact may produce stimulatory factors for B cells which are mitogenic and hence mutagenic.

3. THE GENESIS OF FORBIDDEN CLONES

3.1. The Features of Autoimmune Disease

Never Generalized

From the time of the epochal discovery of thyroglobulin autoantibodies by Doniach and

Roitt (6), it has been found that autoimmunity is never generalized but always involves immune reactivity with a single or very few, probably structurally related autoantigens. This shows that generalized loss of immune tolerance to autoantigens does not occur.

Abnormal Antibodies, Normal Antigens

All autoantibodies so far discovered react with autoantigens present in other, normal individuals, showing that the autoimmune reaction is based on an abnormal specificity of the immunocyte, not the host antigen.

Random Age of Onset

The random age of onset of autoimmune disease is one of its most striking features, familiar to every clinician. Apart from transient, neonatal versions of Graves' disease (93) and myasthenia gravis (94) caused by transplacental passage of maternal autoantibodies, autoimmune diseases are extremely rare in early life, increasing in frequency with advancing age in a manner indicative of involvement of random events, such as somatic mutations (95).

3.2. Burnet's Forbidden Clone Theory

Regarding the *clone* (Section 2.1) as the unit of specificity of the immunity system and autoimmune diseases as defects of immune specificity in which the immunity system, in error, reacts with a normal host antigen, Burnet (9) postulated that autoimmune disease is caused by ''forbidden clones'' of self-reactive immunocytes, absent from unaffected people.

Today, Burnet's forbidden clones are an established reality. In *Graves' disease*, forbidden clones of plasma cells make TSAb, which can be demonstrated in 90% of the patients, in amount proportional to the severity of the disease (96), but which are absent from normal people (93). Similarly, in *myasthenia gravis*, forbidden clones of plasma cells produce autoantibodies, absent from normal people, which disrupt neuromuscular transmission by reacting with the acetylcholine receptor of the neuromuscular junction (152).

In many other autoimmune diseases the causative clones are less clearly established, but this is likely to be due to present limitations of technology, as discussed in Section 4.

Accepting the compelling evidence that forbidden clones of immunocytes exist and cause autoimmune disease (Section 4), one is left with the question of why they occur. Burnet postulated somatic mutation (9) of immunocyte V genes. This also has become increasingly probable and has been supplemented by Jerne's concept that there is a network of interclonal deletions (22) (Section 2.5).

Evidence for Repertoire Alteration by Somatic Mutations and Interclonal Deletions in the Genesis of Forbidden Clones

This is the evidence for a random, "environmental," noninherited component, namely:

1.   The approximately 50% *discordance* of Graves' disease and insulin-dependent diabetes mellitus (IDDM) in monozygotic twins (97).

2.   The juvenile grace gap and characteristic age-specific onset rates (Section 3.1).

3.   The increasing variety of autoimmune features with age, for example, appearance of exophthalmos in a patient originally presenting with hyperthyroidism only, and appearance of TSAb which cross-react with the mouse in a patient previously showing only human-specific TSAb.

4.   The frequent observation of remission in autoimmune disease with reversible lesions, for example, hyperthyroidism, can be accounted for by temporary quiescence of forbidden clones. However, sometimes one sees complete recovery from exophthalmos whereas hyperthyroidism persists. This suggests a specific deletion of the putative forbidden clone reactive with an orbital antigen (98). Presumably such deletion occurs due to the advent of an appropriately specific anti-idiotope clone (Section 2.5).

5.   The frequently observed onset of an autoimmune disease following infection, for example, IDDM following Coxsackie B virus infection (99), could result from presentation to lymph node cells of autoantigen made available through viral cytolysis (Section 2.3) but where the site of the infection is remote from the site of the autoantigen, somatic mutation in the huge population of anamnestically stimulated dividing immunocytes may be involved.

The Effect of Thyroid Tissue Damage

Treating cases of thyrotoxicosis with therapeutic doses of iodine-131, Irvine (100) observed that titers of thyroglobulin autoantibodies (Tg-Ab) and thyroid microsomal autoantibodies (M-Ab) regularly rose, apparently in response to the increased antigenic stimulus resulting from the release of antigen consequent on the irradiation damage to the thyroid cells. However, in some cases, where one of the two autoantibodies was absent, even repeated doses of iodine-131 failed to elicit its appearance. From this, Irvine concluded that autoantibody production requires not only the appropriate antigenic stimulus but also a particular genetic predisposition. Similarly, Volpe (101, 102) and Adams (93) have observed that severe thyroid damage by virus infection is not usually followed by the appearance of thyroid autoantibodies, but if such antibodies are already present then their titer is increased.

Today it seems likely that the necessary predisposition to autoimmunity lies in the specificity of the immune response repertoire and that this is a consequence not only of germ-line genes (V and H) (Section 3.5) but also of somatic events including mutations and interclonal deletions.

Adjuvant-Induced Autoimmune Disease

Chapter 2 describes models of autoimmune disease inducible in certain laboratory animals by immunization with an autoantigen in Freund's adjuvants (103). A water-in-oil emulsion of the water-soluble protein antigen is made, small amounts of killed mycobacteria are added, and the emulsion is injected into various sites in the animal being immunized.

The procedure seems to bypass the normal limitation of antibody production by elimination of antigen and suppressor T cell control. Instead of a brief appearance of antibody, the titer rises steadily for 4 to 6 weeks and remains maximal for months. It seems likely that the mutagenic effect of Freund's adjuvants is a function of this prolonged period of immunocyte stimulation, with inevitable occurrence of somatic mutations during the cell divisions.

When Freund's incomplete adjuvants (lacking the mycobacterial component, which may have plant lectin-like mitogenic property) are used with brain extracts, experimental autoimmune encephalitis is not induced, as it is with the complete adjuvant, and the animals are rendered refractory to subsequent immunization with the complete adjuvant (104). There is some evidence that the protective effect is due to induction of suppressor T cells (104) which could abort the immune response before the requisite somatic mutations have occurred. It also seems possible that the nonautoimmune clones initially reactive with the antigen preparation preempt the second dose of the antigen and so prevent induction of the autoimmune clones obtainable with initial use of the maximally mutagenic stimulus.

3.3. The Lack of Suppressor T Cell Theory

Following the discovery that T cells can inhibit B cell activity, Allison et al. (105) postulated that autoimmunity is caused by a lack of suppressor T cells against forbidden clones. This concept proved extremely popular and a spate of evidence appeared to support it. However, much of this evidence has proved to be spurious.

For example, it was reported that if thymocytes from young, healthy NZB mice were transferred to aging animals of the same strain, the development of their autoimmune anemia was suppressed (106). Stringent studies with much larger numbers of animals have shown no such effect (107).

Again, evidence purporting to show that normal people have clones of B cells reactive with autoantigens is not convincing (108, 109). Thyroglobulin labeled with iodine-125 adheres to an occasional lymphocyte from the blood of normal people, but it adheres to a greater number of lymphocytes from people showing thyroglobulin autoantibodies (109), and there is no evidence that the lesser reaction with normal lymphocytes is specific. Indeed, the labeled cells from normal people could be phagocytic monocytes (110). No functional reactivity, such as uptake of ^{3}H-thymidine or blast transformation was demonstrated in the allegedly thyroglobulin-specific B cells occurring in normal people. In a recent study, Davies (110a) found that patients with autoimmune thyroiditis have circulating lymphocytes which secrete Tg-Ab, in culture, as measured by an indirect plaque-forming cell assay. Normal people have no such cells.

In adoptive transfer studies, De Heer and Edgington (111) have provided clear evidence that NZB mice have forbidden clones of B cells which make their antierythrocyte autoantibodies and are absent from BALB/c, B10-D2, C57BL/Ks, and DBA/2 mice. NZB mice do not have a generalized defect in tolerance to self-antigens and their spontaneously arising antierythrocyte forbidden clones are different from those which can be induced in other strains by repeated immunization with rat erythrocytes (112).

Evidence from Beall and Kruger

Culturing peripheral blood lymphocytes in the presence of plant mitogens, Beall and Kruger have shown that B cells which secrete Tg-Ab are present in patients showing these autoantibodies, but not in normal people (113). The in vitro autoantibody production depends on the presence of T cells and is suppressed by excessive numbers of T cells. Moreover, T-helper and T-suppressor effects occurred with T cells from normal people as well as with the patients' own T cells (114). Beall and Kruger conclude that the abnormality responsible for autoantibody production does not lie in T cells.

3.4. The Nature of Autoantigens

This topic is discussed in Section 4 in relationship to the action of forbidden clones; here it is considered for the light it throws on their genesis.

Never Histocompatibility or ABO Erythrocyte Alloantigens

Although Epstein et al. (115) have perceptively postulated that primary biliary cirrhosis is similar to graft versus host disease in being based on immune reaction against histocompatibility antigens, which are especially dense on the ductal epithelial cells of the biliary tree, the specificity of these postulated forbidden clones against self-histocompatibility antigens has not been demonstrated and unless it is, it will remain a mystery why such autoimmunity does not occur. Everyone has well-developed clones against other people's major histocompatibility antigens, probably to speed defense against virus infection, as explained in Section 2.3. It would be expected that somatic mutants of these clones would occur and would be the commonest cause of autoimmune disease. Similarly, one would expect the A and B erythrocyte alloantigens to be the commonest target for forbidden clones causing hemolytic anemia, but again such autoimmunity does not appear to occur. The significance of this is discussed in Section 3.6.

Mainly Surface Components of Fixed Cells, Internal Components of Cells, and Semi-sequestered Secretory Products

The thyroid-stimulating hormone receptor and the acetylcholine receptor, involved as autoantigens in Graves' disease and myasthenia gravis, are surface components of fixed cells. The microsomal autoantigens, associated with ulcerative colitis, pernicious anemia, and destructive autoimmune disease of the endocrine glands are intracellular, but presumably have surface representation or have structural stimilarity to the surface antigens reactive with the pathogenic forbidden clones. In systemic lupus erythematosus, cells bearing the autoantigens include leukocytes, which circulate, but the autoantigen is entirely within the cell membrane. The proteins, thyroglobulin and intrinsic factor, secreted by thyroid and gastric parietal cells, respectively, are common autoantigens, but are relatively sequestered in the thyroid gland follicles and in the stomach. Thus autoimmunity mainly involves noncirculating, intracellular, or semi-sequestered autoantigens. The significance of this is discussed in Section 3.6.

3.5. The Genetic Predisposition to Autoimmune Disease

Multiple Dominant Genes with Positive or Negative Effect

For decades there has been debate as to whether the genes predisposing to autoimmune diseases, such as IDDM and Graves' disease, are dominant or recessive (116). The regular occurrence of Graves' disease in three successive generations made early investigators think that the genes involved were dominant with incomplete penetrance, but Bartels (117) observed that the prevalence of thyrotoxicosis was greater in the siblings of probands than in the parents, from which he concluded that the genes involved were recessive. Studying diabetics with onset younger than 20 years of age, Simpson (118) also observed a higher prevalence in siblings than in parents of probands, but she found her data best fitted a predisposition by multiple genes.

In animal studies it has been shown that genes active in the heterozygous state (i.e., dominant or codominant) can both cause (40, 119) and prevent (120, 121) a specific immune response, including autoimmune disease (119). The nature of these genes and their mode of action now seem clear, as discussed below after consideration of a previous concept.

The Linkage Disequilibrium Theory

Vladutiu and Rose (122) discovered that major histocompatibility antigen status influences the occurrence of autoimmune disease in mice. Subsequently, an immense research effort has shown that most human autoimmune diseases show a weak positive or negative association with various major histocompatibility antigens (123, 124). The "histocompatibility-linked immune response (H-Ir)" genes, postulated by Benacerraf and McDevitt (40) (Section 2.2), were very attractive candidates for the causative role (123). It was observed that the human major histocompatibility A locus antigen, HLA-A1, occurs unduly frequently with the B locus antigen, HLA-B8, a phenomenon called "linkage disequilibrium," presumably resulting from incomplete chromosomal shuffling of genes in intermarrying people from different populations (125). McDevitt and Bodmer (123) postulated that the observed associations between major histocompatibility antigens and autoimmune diseases were due to a similar linkage disequilibrium between the histocompatibility antigen genes and putative, neighboring, pathogenic "immune response genes." This concept has proved very popular, but has been disappointing in that experimental confirmation has not been obtained. Apart from Ia antigens (Section 2.2), no H-Ir gene product is known. Some evidence suggests that certain Ia antigens are important for the interaction of T cells with B cells and macrophages (47, 48, 126, 127, 128), but evidence from von Boehmer et al. (129) indicates that this is not so in the natural, syngeneic situation. The concept (126) that Ia antigens influence the specificity of the immune response repertoire by modulating the reaction of T cells with other cells is hard to envisage, especially because Ia antigens seem to be insufficiently polymorphic. However, Ia antigens could certainly influence the repertoire by deleting complementary clones and this could possibly be a significant mechanism for defense against autoimmunity, as discussed below.

The V Gene Theory

Because the genetic predisposition to autoimmune diseases is disease specific (e.g., Graves' disease predisposes to itself, as does IDDM), the genes involved clearly influence antibody specificity. Therefore, when the immunoglobulin V genes, coding for antibody specificity, were discovered (20, 25) (Section 2.2), they provided prime suspects for the predisposing role (130), especially as they are codominant genes, working in pairs (heavy and light chain V gene combinations) and so fitted the inheritance patterns suggesting involvement of more than one, codominant gene.

The theory that immunoglobulin V genes predispose to autoimmune disease can be tested by exploiting the tight linkage of V genes with the C genes (Section 2.2, which show allotypic variation. This enables people to be typed for their C genes, similarly to ABO blood group typing. Unfortunately, C gene allotypes are few. There are none for the lambda light chains, only two for the kappa light chains, and whereas the heavy chains show several, most are very common or very rare, so that frequently there is no analyzable variation between members of a family (131). This is quite unlike the situation with histocompatibility typing, where nearly all individuals are clearly distinguishable. Family studies in New Zealand people, testing for associated inheritance of Graves' disease and immunoglobulin allotypes (Gm and Km), by observation of known heterozygous allotypes and also by Penrose's sibling pair method, have failed to show involvement of immunoglobulin genes (131).

In Japan, the heavy chain C gene allotype, Gm1, absent from 50% of Europeans, is reported to be universal (132). Another allotype, Gm2, has been found to have increased prevalence in myasthenia gravis, Graves' disease, and Hashimoto's disease (133). In a family study, it has been found that relatives affected with Graves' disease share heavy chain chromosomes unexpectedly often (134). Confirmation of this last report would suggest that immunoglobulin V genes do play a role in the genetic predisposition to Graves' disease at least in the Japanese people studied. However, the Gm2 effect could possibly be a consequence of racial admixture, mediated by genes on any chromosome.

Further studies are needed to settle the question of whether germ-line V genes are genetic determinants for autoimmune disease.

The alternative, that we all have germ-line V genes equally capable of mutation to autoimmune specificity, seems unlikely, especially interracially.

The H Gene Theory

Making inbred strains of mice to facilitate transplantation of tumors in their cancer research, the Bielschowskies discovered that their New Zealand Black (NZB) strain develops autoimmune hemolytic anemia (135). Studying the genes involved in this disorder, Howie and Helyer discovered that hybrids of the NZB and New Zealand White (NZW) strains develop not anemia, but a classical lupus nephritis, based on the development of forbidden clones which make antinuclear autoantibodies (136). The occurrence of lupus nephritis in the offspring of homozygous parents who themselves lack the disease shows that it is based on at least two genes (one or more from each parent) which are dominant or codominant in that they are active in the heterozygous state. Detecting the presence of renal disease by accurate measurement of urinary protein excretion, Knight et al. (137) made backcross studies which showed involvement of three genes (119), one from the NZB strain and two from the NZW strain. Similar studies on the inheritance of the autoimmune anemia, which is transmitted from

NZB mice to hybrids with the New Zealand Chocolate (NZC) strain, has shown involvement of two further genes (138, 139). Studies of linkage with the MHC, coat color, and immunoglobulin heavy chain allotypes have shown that one of the pathogenic genes is in the MHC, none are linked to allotype, but two are in the neighborhood of minor histocompatibility antigens (139). These findings prompted us to propose the H (histocompatibility antigen) gene theory, which postulates that genes for major and minor histocompatibility antigens can themselves be determinants for autoimmune disease (140).

How Histocompatibility Antigens May Affect the Prevalence of Autoimmune Diseases. Histocompatibility antigens vary between individuals in a population and so the blanks they impose on the immune response repertoire also vary (Section 2.5) (Fig. 6). The nature of the blanks could influence the chance of emergence of a forbidden clone by somatic mutations occurring in V genes and clonal deletions mediated by paratope-idiotope reaction (Jerne's networks) (Section 2.5) (Fig. 7). By deleting anti-idiotope clones, paratope-idiotope deletions can add to the clonal repertoire as well as subtract from it. Figure 8 outlines the clonal events which could enable the presence of the major histocompatibility

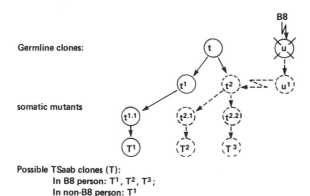

Possible TSaab clones (T):
In B8 person: T¹, T², T³;
In non-B8 person: T¹

Figure 8. A mechanism for the predisposition to Graves' disease by HLA-B8. The germ-line clone, u, is cross-reactive with B8 and is therefore deleted. This prevents the subsequent development from clone u by somatic mutation of clone u¹, which has specificity for the idiotope of a precursor, t^2, of potential thyroid-stimulating clones T² and T³, capable of causing Graves' disease. Thus the presence of HLA-B8, by causing deletion of a precursor of a relevant anti-idiotope clone, increases the risk of occurrence of Graves' disease.

antigen, HLA-B8, to increase the prevalence of Graves' disease.

Protective effects, such as that against IDDM in people with HLA-B7, may result from clonal deletions which reduce the chance of emergence of the pathogenic clone.

How Sex May Affect the Prevalence of Autoimmune Diseases. In addition to offering an explanation for the effect of histocompatibility antigen status on the prevalence of autoimmune diseases, the H gene theory accounts for the effect of sex. Graves' disease is about six times more common in females, the pattern of inheritance excluding a causative role by a gene on the X chromosome (116, 117). The H gene theory explanation is that the clonal deletions imposed by the H-Y antigens, present in males only, increase the chance of emergence of the pathogenic clones by interclonal network reactions and somatic mutations (Fig. 9). If ankylosing spondylitis is an autoimmune disease, which seems probable, the predisposing effect of male sex can be readily explained if the clonal deletions by H-Y antigens reduce the chance of emergence of a protective clone with specificity for the idiotopes of the forbidden clones or their precursors.

Table 1 lists the predisposing and protective effects of HLA antigens and sex on illustrative autoimmune diseases.

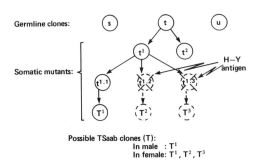

Germline clones:

Somatic mutants:

H–Y antigen

Possible TSaab clones (T):
In male : T^1
In female: T^1, T^2, T^3

Figure 9. A mechanism for the protection from Graves' disease afforded by male sex. Clone $t^{1.2}$ and $t^{1.3}$, potential precursors of thyroid-stimulating clones, are cross-reactive with the male-specific H-Y antigen and are therefore deleted.

Are D Locus Antigens Evolved Restrictors of the Immune Response Repertoire? Whereas the A, B, and C locus antigens of the MHC, with their strongly developed alloreactive clones, seem to have the purpose of speeding defense against viruses (Section 2.3), it seems possible that other MHC antigens (e.g., at the D locus) may have the different function of deleting nascent forbidden clones. Because there is no known autoimmunity against self-histocompatibility antigens, it seems that antigens on circulating lymphocytes may be able to impose a continuing tolerance. Antigens on fixed cells could be protected from autoimmunity if they had cross-reactivity with D locus antigens on circulating lymphocytes. If the D locus has this function, one would expect that most of the antigens involved would be identical between the individuals of a population and so would not show allogeneic variation.

Weaknesses of the Linkage Disequilibrium Theory

The theory that associations between autoimmune diseases and HLA-A and B locus antigens are based on linkage disequilibrium with another gene locus received support when D locus antigens (B cell alloantigens) were found to have stronger associations with some autoimmune diseases than the A and B locus antigens (141). However, the effect is not consistent (142) (Table 1). The highest known relative risk, 87-fold, is imposed by the B locus antigen, B-27, for ankylosing spondylitis. For myasthenia gravis in females the relative risk imposed by B8 is 5.5-fold compared to 2.9-fold for DR3. There does not seem to be any consistency between the magnitude of D locus and B locus effects (142). Being on B cells, D locus antigens might possibly be sets of immunoglobulin idiotopes, in which case they would be multiclonal, repertoire indicators, rather than conventional alloantigens (Section 2.2).

The H gene theory, with or without the V gene theory, which is complementary, seems to offer a more comprehensive explanation

Table 1.   Some of the highest relative risks, both increased and decreased, imposed by various MHC antigens and H-Y antigen

Disease	Antigen	Relative Risk	Type of Clone (or its precursor) Deleted
Ankylosing spondylitis	B27	× 87	anti-idiotope
	H-Y	× 8	anti-idiotope
Reiter's disease	B27	× 37	anti-idiotope
IDDM	DW2	÷ 33	forbidden
	DRW3	× 5.7	anti-idiotope
Ulcerative colitis (Japanese)	AW19	÷ 25	forbidden
	B5	× 3.9	anti-idiotope
Chronic active hepatitis	DRW3	× 13.9	anti-idiotope
Goodpasture's disease	DRW2	× 13.1	anti-idiotope
SLE	H-Y	÷ 10	forbidden
	B8	× 2.1	anti-idiotope
Addison's disease	DW3	× 6.3	anti-idiotope
Graves' disease	H-Y	÷ 6	forbidden
	DW3	× 3.7	anti-idiotope
	B8	× 2.3	anti-idiotope
Myasthenia gravis (females)	B8	× 5.5	anti-idiotope
	DR3	× 2.9	anti-idiotope
Young adult females only	H-Y	÷ 3	forbidden

Relative risks extracted from L. P. Ryder et al., "HLA and Disease Registry. Third Report, Munksgaard, Copenhagen, 1979.

of the genetic predisposition to autoimmunity than does the linkage disequilibrium theory (Table 2).

3.6.   Conclusions

The reason why we develop forbidden clones against some of our antigens, but not against others, remains mysterious. As mentioned in Section 3.4, according to Burnet's original theory (9) of tolerance by clonal abortion in fetal life and subsequent somatic mutation throughout postnatal life, one would expect histocompatibility antigens to be the commonest targets for autoimmunity. The fact that they are not suggests the existence of an infallible, protective mechanism, continuing to act throughout life. Slavin et al.'s (77) induction of permanent tolerance to allogeneic grafts by injection of bone marrow cells after total lymphoid irradiation (see Section 2.4) suggests that histocompatibility antigens on circulating lymphocytes can act in postnatal as well as in fetal life, to impose continuing, absolute tolerance. Nossal and Pike's (66) evidence (Section 2.4) suggests that the mechanism involved is abortion of nascent clones by contact with complementary antigen. However, present evidence on the mechanism falls short of certainty. Some other mechanism, including the presence of specific suppressor T cells, could conceivably be operative. The paradox of consistently absent autoimmunity against self-antigens (MHC and ABO), for which we inherit genes for reactive clones, could be explained by induction of suppressor T cells by these antigens, consistently circulating through the bone marrow and lymphoid tissues. A circulating self-antigen for which there was no complementary clone could not induce suppressor T cells and it is conceivable that in the absence of these, a nascent clone in a lymph node, for example, with the help of macrophages and T cells

Table 2.   Comparison of the linkage disequilibrium theory and the H gene and V gene theory for ability to explain the observed features of the genetic predisposition to autoimmune disease

Explains:	Linkage Disequilibrium Theory	H Gene & V Gene Theory
1. Patterns of inheritance (multiple codominant genes with +ve or −ve effect)	—	✓
2. Nature of "environmental" factors (infection and somatic mutation	—	✓
3. Increased risk from certain MHC antigens (e.g., HLA-A, B, C, D)	✓	✓
4. Decreased risk from certain MHC antigens	✓	✓
5. Synergistic effect of MHC antigen combinations	?	✓
6. Effect of non-MHC genes	—	✓
7. Increased risk from male sex (clonal deletions by H-Y antigens)	—	✓
8. Decreased risk from male sex	—	✓
9. Nature of gene products (alloantigens or autoantibody paratopes)	—	✓
10. Action of gene products (repertoire alteration by clonal deletion)	—	✓

might be triggered to immune response by contact with the autoantigen or a related molecule.

Whatever mechanism protects circulating histocompatibility antigens from immune reaction is clearly not available for antigens on fixed cells or antigens inside the cell membrane. For these antigens it would seem the only protection against autoimmunity is provided by natural selection, acting on germline V genes, H genes, and D locus genes (if they exist) (Section 3.5) and so minimizing emergence of the forbidden clones by somatic mutations and the network of interclonal deletions. The high prevalence of thyroid and islet cell autoimmunity suggests the operation of a balanced polymorphism. The reproductive disadvantage of the genes in the combinations allowing these diseases may be balanced by their value for successful defense against dangerous infectious disease.

Consistent provision of clones reactive with the idiotopes of potential forbidden clones could be an important supplement to clonal abortion, as suggested by Teale and Mackay (143). This seems a probable mechanism protecting against ankylosing spondylitis, which may be based on autoimmunity against antigens in the sacroiliac and paravertebral joints. The powerful predisposing effect of HLA-B27 suggests that this antigen acts in the network toward deletion of the protective clones (Fig. 8). The predisposing effect of the H-Y antigen (male sex) suggests that it too acts toward deletion of protective clones (Fig. 8).

Our understanding of the genesis of forbidden clones is fragmentary and uncertain, but we may have glimpsed the main mechanisms involved.

4.   THE ACTION OF FORBIDDEN CLONES

4.1.   Requirements for Pathogenicity

When Doniach and Roitt (6) made the monumental contribution of discovering autoimmunity in the form of autoantibodies which precipitate with thyroglobulin, it was naturally assumed that the associated Hashimoto's thyroiditis was caused by these autoantibodies, especially since they were absent from 105 cases of thyrotoxicosis and 103 cases of nontoxic nodular goiter. However, Witebsky's team (7), simultaneously discovering thyroiditis, introduced the more sensitive tanned red cell agglutination test of Boyden (144) which revealed TGAb in many cases of thyrotoxicosis and even in many apparently normal people. Similarly, other autoantibodies against the cells of various endocrine glands, demonstrable by the indirect fluorescence test, are often found in healthy people. The upshot of this was that many clinicians came to regard autoimmunity not as a cause of disease, but as an inconsistent, passive consequence of it.

There is now strong evidence that some forbidden clones are pathogenic (Sections 4.2, 4.4, and 4.5), but others, including those making Tg-Ab, appear to be harmless. Whether a forbidden clone is pathogenic or not is likely to depend on the following:

1. Its antigenic target; whether noncellular, intracellular, or cell surface.
2. Whether its autoantibodies fix complement.
3. Whether it includes cytotoxic T cells.

Clones making noncomplement-fixing autoantibodies against noncellular or intracellular antigens are probably invariably nonpathogenic. Complement-fixing clones against intracellular antigens are potential pathogens if their target cells suffer lysis (Section 4.5).

4.2. Interference with Cell Receptor Function

In Graves' Disease
Evidence for Pathogenicity. The TSAb were discovered in a mouse bioassay for thyroid-stimulating hormone (TSH) (145, 93). Only about 30% of cases of Graves' disease show TSAb cross-reactive with the mouse,

but when an elaboration of the bioassay is used, involving reaction of the autoantibodies with human thyroid, 90% of cases are positive (96). The amount of TSAb present shows a correlation with the degree of thyroid overactivity (96), and human-specific TSAb, inactive in the mouse, have been shown to stimulate the human thyroid on intravenous infusion into volunteers (146).

Mode of Action. Because TSAb mimic the action of TSH, the presumptive autoantigen involved was the thyroid cell's receptor for TSH, but this proved difficult to demonstrate experimentally because the purified receptor tends to lose its affinity for TSH. However, Manlcy ct al., using delicately prepared thyroid tissue, were able to show a binding reaction for receptor-purified, ^{125}I-labeled TSH (147), and its inhibition by TSAb (148). On the basis of this work, Smith and Hall (149) have developed a clinically used radioreceptor assay for TSAb. The binding of TSAb to the thyroid receptor, like that of TSH, stimulates the cell by activating adenylate cyclase inside the cell membrane (93).

In Myasthenia Gravis
A perceptive clinician, J. A. Simpson (150) long suspected that myasthenia gravis is based on autoimmune attack on the neuromuscular junction, but confirmation was not possible until the interlacing ramifications of science provided unexpected help. Snake venoms causing paralysis were found to contain neurotoxins which impair neuromuscular transmission by binding to the acetylcholine receptor. An eel that stuns its prey by electric shock was found to have an electric organ with a remarkable concentration of acetylcholine receptors. Patrick and Lindstrom (151) purified acetylcholine receptors from the electric eel, using affinity chromatography with snake neurotoxin, then set out to make antibodies to the receptor by immunizing rabbits, using Freund's complete adjuvants. Unexpectedly, several of the immunized rabbits developed paralysis which could be relieved by the acetylcholine potentiator neostigmine.

Thus an experimental model of myasthenia gravis had been created and the suspected autoimmune mechanism demonstrated. Lindstrom went on to develop a radioimmunoassay which confirmed the pathogenic role of the autoantibodies by showing them to be present in 90% of myasthenia patients but virtually absent from normal people (152).

In Insulin Resistance

For many years it has been observed that rare patients develop a resistance to insulin which may be spectacularly intense. For example, in 1952 in Dunedin (153) a diabetic woman who had been controlled for years by a dosage of about 40 units of soluble insulin per day was admitted in diabetic coma. In the following 18 weeks she required 259,700 units of insulin, the maximum daily dosage being 5000 units, falling to 700 units 4 months later. Antibodies against insulin were not detectable, but tests in rats showed that the patient's blood contained high levels of physiologically active insulin, which was clearly ineffective in the body of the patient. Why? Twenty-three years later Flier et al. (154) provided the answer, in elegantly clear and simple studies on six patients with extreme insulin resistance. Using peripheral blood monocytes as a convenient source of insulin receptors, the investigator showed that the patients had grossly impaired binding of ^{125}I-insulin. Furthermore, immunoglobins in the serum of the patients reacted with normal lymphocytes to inhibit the binding of subsequently added ^{125}I-insulin. Apparently these patients have autoantibodies which react with the insulin receptor, or an adjacent site, to block the action of insulin. Subsequent studies of patients with insulin-receptor autoantibodies have shown that their insulin receptors are entirely normal, functionally and immunologically (155), in accord with the general finding that autoantigens do not show allotypic or other variation (93).

Other Possibilities

Schizophrenia and manic-depressive disorder have features suggesting an autoimmune basis (remission and relapse, random postnatal onset, weak genetic predisposition). Blocking or stimulating autoantibodies against certain neural receptors could be involved in the disruption of normal mental processes which occurs in these disorders.

4.3.   Specific Cell Destruction

In many diseases where there is destruction of particular cells, autoantibodies against the cells are often present. This suggests that the cell destruction is caused by autoimmune attack, but the mechanism of cytolysis is not established. The two main contenders for the pathogenic role are complement-fixing autoantibodies and cytotoxic T cells.

Complement-fixing Autoantibodies

In 1957, Trotter et al. (156) discovered the existence of thyroid autoantibodies, which, unlike TGAb, fix complement. The antigen is a component of thyroid cells, being most abundant in microsomal fractions, which indicates that it is associated with the cell membranes. Every medical student knows that one can apply specific antibodies to washed erythrocytes without any visible effect, but that addition of complement causes cell lysis with release of hemoglobin. Trotter's complement-fixing autoantibodies against a thyroid cell microsomal antigen (thyroid microsomal autoantibodies, TMAb) were therefore strong candidates for the causal role in the autoimmune thyroiditis which leads to myxedema. Clinical studies have confirmed that these autoantibodies have a close relationship with autoimmune thyroiditis (157).

Subsequently, similar autoantibodies specific for the tissue involved have been found (158) in Addison's disease, hypoparathyroidism, pernicious anemia, ovarian failure, testicular failure, hypopituitarism, vitiligo (antimelanocyte) (159), ulcerative colitis (anticolonic epithelial cells) (160), and IDDM (161). These autoantibodies are not confined to people showing the various diseases and are not detectable in all cases. This is discussed in Section 4.6.

IDDM. Yet another monumental contribution from Deborah Doniach was her discovery with Bottazzo and Florin-Christensen of autoantibodies to pancreatic islet cells (161). Are these the cause of IDDM?

The original discovery used Coons and Kaplan's (162) indirect fluorescence method on human postmortem islet tissue. Of 13 positive sera, 10 came from a group of 20 diabetics who had additional glandular disorders and three came from nondiabetics. The 158 negative sera included 39 cases of diabetes uncomplicated by other autoimmune disease. Thus evidence of a causal relationship was scant, but the breakthrough had been made, prompting a massive collaborative study. In 829 children with newly diagnosed diabetes, Lendrum et al. (163) found the islet cell autoantibodies in 38% of cases, compared with 5% of 112 non-insulin-dependent diabetics and 1.7% of 177 nondiabetic subjects.

Rittenhouse et al. (164), using isolated islets from hamsters, found complement-dependent cytotoxic activity in serum from 11 out of 30 IDDM subjects, absent from 28 controls. This could indicate a cytotoxicity universally present in IDDM, but not always cross-reactive with the hamster antigen, analogous to LATS activity in Graves' disease (Section 4.2).

The islet cell autoantibodies react with the α, β, and δ cells of the islet (161), which is anomalous, for only the β cells make insulin and the α cell product, glucagon, does not appear to be deficient in IDDM. The implication of this is discussed in Section 4.6.

Cytotoxic T Cells

Govaerts (165) founded an extensive field of research when he grafted dogs with allogeneic kidneys, then tested the effect of their thoracic duct lymphocytes on donor kidney cells in tissue culture. The lymphocytes became aggregated to the cultured cells which were killed in 24 to 48 hours. Lymphocytes from normal dogs were not cytotoxic. Extensive subsequent studies (166) have confirmed the cytotoxic effect of lymphoid cells with specificity for MHC antigens and have shown similar activity against tumor cells and virus-infected cells (Section 2.2) (166). Is this mechanism involved in the specific cellular destruction of "organ-specific" autoimmune disease? Suggestive positive evidence has been obtained in cell transfer studies on mice with experimental autoimmune thyroiditis (167) and in human studies where lymphoid cells from cases of ulcerative colitis have been applied to cultured colon cells (168, 169). However, I agree with Ivan Roitt (17) that the evidence is not yet conclusive.

K Cells and NK Cells. Perlmann and Holm (166) discovered that, in the absence of complement, a coating with complementary antibodies can facilitate the killing of tissue culture cells by lymphoid cells which apparently react nonspecifically with the Fc ends of the attached antibodies. The lymphoid cells involved are known as K (killer) cells (170) but have not been shown to be a single cell type. The phenomenon is analogous to the enhanced phagocytosis of bacteria by opsonization. It could be involved in autoimmune cytolysis.

NK (natural killer) cells are also lymphoid cells which appear to have cytotoxicity for cells in tissue culture, but they are obtained from animals that have not been immunized against the tissue culture cells. Originally, NK cells served as controls for cytotoxic T cells from immunized animals. If clonally specific (which is not established), NK cells could be virgin clones or thymus-developed clones. Any role of NK cells in vivo is uncertain.

Demonstration of K cell and NK cell activity habitually involves use of a huge excess of the lymphoid (effector) cells over the tissue culture (target) cells, effector cell to target cell ratios being 50:1 or 100:1 (171). This makes the specificity of the reactions uncertain, for the target cells could possibly die due to a nutritional deficiency imposed by the effector cells, or from pollution by their excretory products.

4.4.   Neutralization of a Secretory Product

The pathogenesis of the common autoimmune type of pernicious anemia has been elucidated to a state of beautiful clarity (172). Irvine et al. (173) discovered complement-fixing autoantibodies against a microsomal antigen in the gastric parietal cells (parietal cell autoantibodies, PC-Ab) analogous to thyroid microsomal autoantibodies. Roitt et al. (172) found PC-Ab in 88% of 191 cases of pernicious anemia, which suggests the disorder is based on autoimmune destruction of the parietal cells with loss of their secretory product, intrinsic factor, needed for absorption of vitamin B_{12}. However, autoantibodies to intrinsic factor (IF-Ab) also occur. These are noncomplement fixing, like TGAb, but unlike the latter appear to have a pathogenic role, for they have never been found in patients with simple atrophic gastritis which has not progressed to pernicious anemia (172). It appears that IF-Ab, presumably of IgA class, secreted into the stomach lumen from plasma cells in the gastric mucosa lesions neutralize secreted intrinsic factor to aggravate its deficiency.

4.5.   The Pathogenic Effect of Immune Complexes

Serum Sickness

The humoral immunity system has evolved to provide defense against microbial pathogens, which are of negligible physical quantity. When large amounts of foreign antigen are administered parentally, malfunction may occur. In the days when diphtheria and tetanus were treated by passive immunization, in the form of injection of serum from horses immunized against the bacterial toxins, serum sickness was common. Its incidence ranged from 10%, for small amounts of horse serum, to 90% when the dosage was 100 ml, or

more. Four to ten days after the serum injection, the patient developed a syndrome including rash, itching, edema, arthralgia, myalgia, fever, and lymphadenopathy. In his blood the foreign protein was detectable and complement levels were reduced. Clearly the foreign protein elicited an immune response and because of its great bulk was still circulating in quantity when copious amounts of specifically reactive antibodies appeared. This led to the development of circulating, soluble antigen-antibody complexes, with activated complement-triggering sites on the antibody molecules. The excessive amount of these immune complexes overwhelmed neutralizing mechanisms, resulting in complement-mediated damage in various vulnerable sites.

Immune Complex Nephritis

Lindemann (174) showed that glomerulonephritis can be produced in guinea pigs by injections of antiserum to guinea pig kidney, made in rabbits. These nephrotoxic, cross-species antibodies have autoreactive equivalents in man, occurring in Goodpasture's syndrome where fluorescence microscopy and electron microscopy reveal the antiglomerular autoantibodies lying linearly on the basement membrane. Similar antiglomerular autoantibodies may also occur in some cases of post-streptococcal glomerulonephritis, but more commonly microscopic studies show the discontinuous lumpy pattern of immunoglobulin and complement along the basement membrane, characteristic of immune complex nephritis. Like serum sickness, this is based on the pathogenic action of complement-activating immune complexes, to which the glomerulus is especially susceptible. Unanue and Dixon (175) have produced this type of nephritis in laboratory animals by injecting preformed antigen-antibody complexes.

What antigen is involved in immune complex nephritis? Most cases can be seen to be postinfectious, following infection with a wide range of pathogenic microorganisms including Epstein-Barr virus, hepatitis viruses, staphylococci, and malaria (176). No involvement of an autoantigen is known, so presumably the antigen comes from the invading organism itself, or is an altered host component. Obviously any weakness of complement control mechanisms (e.g., reduced C1 inactivator activity) could predispose to the complement-mediated damage.

The NZB × NZW Mouse. This hybrid of two inbred strains of mice develops a classical, swiftly fatal, immune complex nephritis, with the characteristic lumpy deposits of immunoglobulin along the glomerular basement membrane (136). The source of the antigen appears to be the animals' own cell nuclei since there are antinuclear autoantibodies demonstrable by the Coons and Kaplan (162) technique. Injections of carbon tetrachloride, a liver cell poison, have been shown to hasten the disease process (177), presumably by increasing availability of the intracellular autoantigen by lysis of liver cells. It is not known whether the nuclear antigen is normally made available in the necessary quantity by undiscovered cytolytic forbidden clones or by some other cell-lysing process, for example, the mild, chronic, viral infection which is endemic in the animals.

Systemic Lupus Erythematosus (SLE)

This once sinister disorder, for many years of uncertain entity and mysterious pathogenesis, can now be seen as an autoimmune disease, with its major mysteries stripped away. Thirteen years ago Miescher and Paronetto wrote a classical account of the clinical, pathological, laboratory, and therapeutic features of the disease (178). Today one sees their suspicions regarding the pathogenesis of SLE hardened into near certainty.

SLE, like serum sickness, appears to be based on the pathogenic effects of immune complexes. Clinically there is arthralgia, fever, weight loss, and lymphadenopathy, with localized effects involving skin, red cells, white cells, kidneys, lungs, heart, gut, central nervous system, and liver in decreasing order

of frequency. The basis of the disease appears to be the presence of forbidden clones making complement-fixing autoantibodies against intracellular autoantigens. Some of these autoantibodies can opsonize exposed cell nuclei, facilitating their phagocytosis by polymorphonuclear leukocytes (the L. E. cell phenomenon of Hargreaves et al.) (179). The intracellular autoantibodies are customarily called antinuclear autoantibodies (ANA) but the exact nature of the autoantigen is probably unimportant, provided it is intracellular and elicits autoantibodies which are complement fixing. ANA are usually tested for on non-human tissue, for example, mouse liver cells, which differ slightly from the human counterpart, so there is scope for false positive and negative results. ANA are reported to be detectable in 96% of cases (180) but also occur in many unaffected people. Evidence for involvement of complement in the pathogenesis includes the finding of low serum levels during active phases of the disease and the demonstration of complement proteins in the lesions.

When the disease is spontaneous, some cell lytic process is presumably present to make the intracellular autoantigen available in sufficient quantity. Sun-induced skin lesions seem entirely comprehensible on the basis of epidermal cytolysis by ultraviolet rays, with exposure of the intracellular autoantigen; immunoglobulin is found along the dermal-epidermal junction. Some of the variation between cases may be based on specificity of the autoantibodies for intracellular antigens which are present in certain tissues only.

Drug-Induced SLE. Occurrence of SLE after a severe drug reaction seems likely to be due to exposure of intracellular antigen, by the cytolysis, in a person with a latent forbidden clone of appropriate specificity. This concept is supported by evidence that many patients developing SLE when taking high doses of hydralazine have an antedating lupus diathesis (181). In patients with complement-fixing forbidden clones against an intracellular autoantigen, but no cytotoxic forbidden clones, the SLE episode would be expected to resolve after withdrawal of the drug causing the idiosyncratic or other reaction.

4.6. Conclusions

The pathogenic role and mode of action of autoantibodies reactive with hormone receptors seems clear. In Graves' disease the reaction is stimulating (agonist), whereas in myasthenia gravis and in insulin resistance it is inhibitory (antagonist). Similarly, in systemic lupus erythematosus, clear evidence indicates that the disease is based on complement activation by excessive quantities of immune complexes, composed of autoantibodies and their complementary intracellular autoantigens.

In autoimmune diseases such as myxedema, IDDM, and ulcerative colitis, based on destruction of a specific type of cell, it is not clear how the cell destruction occurs. Cytotoxic T cells, so clearly responsible for lysis of virus-infected cells, could be responsible. Alternatively, or additionally, complement-fixing autoantibodies may be the cytolytic agents, especially since they are demonstrable in many tissue-specific destructive autoimmune diseases. The correlation between these autoantibodies and their diseases tends to be imperfect, as exemplified by the absence of islet cell autoantibodies in about half the cases of IDDM and their reactivity with all the islet cell types, not just the β cells. It may be that the currently demonstrable autoantigens, which are intracellular, but are exposed on frozen sections for the indirect immunofluorescence test, differ somewhat from structurally related molecules on the cell surface and that these latter, not visible with existing technology, are the target for the truly pathogenic autoantibodies.

5. SELECTIVE NEGATION OF FORBIDDEN CLONES

5.1. Particularly Relevant Diseases

Owing to the success of research in endocrinology, most autoimmune diseases of endocrine glands have satisfactory treatments. In this category are both hyperthyroidism and hypothyroidism. However, *exophthalmos*, although helped by treatment with adrenal steroids, is in need of a specific therapy. In *IDDM*, abortion of the autoimmune attack while appreciable β cells remained would be an immense advance over insulin treatment. The *diabetic complications* involving the retina, the kidneys, and the nervous system, which may be based on autoimmune attack, are in sore need of specific therapy. Partial gastrectomy, by removing the source of acid, successfully alleviates *peptic ulcer* but is disabling and would be well replaced by a therapeutic intervention which preserves the gut endocrine cells which regulate digestive function and whose destruction by autoimmune attack is a probable cause of peptic ulcer. *Ulcerative colitis* is another autoimmune disease in urgent need of specific therapy. The nonendocrine list includes multiple sclerosis, SLE, rheumatic fever, glomerulonephritis, myasthenia gravis, rheumatoid arthritis, and ankylosing spondylitis.

5.2. Promising Research Foundations

A forbidden clone has only two features that distinguish it from other clones—the specificity of its paratope and the specificity of its idiotope (Fig. 2). Therefore, selective destruction or inhibition of forbidden clones must be based on a reaction with one of these two structures. Certain research has laid promising foundations.

With powerful theory and ingenious practice, Ramseier and Lindenmann (182) studied the antigenicity of specific "recognition structures (RS)" for antigen. Realizing that specific RS would provide the only foreign antigen when lymphocytes from one of the parental strains were injected into F_1 hybrid animals, Ramseier and Lindenmann were able to make anti-idiotype antibodies. This started a line of research which culminated in Binz and Wigzell's (183) successful prolongation of skin graft survival by induction of specific clones against the idiotopes of the anti-graft clones.

The remarkable success of Kaplan's team (Section 2.4) in achieving permanent acceptance of foreign grafts by total lymphoid irradiation and bone marrow injection is highly relevant to prevention or cure of autoimmune disease, as discussed in Section 5.3.

A third promising avenue is well reviewed by Nisonoff and Greene (184), who have achieved striking inhibition of specific immune responses by induction of suppressor T cells to chemical haptens. Whereas subcutaneous injection of a hapten on a carrier protein induces an immune response, intravenous injection elicits formation of suppressor T cells which specifically inhibit the immune response.

Finally, Ada and Byrt (185), to demonstrate the clonal nature of responsiveness to antigens, selectively inhibited immune response to flagellin by prior treatment of mice with the antigen combined with radioactive iodine in sufficient dosage to kill reactive cells.

5.3. Therapy and Prophylaxis of Autoimmune Disease

The least noxious procedure would seem to be administration to the patient of complement-fixing antibodies against the idiotopes of the pathogenic clones (91), with a view to selective lysis of the injurious immunocytes. The anti-idiotope antisera might be able to be produced in animals. Their Fab portions could be combined with the patients' Fc region to reduce allergic reaction from repeated administration.

For lethal or crippling autoimmune conditions, the use of total lymphoid irradiation (TLI), or a chemotherapeutic equivalent, can be contemplated. TLI has been shown to produce excellent temporary remissions in people with rheumatoid arthritis (186) and in NZB × NZW mice with lupus nephritis (187). The procedure could serve as a basis for achievement of more permanent remission by (1) induction of suppressor T cells specific for the autoantigen, or (2) enabling transfer of heterologous or xenologous clones with specificity for the idiotopes of the pathogenic clones.

6. CONCLUSION

Research in immunology has made uneven progress. Mention has been made of its brilliant start, with discovery and therapeutic conquest of infectious disease, and also of the extraordinary gap inspired by the false "horror autotoxicus" dogma before the discovery of autoimmunity and the gradual realization that it can be pathogenic. Other milestones have been the discovery of the function of lymphocytes; the structure of antibodies and complement; T cells and B cells; the histocompatibility system, its influence on graft rejection and on disease prevalence, and finally, its purpose; suppressor T cells; and anti-idiotope reactions. We must take these clever discoveries, dust them a little, reposition them if necessary, and apply the resultant understanding to guide new research toward the rapidly approaching goal of a general principle of therapy for the common and distressing autoimmune diseases.

REFERENCES

1. R. J. Dubos, *Louis Pasteur*, Gollancz, London, 1951.
2. P. Ehrlich and J. Morgenroth, in F. Himmelweit, Ed., *The Collected Papers of Paul Ehrlich*, Pergamon Press, London, 1954, p. 246.
3. P. Ehrlich and J. Morgenroth, in F. Himmelweit, Ed., *The Collected Papers of Paul Ehrlich*, Pergamon Press, London, 1954, p. 205.
4. W. Dameshek and S. O. Schwartz, *Am. J. Med. Sci.*, **196**, 769 (1938).
5. W. Dameshek, *Ann. N.Y. Acad. Sci.* **124**, 6 (1965).
6. D. Doniach and I. M. Roitt, *J. Clin. Endocrinol. Metab.* **17**, 1293 (1957).
7. E. Witebsky, N. R. Rose, K. Terplan, J. R. Paine, and R. W. Egan, *J. Am. Med. Assoc.* **164**, 1439 (1957).
8. N. K. Jerne, *Proc. Natl. Acad. Sci. USA* **41**, 849 (1955).
9. F. M. Burnet, *The Clonal Selection Theory of Acquired Immunity*, Cambridge University Press, London, 1959.
10. N. K. Jerne, *Eur. J. Immunol.* **1**, 1 (1971).
11. L. B. Brown and B. S. Hetzel, *J. Psychosom. Res.* **7**, 222 (1963).

12. M. G. Weigert, I. M. Cesari, S. J. Yonkovich, and M. Cohn, *Nature*, **228**, 1045 (1970).

13. O. Bernard, N. Hozumi, and S. Tonegawa, *Cell* **15**, 1133 (1978).

14. M. J. Taussig, *Nature* **248**, 236 (1974).

15. M. A. Philip, G. Standen, and J. Fletcher, *Lancet* **1**, 866 (1981).

16. A. C. Allison, *Br. Med. J.* **1**, 290 (1954).

17. I. M. Roitt, *Essential Immunology*, 4th ed., Blackwell, Oxford, 1980.

18. R. R. Porter, *Biochem. J.* **73**, 119 (1959).

19. G. M. Edelman, *J. Am. Chem. Soc.* **81**, 3155 (1959).

20. N. Hilschmann and L. C. Craig, *Proc. Natl. Acad. Sci. USA* **53**, 1403 (1965).

21. T. T. Wu and E. A. Kabat, *J. Exp. Med.* **132**, 211 (1970).

22. N. K. Jerne, *Ann. Immunol. (Inst. Pasteur)* **125C**, 373 (1974).

23. J. A. Gally and G. M. Edelman, *Ann. Rev. Genet.* **6**, 1 (1972).

24. C. M. Croce, M. Shander, J. Martinis, L. Cicurel, G. G. D'Ancona, T. W. Dolby, and H. Koprowski, *Proc. Natl. Acad. Sci. USA* **76**, 3416 (1979).

25. W. J. Dreyer and J. C. Bennett, *Proc. Natl. Acad. Sci. USA* **54**, 864 (1965).

26. M. Robertson, *Nature* **290**, 625 (1981).

27. M. M. Mayer, *Sci. Am.* **229**, 54 (1973).

28. H. J. Müller-Eberhard, in M. Fougereau and J. Dausset, Eds., *Immunology 80*, Academic Press, New York, 1980, p. 94.

29. J. L. Gowans, in R. A. Good and D. W. Fisher, Eds., *Immunobiology*, Sinauer Associates, Stamford, Conn., 1972.

30. J. L. Gowans, D. D. McGregor, D. M. Cowen, and C. E. Ford, *Nature*, **196**, 651 (1962).

31. D. D. McGregor and J. L. Gowans, *J. Exp. Med.* **117**, 307 (1963).

32. N. H. Claman, E. A. Chaperon, and R. P. Triplett, *Proc. Soc. Exp. Biol. Med.* **122**, 1167 (1966).

33. M. Feldman and A. Basten, *J. Exp. Med.* **136**, 49 (1972).

34. T. Tada, K. Okumura, and M. Taniguchi, *J. Immunol.* **111**, 952 (1973).

35. J. Klein, *Biology of the Mouse Histocompatibility-2 Complex*, Springer-Verlag, New York, 1975.

36. V. A. McKusick, *Mendelian Inheritance in Man*, 5th ed., Johns Hopkins University Press, Baltimore, 1978.

37. H. M. Dick, *Immunol. Today* **1**(1), i (1980).

38. R. M. Zinkernagel and P. C. Doherty, *Nature* **248**, 701 (1974).

39. R. M. Zinkernagel, *J. Exp. Med.* **141**, 1427 (1975).

40. B. Benacerraf and H. O. McDevitt, *Science* **175**, 273 (1972).

41. H. McDevitt, B. D. Deak, D. C. Shreffler, J. Klein, J. H. Stimpfling, and G. D. Snell, *J. Exp. Med.* **135**, 1259 (1972).

42. M. E. Dorf, E. K. Dunham, J. P. Johnson, and B. J. Benacerraf, *J. Immunol.* **112**, 1329 (1974).

43. R. Riblet, B. Blomberg, M. Weigert, R. Lieberman, B. A. Taylor, and M. Potter, *Eur. J. Immunol.* **5**, 775 (1975).

44. D. H. Katz, T. Hamaoka, M. E. Dorf, and B. Benacerraf, *Proc. Natl. Acad. Sci. USA* **70**, 2624 (1973).

45. R. J. Winchester and H. G. Kunkel, *Adv. Immunol.* **28**, 221 (1979).

46. J. G. Bodmer, *Br. Med. Bull.* **34**, 233 (1978).

47. M. J. Taussig, *Immunology* **41**, 759 (1980).

48. T. Tada and K. Hayakawa, in M. Fougereau and J. Dausset, Eds., *Immunology 80*, Academic Press, New York, 1980, p. 389.

49. B. Morris, *Aust. J. Sci.* **31**, 13 (1968).

50. J. L. Gowans and E. J. Knight, *Proc. Roy. Soc. B* **159**, 257 (1964).

51. J. G. Hall and B. Morris, *Br. J. Exp. Pathol.* **46**, 450 (1965).

52. J. G. Hall and B. Morris, *J. Exp. Med.* **121**, 901 (1965).

53. A. J. Cunningham, J. B. Smith, and E. H. Mercer, *J. Exp. Med.* **124**, 701 (1966).

54. N. A. Mitchison, *Eur. J. Immunol.* **1**, 18 (1971).

55. M. Feldman and A. Basten, *J. Exp. Med.* **136**, 49 (1972).

56. M. J. Taussig, A. J. Munro, and A. L. Lazzati, in D. H. Katz and B. Benacerraf, Eds., *The Role of Products of the Histocompatibility Gene Complex in Immune Responses*, Academic Press, New York, 1976, p. 553.

57. R. M. Zinkernagel, *J. Exp. Med.* **144**, 933 (1976).

58. R. Finberg, S. Burakoff, H. Cantor, and B. Benacerraf, *Proc. Natl. Acad. Sci. USA* **75**, 5145 (1978).

59. H. von Boehmer, H. Hengartner, M. Nobholz, W. Lernhardt, M. H. Schreier, and W. Haas, *Eur. J. Immunol.* **9**, 592 (1979).

60. G. Ada, Lecture to New Zealand Immunology Society, 1979.

61. F. M. Burnet and F. Fenner, *The Production of Antibodies*, Macmillan, Melbourne, 1949.

62. R. E. Billingham, L. Brent, and P. B. Medawar, *Nature* **172**, 603 (1953).

63. R. E. Billingham and L. Brent, *Transplant. Bull.* **4**, 67 (1957).

64. D. G. Osmond and G. J. V. Nossal, *Cell. Immunol.* **13**, 132 (1974).

65. J. W. Stocker, D. G. Osmond, and G. J. V. Nossal, *Immunology* **27**, 795 (1974).

66. G. J. V. Nossal and B. L. Pike, *J. Exp. Med.* **141**, 904 (1975).

67. N. K. Jerne and A. A. Nordin, *Science* **140**, 405 (1963).

68. P. J. McCullagh, *Aust. J. Exp. Biol. Med. Sci.* **48**, 351 (1970).

69. P. J. McCullagh, *Aust. J. Exp. Biol. Med. Sci.* **48**, 369 (1970).

70. D. Nachtigal, I. Zan-Bar, and M. Feldman, *Transplant. Rev.* **26**, 87 (1975).

71. N. A. Mitchison, *Proc. Roy. Soc. B* **161**, 275 (1964).

72. D. W. Dresser, *Immunology* **5**, 378 (1962).

73. G. J. V. Nossal and J. Mitchell, in G. E. W. Wolstenholme and R. Porter, Eds., *The Thymus, Experimental and Clinical Studies*, Ciba Foundation Symposium, Churchill, London, 1966, p. 105.

74. H. S. Kaplan, *Cancer* **45**, 2439 (1980).

75. H. S. Kaplan, *Hodgkin's Disease*, Harvard University Press, Cambridge, Mass., 1972.

76. S. Slavin, S. Strober, Z. Fuks, and H. S. Kaplan, *Science* **193**, 1252 (1976).

77. S. Slavin, S. Strober, Z. Fuks, and H. S. Kaplan, *J. Exp. Med.* **146**, 34 (1977).

78. S. Slavin, B. Reitz, C. P. Bieber, H. S. Kaplan, and S. Strober, *J. Exp. Med.* **147**, 700 (1978).

79. A. Basten, J. F. A. P. Miller, and P. Johnston, *Transplant. Rev.* **26**, 130 (1975).

80. R. K. Gershon and K. Kondo, *Immunology* **21**, 903, (1971).

81. H. Ramseier and J. Lindenmann, *J. Exp. Med.* **134**, 1083 (1971).

82. H. Binz and H. Wigzell, *Nature* **264**, 639 (1976).

83. J. M. Adams, *Immunology Today* **1**, 10 (1980).

84. P. Leder, E. E. Max, and J. G. Seidman, in M. Fourgereau and J. Dausset, Eds., *Immunology 80*, Academic Press, New York, 1980, p. 34.

85. J. Oudin and M. Michel, *C. R. Hebd. Seances Acad. Sci. Ser. D.* **257**, 805 (1963).

86. H. G. Kunkel, M. Mannick, and R. C. Williams, *Science* **140**, 1218 (1963).

87. H. Cosenza and H. Köhler, *Science* **176**, 1027 (1972).

88. D. A. Hart, A. Wang, L. L. Pawlak, and A. Nisonoff, *J. Exp. Med.* **135**, 1293 (1972).

89. L. Kluskens and H. Köhler, *Proc. Natl. Acad. Sci. USA* **71**, 5083 (1974).

90. H. Binz and H. Wigzell, *J. Exp. Med.* **142**, 1231 (1975).

91. K. Eichmann, *Eur. J. Immunol.* **4**, 296 (1974).

92. D. M. Segal, E. A. Padlan, G. H. Cohen, E. W. Silverton, D. R. Davies, S. Rudikoff, and M. Potter, in L. Brent and J. Holborow, Eds., *Progress in Immunology II*, Vol. 1, American Elsevier, New York, 1974, p. 93.

93. D. D. Adams, *Vitam. Horm.* **38**, 119 (1980).

94. J. S. Scott, *Lancet* **1**, 78 (1976).

95. P. R. J. Burch, *An Inquiry Concerning Growth, Disease and Ageing*, Oliver & Boyd, Edinburgh, 1968.

96. D. D. Adams, T. H. Kennedy, and R. D. H. Stewart, *Br. Med. J.* **1**, 199 (1974).

97. D. D. Adams, *J. Clin. Lab. Immunol.* **1**, 17 (1978).

98. A. Knight and D. D. Adams, *Horm. Res.* **13**, 69 (1980).

99. J. Steinke and K. W. Taylor, *Diabetes* **23**, 631 (1974).

100. W. J. Irvine, *Q. J. Exp. Physiol.* **49**, 324 (1964).

101. R. Volpé, V. V. Row, and C. Ezrin, *J. Clin. Endocrinol. Metab.* **27**, 1275 (1967).

102. R. Volpé, *Clin. Endocrinol. Metab.* **7**, 3 (1978).

103. J. Freund, K. J. Thomson, H. B. Hough, H. E. Sommer, and T. M. Pisani, *J. Immunol.* **60**, 383 (1948).

104. C. C. A. Bernard, *Clin. Exp. Immunol.* **29**, 100 (1977).

105. A. C. Allison, A. M. Denman, and R. D. Barnes, *Lancet* **2**, 135 (1971).

106. M. E. Gershwin and A. D. Steinberg, *Clin. Immunol. Immunopathol.* **4**, 38 (1975).

107. J. G. Knight and D. D. Adams, *J. Clin. Lab. Immunol.* **1**, 151 (1978).

108. A. D. Bankhurst, G. Torrigiani, and A. C. Allison, *Lancet* **1**, 226 (1973).

109. I. M. Roberts, S. Whittingham, and I. R. Mackay, *Lancet* **2**, 936 (1973).

110. P. Byrt and G. L. Ada, *Immunology* **17**, 503 (1969).

110a. T. F. Davies, *Clin. Res.*, in press 1982.

111. D. H. DeHeer and T. S. Edgington, *J. Immunol.* **118**, 1858 (1977).

112. J. Knight, A. Knight, and G. Winchester, *Cell Immunol.* **56**, 317 (1980).

113. G. N. Beall and S. R. Kruger, *Clin. Immunol. Immunopathol.* **16**, 485 (1980).

114. G. N. Beall and S. R. Kruger, *Clin. Immunol. Immunopathol.* **16**, 498 (1980).

115. O. Epstein, H. C. Thomas, and S. Sherlock, *Lan-*

cet, **1**, 1166 (1980).

116. V. A. McKusick, *Mendelian Inheritance in Man*, 5th ed., Johns Hopkins University Press, Baltimore, 1978.

117. E. D. Bartels, *Heredity in Graves' Disease*, Munksgaard, Copenhagen, 1941.

118. N. E. Simpson, *Diabetes* **13**, 462 (1964).

119. J. G. Knight and D. D. Adams, *J. Exp. Med.* **147**, 1653 (1978).

120. D. L. Gasser, *J. Immunol.* **103**, 66 (1969).

121. D. M. Silver and D. P. Lane, *J. Exp. Med.* **142**, 1455 (1975).

122. A. O. Vladutiu and N. R. Rose, *Science* **174**, 1137 (1971).

123. H. O. McDevitt and W. F. Bodmer, *Lancet* **1**, 1269 (1974).

124. J. Dausset and A. Svejgaard, *HLA and Disease*, Munksgaard, Copenhagen, 1977.

125. W. F. Bodmer and J. G. Bodmer, *Br. Med. Bull.* **34**, 309 (1978).

126. B. Benacerraf, in P. A. Miescher, L. Bolis, and G. Torrigiani, Eds., *The Menarini Series on Immunopathology*, Vol. 3, *Immunogenetics*, Schwabe, Basel, 1981, p. 56.

127. D. H. Katz, in P. A. Miescher, L. Bolis, and G. Torrigiani, Eds., *The Menarini Series on Immunopathology*, Vol. 3, *Immunogenetics*, Schwabe, Basel, 1981, p. 88.

128. A. S. Rosenthal and E. M. Shevach, *J. Exp. Med.* **138**, 1194 (1973).

129. H. von Boehmer, L. Hudson, and J. Sprent, *J. Exp. Med.* **142**, 989 (1975).

130. D. D. Adams, *J. Clin. Lab. Immunol.* **1**, 17 (1978).

131. D. D. Adams, Y. J. Adams, J. G. Knight, J. McCall, P. White, R. Parkinson, R. Horrocks and E. van Loghem, *Life Sciences* **31**, 3–13 (1983).

132. Y. Nakao, H. Matsumoto, T. Miyazaki, H. Nishitani, K. Ofa, T. Fujita, and K. Tsuji, *Lancet* **1**, 677 (1980).

133. Y. Nakao, H. Matsumoto, T. Miyazaki, H. Nishitani, K. Takatsuki, R. Kasukawa, S. Nakayama, S. Izumi, T. Fujita, and K. Tsuji, *Clin. Exp. Immunol.* **42**, 20 (1980).

134. H. Ono, T. Sasazuki, H. Tami, and H. Matsumoto, *Nature* **292**, 768 (1981).

135. M. Bielschowsky, B. J. Helyer, and J. B. Howie, *Proc. Univ. Otago Med. Sch.* **37**, 9 (1959).

136. J. B. Howie and B. J. Helyer, *Adv. Immunol.* **9**, 215 (1968).

137. J. G. Knight, D. D. Adams, and H. D. Purves, *Clin. Exp. Immunol.* **28**, 352 (1977).

138. N. L. Warner, in N. Talal, Ed., *Autoimmunity*, Academic Press, New York, 1977.

139. J. G. Knight and D. D. Adams, *J. Clin. Lab. Immunol.* **5**, 165 (1981).

140. D. D. Adams and J. G. Knight, *Lancet* **1**, 396 (1980).

141. L. P. Ryder, E. Andersen, and A. Svejgaard, *HLA and Disease Registry. Third Report*, Munksgaard, Copenhagen, 1979.

142. J. G. Knight and D. D. Adams, in Ciba Foundation Symposium No. 90, *Receptors Antibodies and Disease*, 35 (1982).

143. J. M. Teale and I. R. Mackay, *Lancet* **2**, 284 (1979).

144. S. V. Boyden, *J. Exp. Med.* **83**, 107 (1951).

145. D. D. Adams and H. D. Purves, *Proc. Univ. Otago Med. Sch.* **34**, 11 (1956).

146. D. D. Adams, F. N. Fastier, J. B. Howie, T. H. Kennedy, J. A. Kilpatrick, and R. D. H. Stewart, *J. Clin. Endocrinol. Metab.* **39**, 826 (1974).

147. S. W. Manley, J. R. Bourke, and R. W. Hawker, *J. Endocrinol.* **61**, 419 (1974).

148. S. W. Manley, J. R. Bourke, and R. W. Hawker, *J. Endocrinol.* **61**, 437 (1974).

149. B. R. Smith and R. Hall, *Lancet* **2**, 427 (1974).

150. J. A. Simpson, *Scott. Med. J.* **4**, 419 (1960).

151. J. Patrick and J. Lindstrom, *Science* **180**, 871 (1973).

152. J. M. Lindstrom, M. E. Seybold, V. A. Lennon, S. Whittingham, and D. D. Duane, *Neurology* **26**, 1054 (1976).

153. J. R. Presland, J. Bruckner, F. B. Cousins, and C. M. Todd, *Proc. Univ. Otago Med. Sch.* **30**, 18 (1952).

154. J. S. Flier, C. R. Kahn, J. Roth, and R. S. Bar, *Science* **190**, 63 (1975).

155. M. Muggeo, C. R. Kahn, R. S. Bar, M. Rechler, J. S. Flier, and J. Roth, *J. Clin. Endocrinol. Metab.* **49**, 110 (1979).

156. W. R. Trotter, G. Belyavin, and A. Waddams, *Proc. Roy. Soc. Med.* **50**, 961 (1957).

157. W. W. Buchanan, D. A. Koutras, J. Crooks, W. D. Alexander, W. Brass, J. R. Anderson, R. B. Goudie, and K. G. Gray, *J. Endocrinol.* **24**, 115 (1962).

158. D. D. Adams, in E. J. Holborow and W. G. Reeves, Eds., *Immunology in Medicine*, Grune and Stratton, New York, 1977, p. 373.

159. K. C. Hertz, L. A. Gazze, C. H. Kirkpatrick, and S. I. Katz, *N. Engl. J. Med.* **297**, 634 (1977).

160. R. J. Shorter, K. A. Huizenga, R. J. Spencer, J. Aas, and B. S. Guy, *Am. J. Dig. Dis.* **16**, 673 (1972).

161. G. F. Bottazzo, A. Florin-Christensen, and D. Doniach, *Lancet* **2**, 1279 (1974).

162. A. H. Coons and M. H. Kaplan, *J. Exp. Med.*

91, 1 (1950).

163. R. Lendrum, G. Walker, A. G. Cudworth, C. Theophanides, D. A. Pyke, A. Bloom, and D. R. Gamble, *Lancet* **2**, 1273 (1976).

164. H. G. Rittenhouse, D. L. Oxender, S. Pek, and D. Ar, *Diabetes* **29**, 317 (1980).

165. A. Govaerts, *J. Immunol.* **85**, 516 (1960).

166. P. Perlmann and G. Holm, *Adv. Immunol.* **11**, 117 (1969).

167. A. O. Vladutiu and N. R. Rose, *Cell. Immunol.* **17**, 106, (1975).

168. P. Perlmann and O. Broberger, *J. Exp. Med.* **117**, 717 (1963).

169. D. W. Watson, A. Quigley, and R. J. Bolt, *Gastroenterology* **51**, 985 (1966).

170. Anonymous, *Nature New Biol.* **243**, 225 (1973).

171. J. Penschow and I. R. Mackay, *Ann. Rheum. Dis.* **39**, 82 (1980).

172. I. M. Roitt, D. Doniach, and C. Shapland, in P. Grabar and P. A. Miescher, Eds., *Immunopathology*, Grune and Stratton, New York, 1965, p. 314.

173. W. J. Irvine, S. H. Davies, I. W. Delamore, and A. W. Williams, *Br. Med. J.* **2**, 454 (1962).

174. W. Lindemann, *Ann. Inst. Pasteur* **14**, 49 (1900).

175. E. R. Unanue and F. J. Dixon, *Adv. Immunol.* **6**, 1 (1967).

176. A. G. Hocken, Personal communication.

177. H. D. Flad, J. H. L. Playfair, A. Ghaffer, and P. A. Miescher, *Proc. Soc. Exp. Biol. Med.* **131**, 121 (1969).

178. P. A. Miescher and F. Paronetto, in P. A. Miescher and H. J. Müller-Eberhard, Eds., *Textbook of Immunopathology*, Vol. II, Grune and Stratton, New York, 1968, p. 675.

179. M. M. Hargreaves, H. Richmond, and R. Morton, *Proc. Mayo Clin.* **27**, 419 (1952).

180. P. H. Schur, in P. B. Beeson, W. McDermott, and J. B. Wyngaarden, Eds., *Textbook of Medicine*, 15th ed., Vol. 1, Saunders, Philadelphia, 1979, p. 174.

181. L. E. Shulman and A. M. Harvey, *Arthritis Rheum.* **3**, 464 (1960).

182. H. Ramseier and J. Lindenmann, *Pathol. Microbiol.* **34**, 379 (1969).

183. H. Binz and H. Wigzell, *J. Exp. Med.* **144**, 1438 (1976).

184. A. Nisonoff and M. I. Greene, in M. Fougereau and J. Dausset, Eds., *Immunology 80*, Academic Press, New York, 1980, p. 57.

185. G. L. Ada and P. Byrt, *Nature* **222**, 1291 (1969).

186. B. L. Kotzin, S. Strober, E. G. Engleman, A. Calin, R. T. Hoppe, G. S. Kansas, C. P. Terrell, and H. S. Kaplan, *N. Engl. J. Med.* **305**, 969 (1981).

187. B. L. Kotz and S. Strober, *J. Exp. Med.* **150**, 371 (1979).

2

Genetics of the Autoimmune Endocrinopathies: Animal Models

Kirk W. Beisel
Noel R. Rose

Department of Immunology and Infectious Diseases
School of Hygiene and Public Health
Johns Hopkins University
Baltimore, Maryland

Contents

1. INTRODUCTION

The genetic predisposition toward autoimmune disease was originally inferred from two types of clinical observations. One is the aggregation of several autoimmune thyroid disorders in the same family (1). In addition, Graves' thyrotoxicosis or Hashimoto's thyroiditis, two of the most frequent autoimmune thyroid diseases, overlap with autoimmune diseases of different organs, such as pernicious anemia and Addison's disease of the adrenal (1). The second is epidemiologic investigations, employing disequilibrium analysis, which have demonstrated that many forms of autoimmune diseases are associated with genetic markers; in particular, the human lymphocyte antigen (HLA) complex (2). Within the Caucasian population a significant association is found between the HLA-A1-B8-Dw3 haplotype and Graves' disease, Addison's disease, some forms of chronic thyroiditis, and juvenile onset diabetes mellitus. However, in other populations where there is a different distribution of the HLA haplotypes there are also different haplotypic associations with the autoimmune endocrinopathies. For example, in Japan, HLA-B8 is relatively rare and Graves' disease is associated with HLA-Bw35 (3). Yet some classical forms of autoimmune disease (e.g., the nongoitrous form of chronic thyroiditis) have no significant correlation with the HLA complex (4, 5).

Although these studies all point to a genetic predisposition toward the development of autoimmune endocrine diseases, other interpretations are not excluded. Infectious agents, such as viruses and mycoplasmas, are passed among family members and may also account for familial aggregation. Food habits and exposure to environmental toxicants are also shared in families. One can, in brief, conceive of "cultural heredity" in addition to genetic heredity as a precipitating factor in human autoimmune disease.

To gain insight into the relative roles of environmental and genetic factors we undertook a study of juvenile forms of autoimmune thyroid disease (6). Patients with chronic lymphocytic thyroiditis or thyrotoxicosis were selected from a pediatric endocrine clinic. Their clinically normal siblings and parents were examined for markers of autoimmunity, such as autoantibodies to thyroglobulin, thyroid microsomes, gastric parietal cells, smooth muscle, mitochondria, nuclear antigens, and other common autoantigens. The results of these investigations of children are especially revealing, since the environmental influences seem to be less prominent at younger ages. Evidence of subclinical autoimmunity (in the form of thyroid autoantibodies) was found in 50% of siblings, compared with the presence of these autoimmune indicators in only 10% of children of the same ages drawn from similar families with no history of autoimmune disease. Moreover, the chance of any unaffected sibling having autoantibodies was directly related to the incidence of autoantibodies in their parents: namely, if both parents had autoantibodies, 71% of their children were also positive; if one parent had autoantibodies, 54% of their normal children were positive; and if neither parent had autoantibodies only 29% of the normal siblings were reactors. Since cultural heredity is equivalent in these

three groups, the significant role of genetic inheritance is confirmed. In addition, the incidence of parietal cell and nuclear autoantibodies is elevated in the children with autoimmune thyroid disease.

To understand the controlling factors for autoimmune responses in endocrinopathies, several animal models have been examined in depth. The best defined and most extensively studied example of autoimmune thyroiditis, experimental autoimmune thyroiditis (EAT), is produced by immunization of mice or rats with murine or rat thyroglobulin, respectively, plus an adjuvant. Spontaneous forms of autoimmune thyroiditis appear in the obese strain (OS) chicken and the Buffalo strain (BUF) rat, and these too have provided a means of identifying the genetic components controlling autoimmunity.

Genetic traits have been described which determine the susceptibility of various mouse strains to other autoimmune diseases, including experimentally induced autoimmune encephalomyelitis (EAE) (7) and myasthenia gravis (EMG) (8). These genes interact additively or syngeneically to modulate the susceptibility or resistance to an autoimmune disease. Further detailed genetic analysis employing the

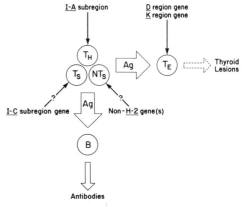

Figure 1. Diagrammatic representation of the genetic control of T cell functions in murine autoimmune thyroiditis: T_H, helper T cell; TS_S, suppressor T cell; NT_S, native (nonspecific) suppressor T cell; T_E, effector cell; B, B cell; Ag, antigen.

inbred strains available should help clarify these issues.

Several mechanisms have been proposed to explain unresponsiveness to self-antigens. One current view is that self-reactive lymphocytes are not eliminated by clonal deletion during fetal life, or by later clonal abortion or anergy, or by receptor blockade. According to this view, autoimmunity to organ-specific antigens of endocrine organs is prevented by active immunoregulatory suppression. Defects in the generation of a distinct subpopulation of suppressor T lymphocytes or a drop in production of anti-idiotypic antibodies, or a combination thereof, will instigate autoimmune disease. This concept has been termed *clonal balance* and is illustrated diagrammatically in Figure 1.

2. AUTOIMMUNE THYROID DISEASE

2.1. Mice

Introduction

Injection of mice with crude mouse thyroid extract or purified mouse thyroglobulin together with a suitable adjuvant, such as complete Freund's adjuvant (CFA), results in lymphocytic thyroiditis. Autoantibodies to thyroglobulin as well as marked infiltration of the thyroid glands by lymphocytes, macrophages, and other mononuclear cells are observed (9). When strains of inbred mice with various H-2 and non-H-2 genes were examined for their responsiveness to thyroglobulin, significant differences were found (10). In some of the strains antibodies to thyroglobulin were detectable by passive hemagglutination within 1 week, and in other strains antibody production was delayed for several weeks although all strains eventually produced significant antibody responses. The thyroid lesions were severe and in some instances virtually the entire gland was destroyed in the mice that responded promptly. In the poor responder strains, where the onset of

Table 1.   Murine H-2-linked response[a] to mouse thyroglobulin

Mouse Strain	H-2 Haplotype	Responder Classification
B10	b	Poor
B10.D2	d	Poor
B10.M	f	Poor
B10.WB	j	Poor
B10.BR	k	Good
B10.F	p	Good
B10.G	q	Good
B10.RIII	r	Poor
B10.S	s	Good
B10.PL	u	Good
B10.SM	v	Poor

[a] *Mice were immunized with 20 μg each of MTg and LPS on days 0 and 7. Titers and pathological indices were obtained on day 28. Strains showing moderate to severe thyroiditis were classified as good responders.*

antibody production was delayed, titers were slightly lower than in the good responder strains, with little or no mononuclear cellular infiltration seen in the thyroid. More recently, studies using lipopolysaccharide (LPS), a weaker adjuvant, have enabled greater distinction between inbred mouse strains in terms of both antibody titer and thyroid pathology (11, 12).

Association with H-2 complex

In the initial genetic studies of Vladutiu and Rose (10), mouse strains were classified as good or poor responders. Only a few strains of the 33 examined were considered as intermediate responders. This study first demonstrated an H-2 association. Mouse strains carrying the H-2[q, s, or k] haplotypes were all good responders, whereas those with the H-2[b or d] haplotypes were uniformly poor responders. Examination of the congenic inbred lines which differ only in regard to their H-2 haplotype supported this H-2 association. Recent investigations in our laboratory of a panel of B10 congenics (Table 1) have provided additional confirmatory evidence for this H-2 control of thyroiditis. The ability of

Table 2. Response of F_1 hybrids between good and poor responder
mouse strains to mouse thyroglobulin

Strains	H-2 Haplotype	Total No. Mice	Antibody[a] Mean Log Titer ± S.E.	Pathology[a] Index ± S.E.
C3H/Anf	k	8	11.2 ± 0.8	1.8 ± 0.3
C57BL/6	b	16	4.8 ± 0.4	0.4 ± 0.1
(C3H/Anf × C57BL/6)F_1	k/b	10	9.0 ± 0.6	1.0 ± 0.2

[a] *Data from day 28. Antibody titer was determined by a hemagglutination assay using erythrocytes coupled to MTg with chromium chloride. The pathology index is expressed as the mean of an arbitrary grading scale from 0 (no infiltration) to 4 (severe infiltration).*

these strains to respond to thyroglobulin was determined using LPS as the adjuvant. Use of LPS as an adjuvant affords greater differences in thyroglobulin antibody titers, permitting easier discrimination between good and poor responders.

F_1 hybrids between a good and poor responder, when immunized with MTg and LPS, produced both antibody titers and pathology indices intermediate between those of the parental lines (Table 2). This is not the case when using CFA, where the response of F_1 hybrids was usually equivalent to the good responder parent (13). These data indicate the subtlety by which the autoimmune response can be manipulated by use of different adjuvants. In the F_2 generation, segregation of responsiveness to MTg was observed, so that all good responders were of the good responder parental H-2 haplotype and all poor responders possessed the genotype of the poor responder parental strain.

Ir-Tg (Fig. 1)

The predominant gene that determines responsiveness to thyroglobulin maps to the H-2 complex (10). Tomazic et al. (14) suggested that this immune response (Ir) gene be called Ir-Tg. The gene controlling susceptibility to EAT was more precisely mapped to the K and/or I-A regions of the H-2 complex. More recently, the Ir-Tg gene has been mapped to

the I-A subregion of the H-2 complex (15). These studies were done using intra-H-2 recombinant strains which were derived from recombination events between the good responder k haplotype and the poor responder b haplotype. The two recombinants principally involved in this mapping study were the B10.MBR and B10.A(4R) (Table 3). Both strains were good responders and shared only the I-A^k region. B10.A(4R) mapped the Ir-Tg gene to the left of the I-B subregion, whereas B10.MBR indicated its location was to the right of the K region.

D-End Influence (Fig. 1)

In the original studies of Valdutiu and Rose (10) the strains which carried the a haplotype were intermediates in response. This haplotype is a recombinant of H-2^k and H-2^d haplotypes, where the poor responder allele, H-2^d, is present at the H-2D-end. Subsequent work by Tomazic et al. (14) also suggested that besides the Ir-Tg gene control the D-end exerted additional influence on the response to MTg in reducing thyroid infiltration. The influence of H-2D-end was explored using intra-H-2 recombinant strains which had similar I region haplotypes but differed in the D-end (16). The three different groups of recombinants examined had the k, s, or d haplotypes at the Ir-Tg gene, respectively. When the Ir-Tg is from the good responder k and s strains,

Table 3.   Genetic mapping of the murine autoimmune response
to mouse thyroglobulin

Strain	H-2 Haplo-type	H-2 Complex K A B J E C S D TL	Antibody[a] Mean Log$_2$ Titer ± S.E.	Thyroid Pathology[a] % Positive	Total No. Mice
B10	b	b b b b b b b b b	1.6 ± 0.3	4	28
B10.BR	k	k k k k k k k k k	9.5 ± 0.4	72	29
B10.A(4R)	h4	k k|b b b b b b b	9.3 ± 0.4	53	19
B10.MBR	bql	b|k k k k k k q a	7.0 ± 0.4	72	29
B10.AKM	m	k k k k k k k q a	7.5 ± 0.7	52	23
B10.A	a	k k k k k d d d a	8.5 ± 0.3	52	24
B10.AQR	yl	q k k k k d d d a	5.4 ± 0.5	70	20

Modified from Beisel et al. (15).
[a] *Data from day 28.*

the degree of mononuclear cellular infiltration is greatly reduced (Table 4) in mice bearing the D-end showed that cellular infiltration is b or q haplotypes at the D end also resulted in reduction of thyroiditis with I^k allele. The D^f allele, however, produced no reduction in the pathology score. The Ir-Tg^s allele was more noticeably influenced by the D^d allele with respect to both a reduction of thyroiditis and the percentage of individuals with disease. Examination of recombinants carrying the poor responder Ir-Tg^d allele and various alleles at the D end showed that cellular infiltration is always minimal. Interestingly, the presence of the k allele at the D end in the C3H.OL strain resulted in a marked reduction of both cellular infiltrate and antibody production. It is apparent from these investigations that the Ir-Tg gene determines a good or poor response to thyroglobulin as such, whereas the D region modifies the severity of the disease. One can speculate that this D region influences a sec-

Table 4.   Influence of the H-2D^d allele on immune response of recombinant
mouse strain to mouse thyroglobulin

Strain	H-2 Haplo-type	H-2 Gene Complex K A B J E C S D TL	Antibody[a] Mean Log$_2$ Titer ± S.E.	Thyroiditis[a] Mean Index ± S.E.
B10.BR	k	k k k k k k k k a	11.2 ± 1.0	2.2 ± 0.2
B10.AKM	m	k k k k k k k|q a	9.8 ± 0.4	1.3 ± 0.3
B10.AM	h3	k k k k k k k|b b	9.0 ± 0.2	1.1 ± 0.2
B10.A	a	k k k k k|d d d a	9.1 ± 0.4	0.6 ± 0.2
B10.M(17R)	aql	k k k k k d d|f a	10.8 ± 0.2	2.2 ± 0.2
B10.S	s	s s s s s s s s b	9.4 ± 0.5	1.3 ± 0.1
B10.S(7R)	t2	s s s s s s s|d a	6.8 ± 0.6	0.7 ± 0.2

Data modified from Kong et al. (16).
[a] *Data from day 28.*

ond-order function which governs the effector mechanisms necessary for thyroid inflammation.

K-End Influence (Fig. 1)

The K-end, like the D-end, influences the expression of the Ir-Tg by modifying the severity of disease. Two lines of evidence support this conclusion. Experiments done by Cohen and co-workers (17–19) have demonstrated that the K^b region, B6.C-H-2^{bml} (20, 21), has a higher incidence of thyroiditis than B6 parent. Since the B6.C-H-2^{bml} is a point mutation (22), it is likely that the H-2K glycoprotein is the H-2 product responsible for facilitating the severity of thyroiditis. These investigators also examined the role of the H-2K product in effector function upon the target thyroid gland (18). In the F_1 hybrids between B6.C-H-2^{bml} and B6 wild type, thyroid glands from each parental strain were implanted under the kidney capsule. Four to five weeks after the induction of EAT, the three thyroids were examined histologically. The thyroids from the bml mice had an incidence of EAT (54%) which was similar to the endogenous F_1 gland (60%). The B6 thyroids, however, had a lower EAT incidence (23%), showing that the attack upon the thyroid target by the effector cells depends upon congruence at the K-end.

Zinkernagel et al. (23) and Bevan (24) have shown that the genotype of the thymus determines the H-2 products that are recognized in association with the antigen by the cytotoxic T cells. Experiments were performed using (C3H/eb × B6)F_1 and (BALB/c × B6)F_1 nude mice (19). Thymuses from various donors were implanted in these mice and the severity of EAT determined. Thymuses from the B6.C-H-2^{bml} (73%) but not the wild type B6 (8%) induced a high incidence of EAT in the (C3H/eb × B6)F_1 nude mice. However, the B6.C-H-2^{bml} thymuses were ineffective in promoting EAT development in the (BALB/c × B6)F_1 nude mice. Antigenic changes in the K^{bml} molecule might be similar to those determinants of the H-2^k gene products that

are recognized in association with thyroglobulin by the invading mononuclear cells. This concept is strengthened by the finding that B6 cytotoxic T lymphocytes directed against B6.C-H-2^{bml} also lyse H-2^k targets (25).

A second line of evidence implicating the K-end in regulating the severity of thyroid lesions comes from studies of intra-H-2 recombinants (15). When the incidence of EAT in good responder strains which differed only at their K region allele was compared, significant differences were observed (see Table 3). Both B10.A (kkkkkddd) and B10.AKM (kkkkkkkq) exhibited a 52% incidence of EAT, whereas B10.AQR (qkkkkddd) and B10.MBR (bkkkkkkq) had an incidence of 70 and 72%, respectively. Thus the presence of K^k results in a lower level of thyroid infiltration than does the presence of K^q and K^b alleles. This observation supports the bml studies suggesting that the K molecule is also involved in the effector phase of EAT. The K and D regions are both responsible for a 45,000 dalton glycoprotein surface molecule, which is associated with β_2 microglobulin. They share similar functions in regulation of the thyroid lesion through yet undefined effector mechanisms.

Non-H-2 Genes

By examining a large panel of independent H-2 haplotypes on C57BL/10 (syn. B10), BALB/c, C3H, and A/J backgrounds for their responsiveness to thyroglobulin using LPS as adjuvant, the effect of genes outside the H-2 region was documented (Table 5). Differences in both antibody titer (11) and incidence of thyroiditis in strains that are identical at H-2 but different at other loci were observed. Besides providing confirmatory evidence of the predominant H-2 role in EAT, an influence of non-H-2 genes was thus demonstrated. A striking example involves differences between the B10.F (H-2^p) and C3H.NB (H-2^p) strains. The B10.F strains develops a poorer response whereas C3H.NB is a good responder in regard to both antibody

Table 5.   Influence of background genes on immune response of congenic mice to mouse thyroglobulin

Strain	H-2 Haplotype	Total No. Mice	Antibody[a] Mean Log$_2$ Titer ± S.E.	Thyroid Pathology[a] % Positive
B10	b	28	2.4 ± 0.3	3
BALB.B	b	9	4.8 ± 1.1	0
C3H.SW	b	23	5.4 ± 0.6	23
A.BY	b	26	4.2 ± 0.1	26
B10.D2	d	17	8.2 ± 0.6	11
BALB/c	d	10	4.0 ± 0.3	0
B10.WB	j	25	1.8 ± 0.3	25
C3H.JK	j	25	6.1 ± 1.0	36
B10.BR	k	29	9.4 ± 0.4	66
BALB.K	k	18	10.2 ± 0.5	50
C3H/Anf	k	7	11.0 ± 0.8	100
B10.F	p	18	5.1 ± 0.4	44
C3H.NB	p	18	10.9 ± 0.7	67

[a] Data from day 28.

titer ($p < .0001$) and the incidence and degree of thyroiditis present ($p < .02$).

In the murine form of EMG, the autoimmune response to nicotinic acetylcholine receptors is determined by at least two distinct loci. One is associated with the H-2 complex and another with the structural genes for the constant region of immunoglobulin heavy chains (IgC$_H$). Because of similarities between the various autoimmune disease in both cellular control and genetic regulation of the immune response, we suggest that the non-H-2 genes controlling EAT may be associated with the immunoglobulin genes.

Cellular Basis of Genetic Control

It has been established that responsiveness of thyroglobulin depends on the presence of thymus-derived (T) lymphocytes (26). Mice depleted of T cells by thymectomy and lethal irradiation followed by reconstitution with anti-thy-and-complement-treated bone marrow cells, as well as athymic (nu/nu) mice, failed to evidence any immunologic response to murine thyroglobulin. Use of the T cell proliferation assay (27) has shown that proliferation differences between good and poor

responders can be determined. The lymphocytes which undergo a proliferative response are T cells, since the response to thyroglobulin is eliminated by pretreatment of the cells with anti-thy-1 serum and complement (27). This in vitro proliferative response parallels thyroid infiltration and may reflect effector T cell activity (28). Response to murine thyroglobulin in mice of different H-2 haplotypes on the C57BL/10 background showed that those strains carrying the H-2^{k,q,r,s} haplotypes were classified as good responders (27). The strains of b, d, f, and j haplotypes were low responders. The results of the T cell proliferation corresponded with those already obtained on the basis of antibody production and cellular infiltration. B10.RIII (H-2^r) was the only exception since this strain appears to be a poor responder in regard to thyroiditis. Since the proliferation appears to measure T effector cell proliferation (29), there may be a high level of suppressor activity which reduced the infiltration of the thyroid.

Examination of recombinant haplotypes in the proliferative response to thyroglobulin has demonstrated that the major Ir-Tg maps to the H-2K-end (27). B10.A(2R), which differs from B10.A(4R) in the I-C subregion and S region, had a stimulation index approximately 50% that of B10.A(4R). This difference suggests that a gene (or genes) mapping in either the I-C subregion and/or the S^d region has a negative influence on the proliferative response. Other H-2 influences were observed when comparing B10.S, B10.S(7R), B10.S(9R), and B10.HTT (Table 6). Recombinant B10.S(7R), which differs from the B10.S in only the H-2D and TL regions, shows a stimulation index of 1.73, thereby suggesting that genes in either D^d or TL^a regions decrease the effectiveness of the Ir-Tg^s genes to respond to thyroglobulin. B10.HTT gives an intermediate response, whereas B10.S(9R), which carries the low responder allele d at the I-C, S, and D regions, is a low responder. These data provide evidence for two "suppressive" genes which map to the right of the I-E subregion. B10.S(9R) has both these genes, while B10.S(7R) and B10.HTT have only one associated with the H-2D end. The two genes with suppressive regulatory effects (Is genes) appear to map to the I-C subregion and the H-2D region.

Evidence from adoptive transfer studies (26) suggests that thymus-generated lymphocytes suppress EAT. A unique function of the intact thymus appears to reduce the development of EAT, most likely through interfering with effector cells responsible for production

of thyroid cellular infiltration. The investigations of Kojima and co-workers (30–32) strongly support this hypothesis. They found that, if mice of certain strains were thymectomized on the fourth day of age, they spontaneously developed autoimmune thyroiditis. Other strains, when treated in a similar manner, developed different forms of organ-specific autoimmune disease such as gastritis (33) and oophoritis (34). Injection of thymocytes from neonates or spleen cells and lymph node cells from older donors prevented the occurrence of post-thymectomy autoimmune thyroiditis. Irradiation of these donor cells destroyed their protective action. It can be postulated that a suppressor cell population arises in the thymus and later migrates to the peripheral lymphoid tissues. Genetic studies by these investigators (35) suggest that the occurrence of post-thymectomy autoimmune thyroiditis is influenced by genetic factors outside the H-2 complex.

Recently, studies of Okayasu et al. (36, 37) demonstrated that injection of aqueous MTg without an adjuvant into mice prevents the development of EAT. Both the timing and dosage of antigen are critical for rendering the mice unresponsive to the immunogenic regimen of murine thyroglobulin with CFA or LPS. This unresponsiveness can be transferred to syngeneic recipients with either spleen or thymus cells for animals pretreated with

Table 6.   Genetic mapping of T-lymphocyte proliferative response to mouse thyroglobulin

Strain	H-2 Haplotype	H-2 Gene Complex K A B J E C S D TL	Proliferative Response[a] (Stimulation Index)
B10.A(4R)	h4	k k b b b b b b b	3.9
B10.A(2a)	h2	k k k k k d d b b	1.7
B10.S	s	s s s s s s s s b	3.0
B10.S(7R)	t2	s s s s s s s d a	1.7
B10.S(9R)	t4	s s ? k k d d d a	0.8
B10.HTT	t3	s s s s k k k d c	1.5

Modified from Christadoss et al. (27).
[a] [^{3}H] thymidine uptake is expressed as experimental mean CPM divided by media control mean CPM.

aqueous MTg. The suppressive effect of these transferred cells is abolished by treatment with anti-thy-1 plus complement showing that the cells responsible for induced immunosuppression are T lymphocytes (Figure 1).

2.2. Rats

Spontaneously Appearing Thyroiditis

BUF rats, a strain which was established by inbreeding in 1931, have been recognized as a model of spontaneous autoimmune thyroiditis (SAT) (38–40). The incidence of this autoimmune disease (41) is related to age and sex. Animals younger than 3 months do not show signs of the disease. However, the incidence of SAT rises to approximately 48% of the BUF rats by 7 months of age. The disease incidence decreased in animals more than 14 months. Females are affected approximately three times more frequently than males.

In the SAT of BUF rats there is an interesting relationship between the occurrence of the circulating antibodies to thyroglobulin and the appearance of thyroid lesions (13). Titers are lowest in animals with little mononuclear infiltration but are highest in those animals displaying intermediate infiltration. However, rats with more severe SAT have lower titers, which may be due to the formation of circulating immune complexes. The histological changes in the thyroid are characterized by dense collections of small and medium sized lymphocytes which sometimes destroy the normal architecture of a large portion of the gland. In more mature lesions, macrophages can make up as much as 12% of the infiltrating cell population. Medium sized lymphocytes predominate and plasma cells are conspicuous (42).

If BUF rats are treated and fed with methylcholanthrene, SAT occurs at a much earlier age. At 3 months 10% of the animals show evidence of SAT (43). In 4-month animals which have been treated with methylcholanthrene, 42% showed histological damage. All other aspects of the drug-induced thyroiditis do not differ from the spontaneous disease. The BUF rats have some genetic propensity to methylcholanthrene-accelerated SAT, since no other rat strain tested developed SAT after methylcholanthrene treatment.

Neonatal thymectomy results in an earlier onset and increased severity of thyroiditis (13, 44). This result suggests that a population of thymus-derived lymphocytes acts to suppress the autoimmune reaction in newborn rats. During aging, the function of this thymic cell population diminishes, as reflected in lymphopenia and the corresponding appearance of SAT (42).

The role of a suppressor cell population in thyroiditis of the rat was examined by Penhale and co-workers (44, 45). They demonstrated that Wistar rats that had been thymectomized and repeatedly irradiated with low dosages developed thyroiditis spontaneously. The animals that were reconstituted with spleen, lymph node, or thymus cells did not develop thyroiditis. As in the mice studied by Kojima et al. (31), anti-T-cell serum and complement destroyed the protective action of the adoptively transferred cells.

EAT in the Rat

The susceptibility of inbred rat strains to EAT has been classified into three categories, high, intermediate, and low (Table 7) (46–48). Disease was induced by immunization of either crude rat thyroid extract emulsified in CFA (46) or purified rat thyroglobulin with both CFA and pertussis vaccine (49). Although the autoantibody response generally correlated well with development of EAT, rats did vary considerably in the severity of thyroid lesions. A significant relationship was observed between both in vivo proliferation and in vivo delayed hypersensitivity to RTg and thyroiditis in good responder rats (48).

Studies of Penhale et al. (46) suggest that strains with the MHC haplotype RTI^c (AgB5) were the most susceptible, whereas the least susceptible strain were of the RTI^w (AgB2) haplotype. However, no linkage studies were done to confirm this relationship between RT1

Table 7.   Strain difference in susceptibility to EAT in inbred strains of rats

Genotype	Strain	Response Category
RT1^l	AS	Intermediate
	CDF	High
	LEW	Intermediate
RT1^w	AO	High
	CAM	Low
	LE	Low
	WAG	Low
	WF	High
RT1^n	BN	Low
RT1^a	ACI	Low
	DA	Low
RT1^c	AUG	High
	HL	Intermediate
	HO	Low
	LH	High
	PVG/c	Low
RT1^b ·	BVF	Intermediate
	M520	Intermediate
	SD	
RT1^k	SHR	Low
	WKY	Intermediate

Modified from Penhale et al. (45), Rose (47), and Lillehoj and Rose (48).

and EAT. Recently our group (48, 50) demonstrated that there was no gross correlation of the RT1 genotype with either autoantibody response to thyroid pathology. However, since RT1 congenic strains have not yet been examined, the possible role of the rat MHC in EAT cannot be completely excluded.

Genetic factors influencing susceptibility to EAT were examined in interstrain F_1, F_2, and backcross animals of the CDF (good responder) and SHR (low responder) strains (50). The pathological indices of the F_1 hybrids were intermediate to the parental strains. The phenotypic segregation patterns of the F_2 and backcross animals suggested the autoimmune response to RTg is under polygenic control. A principal genetic factor controlling response to thyroglobulin in the rat was as-

sociated with the X chromosome. Backcross animals which were homozygous and hemizygous for the CDF X chromosome had a higher incidence of thyroiditis than those that carried the X chromosome from the SHR strain. Furthermore, females of CDF and SHR produced higher levels of anti-RTg antibodies than the males. This observation suggested that antibody production to rat thyroglobulin is a sex-related trait. A relationship was not observed between the severity of thyroid lesions in susceptible and nonsusceptible strains and their response to phytomitogens, phytohemagglutin (PHA), and concanavalin A (ConA). In a more extensive study (51) PHA and ConA responses were recorded in the susceptible CDF strain and nonsusceptible SHR rats. No differences were observed in the ConA response; however, in CDF rats the response to PHA was significantly lower than in the poorly susceptible SHR animals. Intercrosses between CDF and SHR rats demonstrated that a single autosomal gene controls the PHA responses. The PHA gene was not linked to the immune response gene to rat thyroglobulin (Ir-RaTg) genes nor to the RT1 complex.

2.3.   OS Chickens

The obese strain (OS) of white Leghorn chickens was established by Cole (52) by selective breeding of phenotypically hypothyroid chickens of the Cornell strains (CS). At present, OS chickens spontaneously develop the obese phenotype in over 95% of the animals. At 6 to 8 weeks of age the OS thyroid glands are smaller than those of normal chickens. Histologically, proliferation of the thyroid epithelial cells, absence of colloid-containing follicles and the presence of mononuclear cell infiltration are observed. Germinal centers are often seen. Animals over 4 weeks of age have antibodies specific for chicken thyroglobulin. Evidence that the OS chicken thyroid failure is caused by an autoimmune process came from several observations. The presence of the bursa of Fabricius is necessary for development of chicken SAT

(53, 54), and bursectomized animals develop only mild thyroiditis. Also, treatment with cyclophosphamide or testosterone, which induces a bursectomized-like state, causes the mild form of thyroiditis in the OS chickens.

The B Complex

The major histocompatibility complex of the chicken is the B complex. Immunochemical studies demonstrate that, like its mammalian homologue, the B complex controls multiple gene products similar to the products of the H-2K, D, and I genes (55–57). Like H-2, the B complex is highly polymorphic and controls a number of cellular properties necessary for the regulation of the immune system (58, 59).

The heredity of SAT is polygenic in nature and is expressed with a certain degree of dominance (52). The relationship between SAT and the B complex was established by Bacon et al. (60). Offspring of heterozygous B^5B^{13} OS chickens were examined for development of SAT. Chickens with the B^{13} allele, whether present in homozygous form or coupled with B^5, had extensive thyroiditis, whereas B^5B^5 animals displayed only mild SAT.

Additional studies crossing OS with normal Cornell strain (CS) chickens examined (OS × CS)F_1 hybrids with various B genotypes for SAT (61). All offspring with the B^{15} allele, regardless of whether they were in the homozygous or heterozygous state, had the highest relative thyroglobulin antibody titers and the severest disease. It was noted that when B^{13} or B^5 was coupled with B^6 significantly less disease was present. This observation suggests that one or more loci within the B complex are responsible for expression of SAT and that the B haplotypes interact in varying patterns to determine the eventual outcome of disease. In more extensive studies of (CS × OS)F_2 chickens (62), B^6B^6 and B^6B^{15} birds had comparable titers of thyroglobulin antibodies and had lower titers than $B^{15}B^{15}$ birds at 5 and 7 weeks of age. The thyroid pathology scores were greater in the $B^{15}B^{15}$ birds than

the B^6B^{15} animals. The F_2 offspring with B^6B^6 genotype displayed very little cellular infiltration. There may be several genes within the B complex which determine the extent of disease. The first locus is probably the classical Ir-Tg gene which must be present for development of severe thyroiditis. A second locus, homologous to the D-end influence observed in mice, may provide a modulating effect on the severity of disease.

Non-B Complex Influences

Genetic influences of other loci upon the expression of the B haplotype in SAT have been described (63, 64). Evidence that non-B loci affect the disease in chickens was found by assaying the development of SAT in three partially inbred substrains of OS chickens: OSA, OSB, and OSC. When comparing birds of the same B haplotype (B^5B^5, B^5B^{13}, and $B^{13}B^{13}$) from the three substrains, significant differences in both thyroglobulin antibody titer and thyroid pathology were found (Table 8) (64, 65). More recent studies of (CS × OS)F_2 birds provided further evidence that genes outside the MHC control SAT (62). There were significant differences observed among birds with the same B haplotype depending upon how much of the genotype was contributed by the OS or the CS parent.

Role of Thymus-derived Cells

Even though the B complex is an important factor in the development of SAT, other factors do play a role. In the CS chickens, birds rarely develop thyroiditis even if they have the $B^{13}B^{13}$ haplotype. Additional control of susceptibility of OS to the autoimmune disease is mediated through the thymus. Neonatal thymectomy of OS birds results in the production of more severe disease (66, 67). However, little or no effect was observed on the antibody titer to thyroglobulin. These data suggest that natural suppressor cells in the thymus limit the development of disease.

Experiments of Livezey (68) and Sundick et al. (69) demonstrated the direct involvement of OS thymocytes in thyroid infiltration and

Table 8. Influence of background genes on thyroglobulin antibodies in substrains of OS chickens in SAT

	B Haplotype					
	B^5B^5		B^5B^{13}		$B^{13}B^{13}$	
Substrain	n	TgAb $\geq 4^a$ (%)	n	TgAb $\geq 4^a$ (%)	n	TgAb $\geq 4^a$ (%)
OSA	7	0	13	46	4	100
OSB	52	27	103	48	38	42
OSC	6	17	17	76	7	86

Modified from Bacon and Rose (63).
[a] Indicates birds in each group with thyroglobulin antibody titers ≥ 4. These birds were 4 to 5 weeks of age.

production of thyroglobulin antibodies. CS chicks, possessing the same B haplotype as the OS donors, were depleted of T cells by neonatal thymectomy and whole body irradiation. They were reconstituted with thymocytes from 6-day-old OS chickens. Severe thyroiditis was developed in these recipient CS birds. These data show that helper T cells reactive against chicken thyroglobulin are present in the thymuses of OS chickens.

Role of Bursa-derived Cells

The role of the B cells or their antibody products in thyroiditis has also been examined. Passive transfer of high-titered antisera against chicken thyroglobulin has been unrewarding in transferring the disease (70). However, severity of SAT can be dramatically increased by injection of B^5B^5 recipient OS chicks with high-titered serum from $B^{13}B^{13}$ donors. Experiments of Polley and Bacon (71) showed that B cells of CS and OS birds do not differ in their ability to transfer adoptively an autoimmune response, providing they can cooperate with OS T lymphocytes. F_1 hybrids of ($B^{13}B^{13}$) OS and ($B^{13}B^{13}$) CS birds which were bursectomized by cyclophosphamide treatments could be fully restored to antibody responsiveness with either CS or OS bursal cells.

Thyroid Defects

One explanation of the finding that passive transfer of thyroglobulin antibodies causes disease in OS but not CS chickens is that OS birds have a defective thyroid. Newly hatched OS chickens incorporate significantly more iodine-131 into the thyroid gland than thyroids of CS chicken (72, 73). The increased iodine uptake of the OS thyroid appears to be due to an abnormal thyroid gland. In addition, the ratio of mono- to diiodotyrosine in the OS thyroids is significantly increased (74). Thyroids of both OS and CS birds had significantly higher thyroidal incorporation of iodine compared to other strains even after thyroid suppression induced by uptake of throxine (T_4) (75). The unsuppressible hyperactivity of both OS and CS thyroids appears to be intrinsic to the gland itself (75, 76).

3. AUTOIMMUNE DIABETES MELLITUS

3.1. Genetic Influences

Study of autoimmunity in human diabetes mellitus (DM) has permitted a new classification of the various forms of this disease. In Cudworth's classification (77, 78), Type I includes these two principal forms of insulin-dependent diabetes mellitus (IDDM), the classical OS juvenile-onset disease (type Ia), and the form observed mainly in older females (type Ib). Other milder forms of noninsulin-dependent diabetes mellitus (NIDDM) are included in type II. Clinical studies have demonstrated that patients with type I disease have similar HLA haplotypes (see Refs. 77, 79, and 80). Marked increases in relative risk are observed in patients with HLA-Dw3 and Dw4 (or DR3 and DR4) (81). Recently, Solow et al. (82) have suggested that multiple MHC genes may influence the development of type I DM. The primary diabetogenic genes are associated with D or DR alleles, whereas the B15, B40, and Cw3 alleles seem to possess only a secondary influence.

Genetic analyses of experimental models of diabetes are neither as detailed nor as numerous as the clinical investigations. Studies by Kromann et al. (83) used crude extracts of either fetal calf or mice pancreatic islet cells emulsified in FCA to induce experimental autoimmune DM (EADM) in mice. Islet cell surface antibodies (ICSA) were present in the five strains of mice examined and levels increased with repeated immunizations. Examination of glucose tolerance levels in the immunized animal revealed strain differences that can be aligned with differences at the H-2 complex. Heterologous immunization with fetal calf antigen produced a slight abnormality in glucose tolerance in B10.A (H-2^a). Congenic strains B10 (H-2^b) and B10.D2 (H-2^d) had significantly higher levels of glucose tolerance at 2 weeks after the initial immunization, whereas B10.BR (H-2^k) was unresponsive to the heterologous immunizations. Homologous immunizations proved to be the most effective; however, strains differences were difficult to classify into any consistent pattern. Data from the immunizations with foreign pancreatic islet cells suggest that the major histocompatibility complex has some genetic role in development of EADM.

Mouse strains NZB, (NZB × NZW)F$_1$ MRL, and BXSB all develop autoimmune diseases spontaneously. They were examined for evidence of autoimmune reactions against islet cells (84). Infiltrates of lymphocytes and fibroblasts, which were restricted to the islets, were found in all these strains. NZB animals (80%) had the highest incidence, whereas BXSB (20%) had the lowest incidence. All the NZB mice had abnormal glucose tolerance.

In the three other strains abnormal glucose tolerance ranged from 20 to 50% of the animals examined. It is probable that the cellular autoimmune response to the pancreatic islet cells is a consequence of a common immunologic dysfunction in these animals.

3.2. Cellular Influences

Treatment with multiple low doses of streptozotocin induces hyperglycemia in mice (85, 86). Lymphocytic infiltration into the pancreatic islets (insulitis) is also noted. Animals treated in this manner provide a model for studying EADM. Insulitis was transferred using spleen cells from streptozotocin-treated C57BL/6 mice into congenic athymic C57BL 6-nu/nu mice (87). This cell transfer led to lymphocytic infiltrations in 75% of the recipients. However, no hyperglycemia was observed in these recipients. Use of other strains, such as AKR, BALB/c, C3H, and CBA/2, as streptozotocin-treated donors did not lead to significant levels of insulitis in the C57BL/6 nu/nu recipient (88). In the untreated controls insulitis occurred in low incidence.

Other investigations (89) demonstrated that mice undergoing graft-versus-host reactions (GVHR) developed severe insulitis. Histological examination of the pancreas revealed that only the islets contained cellular infiltrations, affecting primarily the beta cells. Infiltrations were not observed in the exocrine part of the pancreas, nor in heart, liver, or kidneys at the early stage of GVHR. It appears that nonspecific dysfunction in immune regulatory mechanism induced by GVHR leads to a cellular autoimmune reaction directed against the beta cells of the pancreatic islet.

4. CORRELATIONS BETWEEN AUTOIMMUNE DISEASE AND LYMPHOID MALIGNANCIES

An increasing volume of literature reports an association between autoimmunity and lymphoid cell malignancies. Clinically this association has been observed with such autoimmune diseases as Sjögren's syndrome (91, 92), Hashimoto's thyroiditis (92, 93), rheumatoid arthritis (94), hemolytic anemia (95), pernicious anemia (96), myasthenia gravis (97), and systemic lupus erythematosus (98). Although it is possible that these reports sometimes represent coincidence of nonneoplastic and neoplastic lymphoid cell abnormalities in the same patients, the frequency of such reports suggests that the association of autoimmune manifestations with lymphoid malignancies is not accidental. Moreover, even in mice, the prime example being the (NZB/NZW)F$_1$ mouse, one sees the association of autoimmune disease and lymphoid malignancy (99, 100).

We offer the working hypothesis that an individual with autoimmune disease or other chronic active immune state, having the appropriate genetic constitution, may be predisposed to the development of lymphoreticular neoplasms. As suggested in Figure 2, self-antigens constantly stimulate the corresponding helper T cells and B cells, leading to long-standing autoantibody production. This process, however, remains under the governance of suppressor T cells. A malignant change in the cycling B cell can render it unresponsive to suppressor T cell regulatory signals. Alternatively, the T$_s$ cell may lose its ability to emit the signal. Either event would lead to a population of autonomous B cells. Indeed, others have suggested that there may be a progression from autoimmune disease to premalignant lymphoproliferation and finally to lymphoma development (101, 102). The malignancies seen with the greatest frequency in human and murine victims of autoimmune disease are reticulum cell sarcomas (also referred to as histiocytic lymphomas or immunoblastic sarcomas). Convincing evidence now places this group of hematopoietic malignancies in the lymphocytic series and probably in the B cell lineage (103).

Only a few clinical studies have reported a genetic correlation between these diseases. Yoiunou and associates (104) evaluated the genetic propensity toward the occurrence of monoclonal gammopathies. Examination of patients and their immediate relatives revealed a correlation with autoimmune diseases (i.e., rheumatoid arthritis, lupus erythematosus, hemolytic anemia, multiple sclerosis, or chronic active hepatitis). The pattern of inheritance in the occurrence of these monoclonal gammopathies was suggestive of dominance. Studies of first-degree relatives of individuals with acute lymphoblastic or acute myeloblastic leukemias showed a significantly increased prevalence of autoimmune disorders (105). Again, a higher incidence in association of autoimmune disease and lymphoid malignancy occurred in these families than was expected in the normal population (105). In patients with Down's syndrome (trisomy 21) a greater incidence of autoimmune thyroid disorders (107) and leukemias (108, 109) was observed. Interestingly, Down's syndrome has been found to be associated with defective T cell function (110).

An association between autoimmunity and leukemia has been described in the NZB mouse strain (111). In a study by Emerit and coworkers (112) using two sublines of NZB

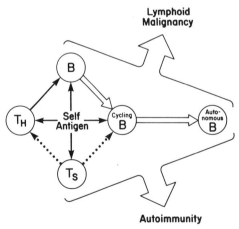

Figure 2. Diagrammatic representation of the common pathways and possible relationship between autoimmunity and lymphoid malignancy: B, B cell; T$_H$, helper T cell; T$_S$, suppressor T cell; →, stimulation; ·······→, suppression; ⇒, transformation.

Table 9.   Genetic control of autoimmune thyroiditis
in rodents and chickens

Species	Model	Genetic Control	
		MHC	Non-MHC
Mouse	EAT	H-2K	Present
		H-2D	
		I-A	
		I-C	
Rat	EAT	None	X-linked; other
	SAT (BUF)	None	Present
Chicken	SAT (OS)	B	Sex-influenced; other

which had either a high (HB) or low (LB) frequency of chromosomal breakage, the incidence of lymphomas as well as other tumors and the positivity of Coombs' tests were compared. Frequencies of both neoplasms and positive Coombs' test were significantly greater and occurred earlier in the HB mice than in either the original NZB or the LB strains. The incidence of lymphoid malignancies in the NZB has been suggested to parallel a specific karyotypic abnormality (trisomy 15) (113). The NZB strain carries Gross leukemia virus and a rapid age-dependent decline in T-lymphocytes (114). Although viruses have been considered in the etiology of both lymphoid neoplasms and autoimmune disease in NZB mice, the work of Datta and Schwartz (115) argues against a viral etiology for the autoimmune diseases. It has been proposed (116) that both the autoimmune and neoplastic processes in the NZB strain are a result of hyperactivity of B cells as well as the loss of effective suppressor T cell function (117, 118).

5. SUMMARY

Clinical and epidemiologic investigations have suggested genetic predisposition toward the development of the autoimmune endocrinopathies. Since formal genetic studies are difficult to carry out in humans, animal models have proved to be useful for exploring the genetic regulation of autoimmune responses. In experimental thyroiditis of the mouse, two levels of immunologic regulation were distinguished. Initial steps in recognition of the thyroglobulin molecule, and in determining the balance of helper or suppressor T cells stimulated, are controlled by genes in the I region of the H-2 complex. The effector anisms that are responsible for the final production of thyroid lesions are controlled by genes at the K or D regions. Non-H-2 genes also modify the response of mice to murine thyroglobulin (Fig. 1).

In the rat, no association between susceptibility to thyroiditis and the major histocompatibility complex could be found. A major gene controlling the development of disease is located in the X chromosome.

Spontaneous thyroiditis of the OS chicken is a genetic disease linked to the avian major histocompatibility complex (B locus). Independent genetic traits influence susceptibility by regulating thyroid function. The aggregation of several different genetic defects may be required for the spontaneous development of autoimmune disease. A summary of the genetic control of thyroiditis in the mouse, rat, and chicken is presented in Table 9.

ACKNOWLEDGMENTS

We thank Ms. Barbara Paton for her excellent secretarial help. This work was supported by NIH grants AM 20023 and AM 20028.

REFERENCES

1. D. Doniach and I. M. Roitt, in P. G. H. Gell, R. R. A. Coombs, and P. J. Lackmann, Eds., *Clinical Aspects of Immunology*, Blackwell Scientific Publications, Philadelphia, 1975, p. 1355.

2. A. O. Vladutiu and N. R. Rose, *Immunogenetics* 1, 305 (1974).

3. Y. Nakao, M. Kishihana, Y. Baba, K. Kama, T. Fukuniski, and H. Imura, *Arch. Intern. Med.* 138, 567 (1978).

4. W. J. Irvine, in N. R. Rose, P. E. Bigazzi, and N. L. Warner, Eds., *Genetic Control of Autoimmune Disease*, Elsevier/North-Holland, New York, 1978, p. 77.

5. N. R. Farid, R. M. Newton, E. P. Noel, J. M. Barnard, and W. H. Marshall, *Tissue Antigens* 12, 205 (1978).

6. C. L. Burek, W. H. Hoffman, and N. R. Rose, *4th Int. Congr. Immunol., Paris, France,* Abs. 14.5.03 (1980).

7. F. J. Waxman, L. E. Perryman, D. J. Hinrichs, and J. E. Coe, *J. Exp. Med.* 153, 61 (1981).

8. P. W. Berman and J. Patrick, *J. Exp. Med.* 152, 507 (1980).

9. N. R. Rose, F. J. Twarog, and A. J. Crowle, *J. Immunol.* 106, 698 (1971).

10. A. O. Vladutiu and N. R. Rose, *Science* 174, 1137 (1971).

11. N. R. Rose, Y. M. Kong, I. Okaysu, A. A. Giraldo, K. Beisel, and R. S. Sundick, *Immunol. Rev.* 55, 299 (1981).

12. P. S. Esquivel, N. R. Rose, and Y. M. Kong, *J. Exp. Med.* 145, 1250 (1977).

13. N. R. Rose, L. D. Bacon, R. S. Sundick, Y. M. Kong, P. S. Esquivel, and P. Bigazzi, in N. Talal, Ed., *Autoimmunity: Genetic, Immunologic and Clinical Aspects*, Academic Press, New York, 1977, p. 63.

14. V. Tomazic, N. R. Rose, and D. C. Shreffler, *J. Immunol.* 112, 965 (1974).

15. K. W. Beisel, C. S. David, A. A. Giraldo, Y. M. Kong, and N. R. Rose, *Immunogenetics* 15, 427 (1982).

16. Y. M. Kong, C. S. David, A. A. Giraldo, M. ElRehewy, and N. R. Rose, *J. Immunol.* 123, 15 (1979).

17. R. Maron and I. R. Cohen, *Nature* 279, 715 (1979).

18. A. Ben-Nun, R. Maron, Y. Ron, and I. R. Cohen, *Eur. J. Immunol.* 10, 156 (1980).

19. R. Maron and I. R. Cohen, *J. Exp. Med.* 152, 1115 (1980).

20. I. F. C. McKenzie, T. Pang, and R. J. Blanden, *Immunol. Rev.* 35, 181 (1977).

21. J. Klein, *Adv. Immunol.* 26, 55 (1978).

22. j. L. Brown and G. S. Nathenson, *J. Immunol.* 118, 98 (1977).

23. R. M. Zinkernagel, A. Althage, S. Cooper, G. Callahan, and J. Klein, *J. Exp. Med.* 148, 805 (1978).

24. M. J. Bevan, *Nature* 260, 417 (1977).

25. M. B. Widmer, B. J. Alter, F. M. Bach, *Nature* 242, 239 (1973).

26. A. O. Vladutiu and N. R. Rose, *Cell. Immunol.* 17, 106 (1975).

27. P. Christadoss, Y. M. Kong, M. ElRehewy, N. R. Rose, and C. S. David, in N. R. Rose, P. E. Bigazzi, and N. L. Warner, Eds., *Genetic Control of Autoimmune Disease*, Elsevier/North-Holland, New York, 1978, p. 445.

28. I. Okayasu, Y. M. Kong, C. S. David, and N. R. Rose, *Cell. Immunol.* 61, 32 (1981).

29. S. S. Alkan, *Eur. J. Immunol.* 8, 112 (1978).

30. A. Kojima, Y. Tanaka-Kojima, R. Sakakura, and Y. Nishizula, *Lab. Invest.* 34, 550 (1976).

31. A. Kojima, Y. Tanaka-Kojima, and Y. Nishizula, *Lab. Invest.* 34, 601 (1976).

32. A. Kojima, O. Taguchi, and Y. Nishizula, in N. D. Reed. Ed., *Proc. 3rd Int. Workshop on Nude Mice*, Gustav Fisher, New York, 1982 p. 245.

33. A. Kojima, O. Taguchi, and Y. Nishizuka, *Lab. Invest.* 42, 387 (1980).

34. O. Taguchi, Y. Nishizuka, T. Sakakura, and A. Kojima, *Clin. Exp. Immunol.* 40, 540 (1980).

35. A. Kojima and R. T. Prehn, *Immunogenetics* 14, 15 (1981).

36. I. Okayasu, Y. M. Kong, N. R. Rose, and C. S. David, *Fed. Proc.* 39, 667 (1980).

37. I. Okayasu, Y. M. Kong, N. R. Rose, and C. S. David, *4th Int. Congr. Immunol.*, Abs. 14.3.42 (1980).

38. E. L. Gover and M. D. Reuber, *Arch. Pathol.* 86, 542 (1968).

39. A. Hajdu and G. Roma, *Experimentia* 25, 1325 (1969).

40. M. D. Reuber, *Arch. Environ. Health* 21, 734 (1970).

41. D. A. Silverman and N. R. Rose, *Proc. Soc. Exp. Biol. Med.* 138, 579 (1971).

42. B. Noble, T. Yoshida, N. R. Rose, and P. E. Bigazzi, *J. Immunol.* 117, 1447 (1976).

43. D. A. Silverman and N. R. Rose. *J. Immunol.* **114**, 145 (1975).

44. W. J. Penhale, A. Farmer, and W. J. Irvine, *Clin. Exp. Immunol.* **21**, 362 (1975).

45. W. J. Penhale, W. J. Irvine, J. R. Inglis, and A. Farmer, *Clin. Exp. Immunol.* **25**, 6 (1976).

46. W. J. Penhale, A. Farmer, S. J. Urbaniak, and W. J. Irvine, *Clin. Exp. Immunol.* **19**, 179 (1975).

47. N. R. Rose, *Cell. Immunol.* **18**, 360 (1975).

48. H. S. Lillehoj and N. R. Rose, *Clin. Exp. Immunol.* **47**, 661 (1982).

49. F. J. Twarog and N. R. Rose, *Proc. Soc. Exp. Biol. Med.* **130**, 434 (1969).

50. H. S. Lillehoj, K. Beisel, and N. R. Rose, *J. Immunol.* **127**, 654 (1981).

51. H. S. Lillehoj and N. R. Rose, *Cell. Immunol.* **62**, 156 (1981).

52. R. K. Cole, *Genetics* **53**, 1021 (1966).

53. R. K. Cole, J. H. Kite, Jr., and E. Witebsky, *Science* **160**, 1250 (1968).

54. G. Wick, J. H. Kite, Jr., R. K. Cole, and E. Witebsky, *J. Immunol.* **104**, 45 (1970).

55. J. R. L. Pink, *Folia Biol. (Praha)* **25**, 333 (1979).

56. C. H. Brogren and S. Bisati, in H. Peeters, Ed., *Protides of the Biological Fluids*, Pergamon Press, Oxford, 1980, p. 356.

57. M. Crone, J. Jensenius, and C. Koch, *Immunogenetics* **13**, 38 (1981).

58. F. Pazderka, B. M. Longenecker, G. R. L. Law, and R. F. Ruth, *Immunogenetics* **2**, 101 (1975).

59. M. Simonsen, in M. B. Zaleski, Ed., *Proc. Seventh Int. Convoc. Immunol.*, Karger, Basel, 1981 (in press).

60. L. D. Bacon, J. H. Kite, Jr., and N. R. Rose, *Science* **186**, 274 (1974).

61. L. D. Bacon, *Fed. Am. Soc. Exp. Biol.* **35**, 713 (1976).

62. L. D. Bacon, C. R. Polley, R. K. Cole, and N. R. Rose, *Immunogenetics* **12**, 339 (1981).

63. L. D. Bacon, R. S. Sundick, and N. R. Rose, in A. A. Benedict, Ed., *Avian Immunology*, Plenum Press, New York, 1977, p. 305.

64. L. D. Bacon and N. R. Rose, *Proc. Natl. Acad. Sci. USA* **76**, 1435 (1979).

65. L. D. Bacon, R. K. Cole, C. R. Polley, and N. R. Rose, in N. R. Rose, P. E. Bigazzi, and N. L. Warner, Eds., *Genetic Control of Autoimmune Disease*, Elsevier/North-Holland, New York, 1978, p. 259.

66. G. Wock, J. H. Kite, Jr., and E. Witebsky, *J. Immunol.* **104**, 54 (1970).

67. P. Welch, N. R. Rose, and J. H. Kite, Jr., *J. Immunol.* **110**, 575 (1973).

68. M. Livezey, Ph.D. dissertation, Wayne State University, Detroit, MI, 1980.

69. R. S. Sundick, M. D. Livezey, and N. R. Rose, in J. R. Stockigt and S. Nagataki, Eds., *Thyroid Research VIII*, Australian Academy of Science, Canberra, 1980, p. 773.

70. J. Jaroszewski, R. S. Sundick, and N. R. Rose, *Clin. Immunol. Immunopathol.* **10**, 95 (1978).

71. C. R. Polley and L. D. Bacon, *Poult. Sci.* **55**, 2081 (1976).

71. R. S. Sundick and G. Wick, *Clin. Exp. Immunol.* **18**, 127 (1974).

73. G. Wick, R. S. Sundick, and B. Albini, *Clin. Immunol. Immunopathol.* **3**, 272 (1974).

74. N. R. Rose, L. D. Bacon, and R. S. Sundick, *Transplant. Rev.* **31**, 264 (1976).

75. M. D. Livezey and R. S. Sundick, *Gen. Comparative Endocrinol.* **41**, 243 (1980).

76. R. S. Sundick, N. Bagchi, M. D. Livezey, T. R. Brown, and R. E. Mack, *Endocrinology,* **105**, 493 (1979).

77. A. G. Cudworth, *Diabetologia,* **14**, 281 (1978).

78. A. G. Cudworth, in A. J. Bellingham, Ed., *Advanced Medicine*, vol. 16, Pitman Medical, Tunbridge Wells, 1980, p. 123.

79. J. Nerup, C. Cathelineau, J. Seignalet, and M. Thomsen, in J. Dausset and A. Svejgaard, Eds., *HLA and Disease*, Munksgaard, Copenhagen, 1977, p. 149.

80. G. F. Bottazzo, R. Pujol-Borrell, and D. Doniach, *Clin. Immunol. Allergy* **1**, 139 (1981).

81. J. A. Sachs, A. G. Cudworth, D. Jaraquemada, A. N. Gorsuch, and H. Festenstein, *Diabetologia* **18**, 41 (1980).

82. H. Solow, R. Hidalgo, and D. P. Singal, *Diabetes* **28**, 1 (1979).

83. H. Kromann, A. Lernmark, B. F. Vestergaard, J. Egeberg, and J. Nerup, *Diabetologia* **16**, 107 (1979).

84. H. Kolb, G Freytag, U. Kiesel, and V. Kolb-Bachofen, *Diabetologia* **19**, 216 (1980).

85. A. A. Like and A. A. Rossini, *Science* **193**, 415 (1976).

86. A. A. Rossini, M. C. Appel, R. M. Williams, and A. A. Like, *Diabetics* **26**, 916 (1977).

87. U. Kiesel, G. Freytag, J. Biener, and H. Kolb, *Diabetologia* **19**, 516 (1980).

88. U. Kiesel, H. Kolb, and G. Freytag, *Clin. Exp. Immunol.* **43**, 430 (1981).

89. H. Kolb, and G. Freytag, U. Kiesel, and V. Kolb-Bachofen, *Clin. Exp. Immunol.* **43**, 121 (1981).

90. L. G. Anderson and N. Talal, *Clin. Exp. Immunol.* **10**, 199 (1972).

91. J. Zulman, R. Jaffe, and N. Talal, *N. Engl. J. Med.* **299**, 1215 (1978).

92. J. S. Burke, J. J. Butler, and L. M. Fuller, *Cancer* **39**, 1587 (1977).

93. J. Compagno and J. E. Oertel, *Am. J. Clin. Pathol.* **74**, 1 (1980).

94. P. M. Banks, G. A. Witrak, and D. L. Conn, *Mayo Clin. Proc.* **54**, 104 (1979).

95. M. C. Rosenthal, A. V. Pisciotta, Z. D. Komninos, H. Goldenberg, and W. Dameshek, *Blood* **10**, 197 (1955).

96. A. C. Parker and M. Bennett, *Scand. J. Haematol.* **17**, 395 (1976).

97. J. M. Vogel, P. P. Kornfeld, F. A. Forte, R. A. Jones, G. Genkins, A. E. Papatestas, and S. H. Horowitz, *NY State J. Med.* **77**, 2252 (1977).

98. R. Wyburn-Mason, *Lancet* **1**, 156 (1979).

99. J. East, P. R. Prosser, and E. J. Holborow, *Lancet* **1**, 755 (1967).

100. R. C. Mellors, *Blood* **27**, 435 (1966).

101. N. Talal, in N. Talal, Ed., *Autoimmunity: Genetic, Immunologic, Virologic and Clinical Aspects*, Academic Press, New York, 1977, p. 183.

102. H. H. Fudenberg, *Am. J. Med.* **51**, 295 (1971).

103. K. Lennert, N. Mohr, M. Stein, and E. Kaiserling, *Brit. J. Haematol.* **31**, suppl. 193 (1975).

104. P. Youinou, P. LeGoff, J. P. Saleun, L. Rivat, J. F. Morin, C. Fauchier, and G. LeMenn, *Biomedicine* **28**, 226 (1978).

105. M. Till, N. Rapson, and P. G. Smith, *Br. J. Cancer* **40**, 62 (1979).

106. C. L. Conley, J. Misiti, and A. J. Laster, *Medicine* **59**, 323 (1980).

107. D. Aarskog, *Arch. Dis. Child.* **44**, 454 (1969).

108. A. Stewart, J. Webb, and D. Hewitt, *Br. Med. J.* **1**, 1495 (1958).

109. W. W. Holland, R. Doll, and C. V. Carter, *Br. J. Cancer* **16**, 177 (1962).

110. A. I. Sutnik, W. T. London, B. S. Blumberg, and B. J. S. Gerstley, *J. Natl. Cancer Inst.* **47**, 923 (1971).

111. M. C. Holmes and F. M. Burnet, *Ann. Int. Med.* **59**, 265 (1963).

112. I. Emerit, J. Feingold, A. Levy, E. Martin, and E. Housset, *J. Natl. Cancer Inst.* **64**, 513 (1980).

113. P. J. Fialkow, G. R. Paton, and J. East, *Proc. Natl. Acad. Sci. USA* **70**, 1094 (1973).

114. A. Ghaffar, M. Krsiakova, and J. H. L. Playfair, *Transplantation* **10**, 432 (1970).

115. K. S. Datta and R. S. Schwartz, *Nature* **263**, 412 (1976).

116. M. E. Gerschwin and A. D. Steinberg, *Lancet* **2**, 1174 (1973).

117. N. L. Gerber, J. A. Harden, T. M. Chused, and A. D. Steinberg, *J. Immunol.* **113**, 1618 (1974).

118. R. S. Krakauer, T. A. Waldman, and W. Strober, *J. Exp. Med.* **144**, 662 (1976).

3

Autoimmune Endocrine Disorders and the Major Histocompatibility Complex

NADIR R. FARID

Division of Endocrinology and Metabolism
Department of Medicine and Thyroid Research Laboratory
Memorial University of Newfoundland
St. John's, Newfoundland, Canada

JOHN C. BEAR

Division of Community Medicine
Faculty of Medicine
Memorial University of Newfoundland
St. John's, Newfoundland, Canada

Contents

1. INTRODUCTION

The explosive development of knowledge of the molecular genetics, immunology, and function of the genes located in the major histocompatibility complex (MHC) has propelled this portion of the genome to the forefront of scientific attention (1). Associations of diseases, particularly endocrine diseases, with genetic variation in the MHC require consideration of these developments by the clinician.

In this chapter we offer an overview of the MHC, its role in determining immune responses in mouse and man, the possible mechanisms of association of human disease with the system, and a brief discussion of individual autoimmune endocrine disorders. The literature on these topics is voluminous; to keep the number of citations within reasonable bounds, we refer where possible to recent reviews and books.

2. THE MAJOR HISTOCOMPATIBILITY COMPLEX

The major histocompatibility complex (MHC) of man is located on the short arm of chromosome 6 (2–4). It includes several groups of genes. These code for two types of polymorphic cell surface glycoproteins, the human leukocyte antigen (HLA) transplantation antigens; three components of complement, C2 and C4 of the classical pathway and properdin factor B (Bf) of the alternate pathway; and two enzyme systems, red cell glyoxalase I (Glo) and adrenal 21-hydroxylase (Fig. 1). MHC loci also control some immune responses.

The transplantation antigens are controlled by at least four loci, HLA-A, B, C, and D (DR), at each of which segregate a large number of alleles (Table 1). These loci are usually transmitted on a parental chromosome *en bloc* as a haplotype; recombinations between adjacent loci occur at frequencies of

less than 0.01. Expression of HLA alleles is codominant; an individual can have two antigens of each series.

The antigens coded for by the D locus are identified by functional assay of lymphocytic interaction (mixed lymphocyte culture, or MLC). In recent years, it has proven possible to identify antigenic specificities related to HLA-D antigens (D-related or DR) serologically, as are A, B, and C alleles, on bone marrow-derived (B) peripheral lymphocytes (2, 3). The exact relationship of these HLA-DR antigens to the corresponding D specificities, as well as the number of loci controlling their expression, remains to be determined. Examples of differences in the same individual between HLA-D and DR gene products have been reported (5).

There is evidence to suggest that DR gene products may be controlled by more than one locus (6, 7), and a monoclonal antibody which identifies an Ia-like polymorphic system linked to but distinct from HLA-DR has been described (8) (see Fig. 1 and Chapter 2).

A series of cell-surface antigens structurally related to HLA-A, B, and C antigens have been identified (9, 10), some of which are restricted to T cell blasts or T lymphoblastoid lines; these antigens may well include the human homologues of murine TL and Qa antigens.

The H-2 system of the mouse is homologous with HLA (Fig. 1); much of the investigation of the human MHC is based on this homology. As this chapter amply illustrates, inferences about functional relationships of MHC loci can be based on this homology, though caution is obviously necessary in their interpretation. HLA-A and B are analogous to the K-D region of the mouse H-2 system, whereas HLA-D/DR is broadly equivalent to the mouse I region. Many genes determining immune response map to the I-A region and a few to the I-E region. A number of suppressor genes have also been mapped to the I-E subregion. Interestingly, HLA-DR is considered to be homologous to I-E. Critical review (11) based on recent information suggests

Table 1. HLA-A, B, and C antigens recognized by the WHO committee on HLA nomenclature (1980)[a]

HLA-A	HLA-B		HLA-C	HLA-D/DR	
				HLA-D	HLA-DR
HLA-A1	HLA-B5	HLA-Bw44(12)	HLA-Cw1	HLA-Dw1	HLA-DR1
HLA-A2	HLA-B7	HLA-Bw45(12)	HLA-Cw2	HLA-Dw2	HLA-DR2
HLA-A3	HLA-B8	HLA-Bw46	HLA-Cw3	HLA-Dw3	HLA-DR3
HLA-A9	HLA-B12	HLA-Bw47	HLA-Cw4	HLA-Dw4	HLA-DR4
HLA-A10	HLA-B13	HLA-Bw48	HLA-Cw5	HLA-Dw5	HLA-DR5
HLA-A11	HLA-B14	HLA-Bw49(w21)	HLA-Cw6	HLA-Dw6	HLA-DRw6
HLA-Aw19	HLA-B15	HLA-Bw50(w21)	HLA-Cw7	HLA-Dw7	HLA-DR7
HLA-Aw23(9)	HLA-Bw16	HLA-Bw51(5)	HLA-Cw8	HLA-Dw8	HLA-DRw8
HLA-Aw24(9)	HLA-B17	HLA-Bw52(5)		HLA-Dw9	HLA-DRw9
HLA-Aw25(10)	HLA-B18	HLA-Bw53		HLA-Dw10	HLA-DRw10
HLA-Aw26(10)	HLA-Bw21	HLA-Bw54(w22)		HLA-Dw11	
HLA-A28	HLA-Bw22	HLA-Bw55(w22)		HLA-Dw12	
HLA-A29	HLA-B27	HLA-Bw56(w22)			
HLA-Aw30	HLA-Bw35	HLA-Bw57(17)			
HLA-Aw31	HLA-B37	HLA-Bw58(17)			
HLA-Aw32	HLA-Bw38(w16)	HLA-Bw59			
HLA-Aw33	HLA-Bw39(w16)	HLA-Bw60(40)			
HLA-Aw34	HLA-B40	HLA-Bw61(40)			
HLA-Aw36	HLA-Bw41	HLA-Bw62(15)			
HLA-Aw43	HLA-Bw42	HLA-Bw63(15)			
	HLA-Bw4				
	HLA-Bw6				

[a] The prefix "w" before an antigen number indicates provisional assignment ("workshop"). All antigens of C series have been assigned w to separate them from complement factors. With the availability of more specific sera, some antigens, for instance, A9 and A10, have been split through assignment to either Bw4 or Bw6 superspecificities. DR antigens DR1–5 and DR7 have been accepted as established specificities in the 8th International Histocompatibility Workshop.

61

MOUSE H-2

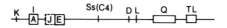

HUMAN HLA

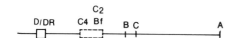

Figure 1. Schematic representation of the MHC regions of mouse chromosome 17 and human chromosome 6. The I region of the mouse comprises a number of genes (12); only those whose existence has been definitely established (A and E) are shown; J-region mapping is tentative (11). The genes in the I region code for I-associated (Ia) cell surface antigens. Likewise loci for complement components C2, C4 and properdin factor B (Bf) map in the MHC region, but their exact location in the B-D interval is tentative (broken squares). Mouse K-D loci are quivalent to human A/B; the D/DR region, the human equivalent of the mouse I region, maps to the outside of B instead of between A and B.

that subdivision of the I region into subregions is either artifactual (for I-B) or based on limited data (for I-J and I-C) and must thus remain tentative. The S-region codes for C4 and its carrier proteins Ss and Slp. Nearby loci (reviewed in Ref. 12) considered to be outside the mouse MHC proper include TL and Qa beyond the D end of the region; the antigens they code for are expressed on T cell lines. The T/t system, outside the K end, influences cell interaction during embryogenesis.

3. HLA

3.1. Tissue Distribution

HLA-A, B, and C antigens are expressed on the surface of all nucleated cells. HLA-(D)DR antigens are more restricted in tissue distribution, being found on B lymphocytes, monocytes (macrophages) (13), sperm (14), Langerhan cells of skin (15), and a small population of nonstimulated T cells (16). Upon activation in mixed lymphocyte culture or following mitogenic stimulation (16), a large proportion of T cells express D/DR antigens on their surface. Cells of the endocrine pancreas have recently been found to express HLA-DR-like antigens (17).

3.2. Structure

The MHC transplantation antigens are heteropolymeric glycoproteins of two types (12). Class I molecules are composed of a polymorphic 43,000 M.W. glycosylated polypeptide, noncovalently linked to an invariant nonglycosylated 12K chain (β_2-microglobulin). The heavy chain is coded for by K, D, and Qa/Ta genes of H_2 and the A, B, and C genes of HLA; the β_2 microglobulin gene is on chromosome 15 in humans and probably chromosome 2 in the mouse (11, 18). Class II molecules are composed of 28K (β) light and 24K (α) heavy chains noncovalently linked. Both chains are controlled by MHC I-A and I-E genes in the mouse; both are probably controlled by D/DR and related loci in humans. The β chain is the more polymorphic, but it is possible that both chains contribute to alloantigenicity (4, 11).

For both class I and class II molecules intracellular posttransitional association of light and heavy chains is necessary for their insertion into cell membrane (18). This requirement is the basis of lack of expression of E$\alpha\beta$ Ia molecules in mice carrying a null (Eα°) gene; if such a mouse is crossed with a strain that expresses such a gene (Eα^+), some of the progeny express both chains (the phenotype is "complemented") (11, 19). There is evidence that this phenomenon occurs with other I-coded genes, giving rise to new composite Ia molecules (11).

Some generalizations are possible concerning the structural basis of allogenicity of these molecules: (1) Serologically similar antigens are also structurally similar; gene products controlled by separate loci are less similar. (2) There are apparently two regions of high variability, other differences being more or less randomly distributed; mutations occur in these portions in mice at the H-2K locus (18). In the absence of a detailed knowledge of the three-dimensional structure of histocompatibility antigens, it is impossible to say whether the regions of variability constitute a single antigenic region or whether there are physically discrete sites on the molecule, each of which is alloantigenic.

The HLA-A, B, C, and DR antigens are inserted into the lipid bilayer at right angles to the plasma membrane (20). Such an orientation is suited to transfer or information from the surface to the cell interior and may be essential for biological function as a receptor site.

Structural homologies exist between HLA, immunoglobulins, and β_2 microglobulin molecules. The intrachain disulfide bridge of the β_2 microglobulin chain shows marked homology with C_H3, the third constant region of the immunoglobulin heavy chain (21). Similarly, the heavy chains of HLA-A, B, and C molecules have two intrachain disulfide bridges which resemble immunoglobulin domains. On the other hand, the HLA heavy chains are more similar to β_2 microglobulin than they are to immunoglobulin domains (22); Orr et al. (23) concluded the HLA heavy chain and β_2 microglobulin divergences occurred around the time of the divergence of the constant regions of the heavy and light chains of immunoglobulin, and the duplication of the genes for the constant region of the heavy chain.

The three complement factors known to be coded for by genes in the MHC region are C2, C4, and factor B (Fig. 1). The allotypic variants of all three components have been linked to HLA, as have C2 and C4 deficiency (reviewed in Ref. 24).

It has been suggested that the genes of the HLA system originated by a series of duplications (25). Biochemical and structural analysis (20) strongly suggests that at least HLA-A, B, and C genes arose from a common ancestral gene by duplication. Similarly, C2 and Bf, controlled by closely linked genes

between the B and D (DR) loci (Fig. 1), are highly homologous and likely to have originated from duplicated genes (24). There is no apparent relationship between these two sets of products or between either of them and D/DR locus gene products. Moreover, the relationship of the C4 gene to other genes so far mentioned is unclear. Structurally, C4 is unlike C2 and Bf (24). O'Neill et al. (26) provide evidence that the C4 gene is duplicated, the fast (F) and slow (S) components being produced by two separate C4 genes on each parental chromosome, one or the other of which may be silent (Fig. 1). It is possible, of course, that the HLA region represents a diverse collection of genes, each duplicated to a different extent (27).

4. FUNCTIONAL CONSIDERATIONS

4.1. Basic Function

Immune receptors must be specific and effective in terms of the biological fitness of the whole organism. In modern immunologic terms, specificity implies that the immunocompetent cells have antigen-specific recognition sites and the genetic and synthetic machinery to secrete humoral factors including antibodies which are specific for that antigen. An effective immunologic reaction should be controlled and should not spill over against other potential immunogens including self-antigens. Control seems to be achieved through a requirement for the participation of more than one cell type within the context of "self." Communicating cells participating in the immune reaction share restricting determinants specific to self, either as cell receptors or as an integral part of the humoral factor. The requirement of simultaneous recognition of antigen and H-2 molecules restricts the specificity of the T lymphocyte; this restriction is probably the basic function of the HLA and H2 antigens. Such dual or associative recognition may well be the only way for organisms to distinguish nonself from self. For the immune reaction to be specific to different forms of nonself (antigens), stereospecific acceptor sites need to be expressed on specific presenting cells. The generation of repertoire for these receptors represents another avenue of selection; the structural constraints of antigen-acceptor sites are a separate mode of communication among immunocompetent cells which may impose control of the immune reaction.

Jerne (28) suggested that during their early development, T lymphocytes specific for self-MHC are selected in the thymus to differentiate and proliferate. Subsequently, only those with low affinity to self-antigen are allowed to mature and leave the thymus as functional T cells. Such T cells, having low reactivity to self-antigens, have high affinity to variants of self-MHC antigens. The expectations from the hypothesis have been amply confirmed. That MHC antigens signal change in self to the immune system was demonstrated by Zinkernagel and Doherty (29), who found that cytolytic T cells from mice immune to specific viruses only lysed virus-infected target cells that shared H-2 antigens with the killer T cell. The restricting elements in the mouse were found to be class I antigens: K/D in the mouse and HLA-A, B in humans.

Such a cell-mediated cytotoxicity mechanism may well explain the extreme genetic polymorphism found in the MHC system. Because T cells which detect altered self are clonally restricted, and recognize gene products of only one parental chromosome, the survival advantage of heterozygotes is apparent. New allelic forms of MHC antigens were presumably favored when they arose by mutation because they enabled the restricted killing of cells infected by a wider range of organisms. In theory, some antigens might be more efficient in this process or might happen to interact with more common pathogens and become frequent in the population. Loci closely linked to these advantageous alleles would also be favored in a "piggyback" manner merely because of their proximity.

The polymorphism of class II (Ia-like) molecules in mouse and man suggests selective pressures probably different from those giving rise to class I antigen polymorphism, resulting in a different type of immunologic competence within the context of self (30). The generation of cytolytic cells specific to nonself and class I antigens is influenced by class II molecule determinants (11). Moreover, these determinants are important in antigen recognition and communication between regulatory and effector cells.

In human populations polymorphism of class I and II molecules and the predominance of certain gene products in some populations but not in others strongly suggest that polymorphism is or was maintained by selective pressures. Most of the diseases for which HLA association has been demonstrated have little effect on reproductive or genetic fitness, but associations may also exist with important infectious diseases. Though investigation is now difficult, there are suggestions of HLA associations with, for example, leprosy, typhoid, tuberculosis, and malaria (reviewed in Ref. 13). Such associations indicate MHC polymorphism may have had considerable selective significance in the history of human populations.

4.2. Polymorphism

At least 56 alleles at H2-K and 45 at the H2-D locus have been identified in the house mouse (12); considering that I region-controlled and other gene products not yet identified are not included in this count, and that heterozygosity is probably favored at each locus, the variability of natural populations at this locus is extraordinary.

In man, the frequencies of HLA antigens also vary from one population to another, as is true for most genetic polymorphisms (13, 25); in all human populations studied a high degree of polymorphism has been observed. Alleles may be divided into three categories as regards population distribution. The first includes antigens found at high frequency in all populations, for example, HLA-A2. The second includes those antigens present in most populations but conspicuously absent in one or more groups; for example, A1, A3, A29, Aw30, and Aw32 are absent in Japanese and A11 in Africans. Finally, there are antigens specific to one population, for example, Aw42 and Aw43 to Africans and Dw12 to Japanese. As more sera become available from black and Japanese populations, more population-restricted antigens will be identified.

*　　*　　*　　*　　*　　*

Linkage, Linkage Disequilibrium, and Relative Risk

A digression is required to introduce the statistical genetic concepts of linkage, linkage disequilibrium, and disease association, because they feature prominently in descriptions of possible genetic relationships of MHC loci with disease susceptibility. Each is elaborated in the main course of the narrative when specific examples are discussed.

Because genetic loci are arranged sequentially on chromosomes, and chromosomes are normally transmitted entire from parents to offspring, neighboring alleles on chromosomes are usually transmitted together rather than independentiy, and are termed *linked*. During the first meiotic division crossovers occur; that is, segments are exchanged between homologous chromosomes. The nearer two loci are on a chromosome, the lower the frequency of such recombinations between them; crossovers in the MHC, for example, are uncommon. In practice, the distance between loci is in fact measured in units of recombination fraction, designated θ, observed from the frequency of recombinant individuals detected in family studies. The relationship of physical distance along the chromosome to recombination fraction is not perfect; if two loci are far apart on a chromosome, crossovers between them occur sufficiently often that their alleles segregate (are transmitted independently) as if the loci were on different chromosomes.

Genetic linkage in itself provides no permanent association between specific alleles at neighboring loci; over many generations crossing-over is expected to randomize the combinations of alleles. Nonetheless, striking departures from the expected random combination of alleles are observed for some loci very close to one another, and alleles at these loci occur together on the same chromosome (in the same haplotype) more often than would be expected by chance. Such *linkage disequilibrium* may indicate that one of the alleles in question has arisen by mutation relatively recently and insufficient time elapsed for crossing-over to randomize its association with the alleles of neighboring loci; that specific combinations of alleles are maintained due to a selective advantage they confer; that migration, admixture, inbreeding, or random drift has influenced the genetic structure of the population under study; or that sampling is biased (31).

Possession of specific alleles at MHC loci has been found to be associated with susceptibility to certain diseases. The degree of *association* between a specific allele and a disorder is commonly expressed in terms of *relative risk* (RR), that is, the ratio of allele frequency in patients to that in controls (32–34). RR values greater than 1 indicate increased disease risk associated with possession of an allele; values less than 1 indicate a decreased risk and suggest a protective effect. Two refinements are necesary in RR calculations involving MHC markers. First, in the comparisons between disease and control groups for each allele at HLA loci, numerous comparisons are usually made at the same time and some spurious significant associations are thus expected to occur by chance. Statistical significance values can be multiplied by the number of comparisons made, reducing them to make allowance for the multiple comparisons. (Follow-up investigations to test the specific hypothesis that a particular disorder is associated with possession of a particular allele are not subject to this qualification.) Second, because linkage disequilibrium between two alleles at MHC loci is in some cases considerable, disease association with a particular allele may result in further associations with alleles in disequilibrium with it. To determine the primary association, patients and controls may be divided into groups positive and negative for one allele, thus neutralizing its effect, the RR conferred by the allele at the other locus evaluated, and the process then reversed (35). To evaluate the effects of several loci or other risk factors alone and in combinations, log linear models may be fitted to the data (36, 37).

Linkage disequilibrium has other implications for determining primary associations. An illustrative example is the reported association of psoriasis with HLA-B13, B17, and B37. When Cw6 typing became available it was found that psoriasis was associated with Cw6 in all racial groups studied. The earlier observation of an association with HLA-B antigens was due to their strong linkage disequilibrium with Cw6 in Caucasoids. As a secondary effect of primary associations linkage disequilibrium may imply associations with entire haplotypes; thus linkage disequilibrium between A1 and B8 and between B8 and DR3 implies a disease which is primarily associated with DR3 and may show an increase in the whole haplotype A1, B8, DR3.

The RR statistic appropriately measures the importance of an allele as a risk factor at the population level. It is, however, sensitive to the frequency of the allele with which association is detected. Disease association with a rare allele can result in a higher RR value than association with a more common allele even though absolute risk conferred by possession of the rare allele remains small, and even though the absolute excess of the rare allele among affected is less than the excess of the common allele. For this reason, RR values for disease, associated with possession of a particular allele, do not indicate the *genetic* importance of the association (for discussion see Ref. 38).

Disease associations are no more or less than statistical observations; several plausible genetic explanations may be offered to explain them (see Section 6).

* * * * * *

Selective pressure may explain the linkage disequilibrium observed in the MHC. Not all alleles of the different HLA loci are involved in significant associations (27); thus, of nearly 300 possible pairwise combinations of HLA-A and B locus alleles, only eight or nine show significant linkage disequilibrium in Caucasoids. The best known are the pairs A1, B8 and A3, B7 in North Europeans. For example: in a North European population it may be found that 17% of individuals carry the A1 and B8 haplotype. If there were no association between these two alleles, the frequency of such haplotypes would be the product of the separate frequencies of the antigens, 0.31 for A1 and 0.21 for B8, or only 0.065 (6.5%). The difference between this and the observed frequency of A1, B8 is the measure of linkage disequilibrium.

Each of the three major racial groups shows distinctive HLA combinations; indeed, haplotypes show greater variation among racial groups than do single alleles. B-C linkage disequilibrium is stronger than A-B and B-DR disequilibrium in the major racial groups, as expected since B and C map closer together than A and B, and B and DR loci (Fig. 1). Linkage disequilibrium may persist because the whole haplotype confers a selective advantage *or* one part of the haplotype compensates for the harmful effects of another part. A clue as to the second mechanism was recently provided by Welsh et al. (39). Linkage disequilibrium may occur also between HLA alleles and putative disease-related genes (see Section 6), and might partly explain some MHC disease associations.

4.3. Immune Responsiveness, Ir genes and Ia

It is a common observation that certain individuals respond poorly to specific antigens but not to others. Using simple synthetic polypeptides, it was first demonstrated that immune response was controlled by a single autosomal dominant gene in guinea pig strains (19, 40). Studies in other species, including the mouse, with similar or more complicated polypeptides and with isologous and foreign antigens emphasized the generality of this phenomenon. Using inbred mouse and guinea pig strains these Ir genes were mapped to the MHC; with congenic resistant mouse strains recombinant within the H-2 complex even finer localization was accomplished. Most murine Ir genes map in the I region of H-2 at I-A or I-E, although some genes (notably that for thyroglobulin) have been mapped to the K region. A common feature of the antigens under Ir gene control is that they are all T lymphocyte dependent (19).

Early observations on cellular and humoral immune response to a hapten-protein conjugate suggested that whereas the antibody response was hapten specific, delayed-type (T-cell-mediated) hypersensitivity was carrier specific. This and later observations indicated that T and B lymphocytes may not be specific for the same determinants and that T cells react preferentially with sequential determinants on protein. This distinction in recognition sites of T and B cells probably places structural (in addition to genetic) constraints on the overall response to an antigen (reviewed in Ref. 19).

Macrophages (M∅) play a central role in the expression of Ir gene action. They take up an antigen, process it, and present it to immunocompetent cells in the context of MHC antigens (41). Whereas lymphocytes associate randomly with M∅, antigen-reactive T cells sharing MHC determinants with an antigen-presenting macrophage form a tight association which subsequently results in proliferation of the bound lymphocyte (42), to generate antigen-specific MHC-restricted regulatory and effector T cells. When T cells are harvested from an animal immunized a few days earlier and mixed with antigen-pulsed M∅, the T cells proliferate to a degree consonant with the degree of immune responsiveness of the donor in vivo. This proliferation assay has demonstrated the importance of MHC antigen restriction in all species studied including man

(43), the clonal nature of such restriction, and the fact that the restricting elements are class II (Ia-like) MHC antigens (11, 19). A key role of M∅ in the control of Ir gene action is selection of discrete regions of the antigen molecule for recognition with self. Guinea pig strains 2 and 13 T lymphocyte responses to angiotensin II and its synthetic analogues show random fluctuation between the two strains and neither strain responds to the same peptide antigen (44). The basis for antigen/MHC recognition and epitope specificity is discussed below. The basis of this Ir gene phenomenon is that certain combinations of MHC molecules and antigens fail to stimulate T cells (11). There are at least two possible reasons for this failure; T cells may not recognize the complex, or suppressor as well as helper T cells may be induced so that a positive response cannot be induced. Lack of T cell recognition may result if the recognition site, the antigen acceptor site, or the combination do not include the antigen in their vocabulary.

There is mounting evidence that class II MHC (Ia-like) molecules are products of Ir genes. This was initially inferred because Ir genes mapped in precisely the same I subregions (I-A, I-E) as those for the p. 29, 34 glycoprotein heteropolymer; because there are no instances of recombination between Ia and Ir loci in the same I region; and because polyclonal and monoclonal antisera, especially those directed to I-A, block the response at the level of the M∅ (see Ref. 19 for review). Furthermore, the cells involved in mediation of Ir gene phenomena bear Ia antigens, as do many of the factors involved in the regulation of Ir gene response (45). More direct new evidence for Ia-like molecules being the expression of Ir genes has been provided by relating the expression of the antigen Iaw39 on M∅ to that of beef insulin Ir gene function (46), and by the reconstitution of functional Ir genes and Ia antigens by gene complementation (47). The association of Iaw39 with specific immune response is all the more interesting in that its membrane expression is regulated by an X-linked gene (46).

The concept of gene complementation arose from the observation that the response to terpolymer GLØ is determined by two genes mapping respectively in the I-A and I-E regions. Neither alone can confer responsiveness but when present together on the same chromosome (cis) or homologous chromosomes (trans) a response is observed (reviewed in Refs. 11 and 19). The physical basis of this phenomenon is as follows: the I-A region codes for at least three polypeptide chains, two β and one α. One α and one β chain combine to form a heterodimer (Aαβ), which is then integrated into plasma membranes. The second β chain, although expressed intracellularly, can enter a heterodimer only if a locus encoded in I-E directs the synthesis of an Eα chain; strains mutant at the Eα locus (Eα°) are unable to make Eαβ molecules (48). If the response to an antigen is controlled by E or more specifically by the Eβ chain which maps to I-A, the responder phenotype cannot be expressed unless Eβ combines with Eα encoded for by I-E, hence the apparent control by two genes and the concept of gene complementation. As a variation on this theme, for certain antigens the generation of helper T cells is controlled by 1-A, whereas that of suppressor cells is controlled by the I-E locus. If the gene product (Eαβ) of the latter is expressed, suppression results and a low-responder phenotype is seen; on the other hand, in a strain such as Eα° which cannot express Eαβ, only T helper cells are generated and a high responder phenotype is seen (11). It is noteworthy that T cells recognize the complex of α and β chains rather than either of the chains alone (47).

Data accumulated by Rose et al. (49) suggest that spontaneous and experimental murine thyroiditis result from thyroglobulin Ir genes mapping at the K end of the H-2 (? I-linked) and from a gene at the D end of the complex, which apparently determines the severity of lymphocytic infiltration. The influence of non-H-2 phenotype on the magnitude of the humoral response to thyroglobulin is also significant (49).

There is considerable debate as to whether T lymphocytes recognize class II molecules and antigens through one or two separate receptors (44, 50–52). Although it is unlikely that the Ia molecules themselves comprise specific antigen-binding determinants, recent evidence suggests that the expression of MHC acceptor site is tightly linked to that of the antigen recognition site. This evidence includes the lack of independent recognition of antigen and MHC antigens by T cell hybridomas (53), the reactivity of anti-idiotypic antibodies raised against MHC-restricted virus-immune cytotoxic T cells (51), and the fine specificity of the regulation of T lymphocyte responses to chemically defined antigens (44). Though a two-receptor model cannot be completely excluded, current data are best accommodated by a model wherein the antigen combining site is due to the physical interaction between T cell receptor and stimulator cell class II antigens (44). This Ia/T cell receptor interaction would define the spatial and contact restraints within this composite recognition site that result in specificity of T cell recognition and restriction of Ir gene action. Much of the contact specificity would be contributed by the *clonally* expressed T cell receptors, whereas stimulator cell Ia antigens may primarily stabilize the T cell receptor and determine the spatial constraints of the combining sites. In contrast to the determinant selection model (50), this model requires (44) that antigen be bound only after the stabilization of the combining site by Ia-T cell receptor interaction and that much of the Ir specificity reside with the T cell antigen acceptor site. In this manner, the same Ia antigen may act as the restricting factor for a number of antigens whereas T acceptor, being specific for a limited number of amino acids, provides for a degree of specificity. Since B cells recognize other antigenic determinants in three dimensions, the overall perception of the immune system of an antigen or a determinant is similar to that of a neuroanatomical homunculus with larger and thus more perceptible parts being seen by T cells.

4.4. Immunoregulatory Circuits

Once antigen determinants have been selected and recognized, a cascade of events is set in motion, leading to the participation of other immunocompetent cells in amplifying this message and the recruitment of yet others to effect and regulate the magnitude of the response. Whether a predominantly helper or suppressor pathway is selected depends on the specific antigen determinants presented, whether or not they are associated with cells, and the particular Ia molecules with which the antigens are presented (Fig. 2).

Progress in the identification of T cell markers in the mouse has allowed the demonstration that certain subsets with specific markers are programmed to subserve different control or effector functions (54, 55). Thus Ly-1$^+$, 2$^-$ T cells are poised to develop into inducer cells even before immunization. They can induce helper T cells, which in turn trigger B cells to make antibodies, and induce MØ and nonspecific inflammatory cells to participate in delayed-type hypersensitivity reaction to induce effector activity from killer cell precursors, and can induce presuppressor cells to develop into antigen-specific suppressor cells. Not all these functions are subserved by exactly the same Ly-1$^+$ cells; Ly1$^+$, 1-J$^+$ cells specialize in inducing suppressor activity whereas 1-J$^-$ cells specialize in inducing B cell activity. These and other inducer cells, through soluble factors, work on Ly1$^+$, 2$^+$ regulatory cells, which possess acceptor for antigen-specific factors; through the amplifier class of T cells terminal effector cells are triggered. For the expression of T helper function a subpopulation of Ly1$^+$, Ia$^+$ is necessary, which acts optimally in the presence of Ly1$^+$, 1a$^-$ cells (54).

Two generations of T cells develop from precursor cells under the influence of soluble factors—the first generation is restricted by MHC products whereas the second is not (Fig. 2).

Like the Ly1$^+$ cells, the Ly-2$^+$ cells appear to be heterogeneous—thus the Ly-2$^+$, 1-J$^-$ fraction contains effector cells which can suppress Ly1$^+$Th activity induced by antigens (56). The feedback inhibition circuit ensures that the Th circuit is controlled. The Ly-2$^+$, 1-J$^+$ cells contain at least two subsets: one is involved in the mediation of suppression and is Qa-1$^-$; the other is Qa-1$^+$ and instead of being a suppressor interacts with Ly1$^+$, 2$^+$ T cells to inhibit the Ly-2 mediated suppressor cell activity. The operation of such an immunoregulatory circuit involving at least two cell subsets communicating with a soluble product is known as contrasuppression. The contrasuppressive circuit works more rapidly than feedback suppression, and is probably important in the maintenance of immunologic memory, local control of immune reaction, and the continuation of a primary immune response (56). The 1-J linked determinants of the contrasuppressive cells are different from those expressed on the suppressive cells (56). The expression of Ia antigens and I-J determinants on suppressor and contrasuppressor cells and factors and the expression of Ia on helper T cells and factors (but not Ly antigens) show the intimate association of MHC with immunoregulatory circuits.

There is growing evidence in humans for the existence of inducer and suppressor T cells, each with a distinctive phenotype (57). Undoubtedly the missing populations of regulator and amplifier cells will be identified in the near future. Meanwhile a ubiquitous mature T cell marker OKT3 appears to be closely linked if not identical to invariant determinants of the antigen-recognition site (58). Patients with a number of autoimmune disorders have been found to have an increased population of Ia$^+$T lymphocytes, probably indicating these T cells are activated (reviewed in Refs. 57 and 59).

The T cell antigen receptors are under the control of V$_H$ immunoglobulin genes and these cells are known to share idiotypic determinants with B lymphocytes specific for the same antigens. Apparently collaboration between T and B cells requires identity of VH genes (60, 61). Moreover, at least the acceptor site

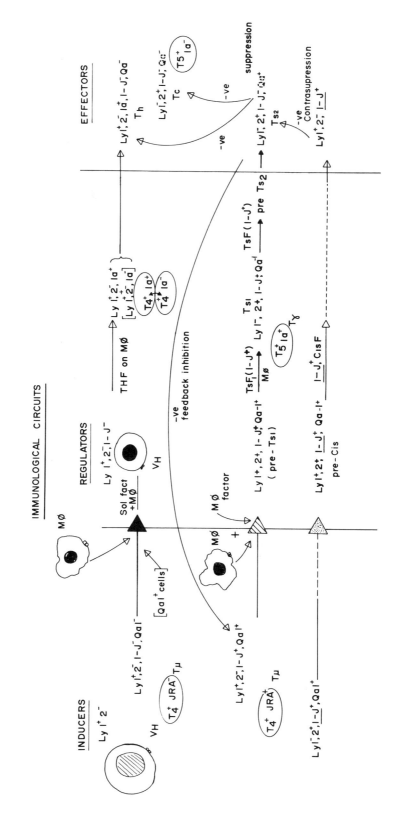

IMMUNOLOGICAL CIRCUITS

for suppressor T factor is encoded by a locus linked to IgH (62). These observations, quite apart from idiotype-, allotype-, and Ig class-restricted help and suppression (63–66), emphasize the participation of another immunologic system in dual recognition of self/nonself. We do not discuss further the role of idiotype/anti-idiotype interactions except to state that they may be relevant to the triggering of antigen-specific regulatory cells and in the modulation of humoral responses.

For an effective immune response to take place, these complicated immunologic circuits must function; a number of defects have been demonstrated in them. Lack of induction of suppressor T cells, and lack of perception by the target cells of the suppressive message of the activation of the feedback control circuit, resulting in an uncontrolled reaction leading to autoimmunity, have been described in a number of mouse strains suffering from lupus-like syndromes (54, 67). These studies emphasize the multiplicity of possible defects in the immunoregulatory circuits and genes contributing to the autoimmune phenotypes.

It is, however, important to note that regulation of antigen-specific response is normal in these mice, at least early on, the major abnormality being in antigen-nonspecific factors. This situation is in contrast to that of organ-specific autoimmunity (67). In contradistinction, disturbance in the induction of Th cells can result in disorders characterized by poor antibody production, and in defective cell-mediated immunity. Rare patients have been described with immunodeficiency and T cell leukemia; they lacked T inducer cells (57, 68, 69).

Curiously, patients who do not express HLA antigens on the lymphoid cells ("denuded lymphocyte syndrome") suffer from a form of severe combined immunodeficiency (70) (see Section 4.7).

4.5. Soluble T Cell Factors

Viewed narrowly, it is unlikely that T cells would release antigen-specific molecules other than the T cell surface recognition factors (45). At least one class of helper and suppressor factor is composed of two distinct polypeptides, one which binds antigen and is controlled

---

Figure 2.   Immunoregulatory circuits as characterized in the mouse with pertinent human data inserted at appropriate points in circles.

JRA$^+$ = T cells reacting with sera from patients with juvenile rheumatoid arthritis; 35% of T_4^+ cells are JRA$^+$. M0 = macrophage. Tc, Th, and Ts = T cytotoxic, helper, and suppressor T cells, respectively; subscripts on Ts signify successive generations of suppressor cells. THF and TSF are suppressor and helper soluble factors, respectively, and CisF is the soluble factor involved in the contrasuppressive circuit. V_H = variable heavy chain gene products; □ and ○ represent cell surface Ia and antigen receptors, respectively—the latter is probably identical to that on T cells and coded for by V_H genes. A distinction is made between I-J molecules detected on T cells subserving the contrasuppression circuit and those detected on suppressor T cells.

Inducer cells for both helper circuit (⎯⎯⎯▶) and suppression circuits (⎯⎯⎯▷) are Ly1$^+$, 2$^-$; contrasuppression inducer cells (⎯ ⎯ ⎯▷) are apparently Ly1$^-$, 2$^+$. Qa1$^+$ cells interact with Ly1$^+$, 2$^-$ inducer cells to activate helper regulatory cells; likewise an Ly1$^+$, Ia$^-$ population is probably necessary to produce optimal help. The Ly system of markers is not linked to the MHC; the I region and Qa genes are. Where Qa are shown in broken line, the phenotypes of the cells concerned with respect to this marker are uncertain.

Although human T cell subsets can be characterized by distinctive monoclonal antibody reactions (OKT series, T in this figure), several qualifications are necessary. All peripheral blood leukocytes are OKT1 and 3 positive; OKT3 reacts with an invariant determinant of the antigen binding site. Furthermore, T amplifier cells are part of a subset with Fc receptor for IgM (Tμ); suppressor cells, on the other hand, are Tγ positive (72). Likewise, SRBC rosette formation is inhibited by 3 mM theophylline in the suppressor T cell subset, though SRBC rosette formation by Tα is resistant to theophylline (73). Although once in doubt (71), T4 have been firmly established as belonging to the T cell lineage (74).

Within the 75 cells further subsets are distinguishable. Suppressor effector cells are Ia$^+$ whereas cytotoxic effector lymphocytes are Ia$^-$ (37).

Under appropriate conditions Tμ can be made to act on a subpopulation not yet identified which subserves feedback loop function.

by V_H genes and a second I-encoded chain; the two chains are covalently linked with disulfide bonds (45, 75). Another, less well-described, antigen-specific factor is a glycoprotein which consists of two regions, one that binds antigen and a second that mediates suppression; this factor has neither Ig nor MHC-coded determinants (76). These antigen-specific factors work on the regulatory and amplifier cells (Fig. 2). Recruitment of distinct T cell subsets into the respective effector pools by other soluble factors seems to be antigen-nonspecific and is MHC restricted in some instances but not others (77, 78). If T factors are indeed shed membrane recognition sites, their apparent heterodimer composition, although it argues strongly for an intimate relationship of MHC and antigen, does not help in judging between the one- versus two-receptor models.

Lymphocytes, in addition, make a large number of factors, collectively known as lymphokines, which act on M0, polymorphonuclear cells, fibroblasts, osteoclasts, and bone marrow precursors. Clearly the influence of these factors extends beyond modulating the immune response and the consequent tissue reactions. Indeed one of these, a type of interferon, can influence the immune process at different points (75).

4.6.   The B Cell Problem

Comparatively less is known about the mechanisms controlling the triggering of B cells to secrete antigen-specific antibodies. B lymphocytes carry surface immunoglobulin which has antigen-binding specificity identical to that of the antibody molecules secreted by their progeny, and share idiotypic determinant with regulatory T cells. Most B cells bear two Ig isotypes, sIgM and sIgD, which share the same idiotype on a given cell clone (see below). B cells bear Ia antigens and Fc receptors as well as receptors for C3 and antigens specific to this cell lineage. The functions of the C3 and Fc receptors are unknown. It is possible that binding of ligand to complement receptor is pertinent to the programming of

the cell for subsequent function. It has been reported that at least a portion of Fc receptors of murine B cells are coexpressed with Ia antigens (reviewed in Ref. 79); similar results are reported for humans (80). Whether this finding is relevant to B cell function is unknown.

The manner and context in which antigens are presented to B cells are unclear. After processing, antigens may well be presented by M0. Whether they are presented in the context of Ia and, if so, whether dual recognition is relevant at the level of B cells, are unknown. If genetic restriction in recognition at the B cell level is not necessary, it is possible that unprocessed antigens are bound by antigen-specific clones (81).

The mere binding of antigen to sIg receptors of B cells does not lead to stimulation unless the antigen comprises determinants which can trigger B cells in a nonspecific manner (polyclonal B cell activators, PBA) or a second mitogenic message is delivered to the B cells (82). Antigen-nonspecific soluble factors secreted by T cells have been shown to act as PBAs; in submitogenic concentration they preferentially trigger antigen-binding B cells whereas in higher concentrations they recruit B cells nonspecifically to the immune reaction (77, 83). In contrast, another subset of T cells secretes an antigen-specific soluble factor which carries idiotypic and Ia-like determinants (see above). We suggest that this factor acts not only on intermediate regulatory T cells but also on B cells. It is possible that early in the immune reaction antigen-specific Ia-restricted clones are recruited and the reaction subsequently expanded; the biological relevance of nonspecific recruitment of B cells is unclear.

T cells also produce suppressor factors, antigen-specific allogenically restricted factors inducing T effector cells which, in man, are not genetically restricted (77, 83). The evidence suggests that only the non-MHC-restricted factors influence B cells.

Apparently, the dual expression of IgD and IgM receptors subserves important regulatory functions at the B cell level (84). IgG prevents inactivation (or tolerance) of B cells at low antigen concentrations in man; T helper cell products seemingly act in synergy to prevent B cell tolerization. By analogy with the mouse, it may be this receptor that triggers and aborts B cell differentiation upon contact with antigen, with the relative densities of two Igs and the state of maturation or the immunologic experience of the B cell determining the outcome (73). Since antigen has a bimodal dose-effect relationship, this implies an intricate system for initiation or abortion of B cell activation (73).

The role of Ia antigens in the antigen-induced activation of B cells is unclear. At least in the mouse, they appear to be involved in the IgG/IgM switch in the course of a *secondary* immune response (85); such a relationship has yet to be shown in humans. If, as we postulate above, Ia$^+$, idiotype-positive helper factors are involved in B cell activation, the antigens on the surface of these cells may be involved in activation through *homologous* rather than complementary interaction. On the other hand, complementary interactions may be relevant if B cells with Ia receptors make physical contact, as they might well do in lymphoid tissue in the course of an immune reaction.

In any event, B lymphocytes are capable of processing certain antigens and presenting them to T cells in the context of Ia (81); the generality of this phenomenon is unknown. In the mouse, B cell-bound antigens may also trigger (directly?) Ly1$^+$ helper cells which are restricted by IgV$_H$ structures; these lymphocytes may in turn impose Ig isotype, allotype, and idiotype selection on potentially responsive clones (86, 87).

Despite the gaps in knowledge, it seems reasonable to generalize as follows: the recognition of nonself and communication between inducer, amplifier, and effector T cells are predominantly restricted by MHC-encoded genes, whereas the terminal controls imposed upon B cell activation are largely determined by IgV$_H$ genes. Because, however, recognition

of nonself occurs within the framework of IgV$_H$, the intimacy rather than dichotomy between these two networks must be stressed.

4.7. Other Functions of the MHC

A large number of loci map in the vicinity of MHC chromosomal regions of mouse and man. These include complement factors C2, C4, and Bf in man and C3 and C4 in the mouse; a number of enzymes including 21β-hydroxylase for the mineralocorticoid and glucocorticoid pathways in man; and antigen systems essential for cellular interactions including TL essential for proper embryogenesis (88). An argument has been advanced (11) that at least some of these loci, for example, the S region in H-2, are unrelated to MHC function. The MHC is by far the best-mapped part of the mouse and the human genome, and thus likely to contain functionally unrelated loci, but understanding of MHC function is tentative. Thus any arguments for functional independence must be tentative. Consider the case of the complement loci in man. C2 and Bf are structurally similar and alleles at each locus show tight linkage disequilibrium with each other and with C4 and HLA alleles. The close proximity of these loci might result from their involvement in the immune response, or it might be inferred that linkage disequilibrium over a time span sufficient for gene duplication results simply from the proximity of loci to one another; indeed, null alleles for C2 and C4 maintain such linkage disequilibria, possibly as a result of duplication of a single mutant (although the age of these genes is unknown). The mapping in man of prolactin to chromosome 6 at some distance from the MHC (89) is almost certainly irrelevant to the function of MHC antigens.

The gene for adrenal 21β-hydroxylase is in all human populations inseparable from the HLA-B locus, which links the MHC to mineral and water metabolism (90).

We have recently reviewed (13) some of the nonimmunologic traits influenced by the MHC. In the mouse these include levels of serum testosterone, response of accessory organs to testosterone, density of uterine estrogen receptors, mating preference, and transduction of glucagon effect on liver adenylate cyclase. In man effects upon β-adrenergic receptors, effects on serum glucocorticoid binding protein, as well as association of HLA alleles with certain nonimmunologically mediated diseases have been described (See Ref. 13 for review; 91). These associations might well be due to segregation with MHC haplotypes of regulatory genes such as that for neuraminidase, which acts on a number of hydrolases and thus influences post-transcriptional modification of glycoproteins (92).

Alternatively, MHC gene products may themselves be influenced by separate loci elsewhere in the genome. Examples follow:

1. An X-linked locus influencing Ia expression (46).
2. The response of tissues to enzymes or ligands (93).
3. Expression or function of receptors such as the Fc receptor (94).

Whatever the mechanism, some of these MHC-related traits affect biological and reproductive fitness.

The fact that Semliki forest virus binds avidly to MHC suggests that MHC gene products can act as receptors for viruses and ligands (95). This is probably an indirect result of the function of MHC in the dual recognition of nonself, due to chance complementarity of MHC to some ligands (96). As a result of structural complementarity, MHC products may well hinder or enhance (modulate) binding of ligands. On the other hand, free or ferritin-bound iron has been found to interfere with cognitive function of T cells and MØ; this may indicate interference with the expression of surface markers, in that inhibition is less pronounced for HLA-A2 individuals (97). Since T cells themselves make ferritin, an auto- and heteroregulatory mechanism through immune recognition may be involved (98).

Reviewing the role of MHC in cell-to-cell interaction, Dausset and Contu (99) suggest that the MHC may be a general self-recognition system. MHC-linked genes were noted to influence the ability of lymphocytes to form rosettes with auto-RBC, the adhesion of trypsinized fibroblasts in monolayers, lymphoid cell homing, contact inhibition between two explants of mouse fibroblasts, and autologous mixed lymphocyte reactions. Except for autologous MLR, these cell-to-cell interactions are determined by class I antigens; auto-MLR is activated by gene products linked to HLA-DR antigens. Besides MHC gene products, other, as yet unknown factors are probably involved in self-recognition. The MHC background of the thymic environment (through education of T cells by large epithelial "nurse" cells) influences the commitment of T cell receptors for MHC determinants (19, 100).

The relevance of MHC and neighboring chromosomal regions as differentiation antigens is stressed by the profound influence on embryogenesis of the T/t complex, the products of which are structurally similar to class I antigens (88) and, less so, by the reported association of HLA antigens with embryonic testicular tumors (101) and hypertrophic cardiomyopathy (102). If HLA antigens act also as differentiation antigens, the suggestion that polymorphism of MHC loci may exist at the tissue level in the same individual is reasonable (103).

5.   FACTORS CONTRIBUTING TO ORGAN-SPECIFIC AUTOIMMUNITY

The emergence of the autoimmune phenotype is influenced by a number of genetic and nongenetic factors, some of which are detailed in Table 2. In autoimmune thyroiditis (49), genetic controls separate from those influencing immunoregulatory T cells determine the severity of the thyroid lesions in the presence of a high responder Ir gene. Target organ susceptibility to autoimmune injury may be

Table 2.   Potentially interacting factors
in autoimmunity[a]

1. Genes: Ir, V_H, others
2. Defects in immunoregulatory circuits
3. Hormonal milieu
4. Nonspecific tissue responses, e.g., interferon
5. Target organ factors
6. Environment: infections, toxins, etc.

[a] *In a specific disorder, not all these influences may be necessary to sustain an autoimmune reaction.*

influenced by MHC-linked, that is, allotypic, tissue-restricted determinants, and non-MHC linked factors as well as tissue-specific antigens.

Genes controlling Ig or Ig-like structures are important in communication between regulatory cells and between regulatory and effector cells (see Section 4.4). Similar Ig genes determine V_H backbone structure and thus contribute to antibody specificity and affinity (104). It may be inferred that MHC and Ig genes may interact to predispose to autoimmunity (104, 105), probably due to the need to recognize "nonself" (through Ig-type receptors) in the context of MHC (see Section 4.1).

Infections and toxins may trigger an autoimmune response by inducing tissue injury or by altering "self" when viewed by T cells in conjunction with surface tissue antigens. Viruses or bacterial products may also act as polyclonal B cell activators and thereby bypass the tolerogenic signals which would otherwise be mediated through T regulatory cells (82). Under normal circumstances immunoregulatory circuits counteract the tendency to autoaggression, but not if a defect in any of these circuits is present.

Interferon, as an example of nonspecific tissue factor, may influence the immune response either by suppressing immunocompetent T cell function (106) or by modulating the tissue responses to viral infections (107), which would in turn trigger autoimmunity. Thus it was shown that the propensity of mouse strains to exhibit pancreatic damage

and carbohydrate intolerance was related to their corresponding capacities to make interferon and thus limit viral replication (107).

Sex hormones influence immune responses, particularly autoantibody production, in several mouse strains susceptible to autoimmunity. In other strains sex hormones have little role in modulating autoimmune injury (reviewed in Ref. 67). The greater involvement of females in susceptible strains is related to the lack of suppressive effects of testosterone. It was recently demonstrated that the thymus has sex hormone receptors (108) and that cells of the T cell lineage exhibit 20α-hydroxysteroid dehydrogenase activity; this enzymatic activity appears to be regulated by testosterone (109). By this route testosterone may influence the thymic and bone marrow environment for T cell maturation. Whether the influence of testosterone on T suppressor cell activity is exerted through this or some other mechanism is unclear (109).

The relationship between the onset of autoimmune disorders and pregnancy and the postpartum period is discussed in Chapters 12 and 13.

6.   MECHANISMS OF HLA-DISEASE ASSOCIATIONS

The list of diseases found to be associated with HLA is lengthy (2, 110), and is steadily enlarging. Studies of the associations and linkage of diseases with HLA have provided important clues as to their heterogeneity, for example, myasthenia gravis (111); modes of inheritance, for example, idiopathic hemochromatosis (112); and on occasion, the possible nature of disease liability, such as the interaction of *Klebsiella* products with B27 in anklyosing spondylitis (113). Studies of associations in different races, by drawing attention to the functional similarities between various HLA antigens found to be increased in the same disorder, have started a quest for the molecular basis of these associations (114). These results are all the more interesting because many of the diseases for which HLA associations have been described are of poorly or incompletely understood etiology, run subacute or chronic courses, and show familial aggregation but are apparently not controlled by single genes (110).

The HLA associations with disease found so far are not absolute (27). For example, more than 90% of patients with anklyosing spondylitis have B27 compared to 8% of controls, but only a small proportion of persons with B27 ever get the disease. There are several possible reasons for this lack of complete association:

1. The most obvious is that environmental factors including predisposing infections may determine whether susceptible individuals actually contract the disease or not.

2. Association may be due to linkage disequilibrium between the marker locus and as-yet-undetectable loci influencing susceptibility.

3. Genetic factors not related to the HLA system may also contribute to disease susceptibility.

4. The disease studied may be heterogeneous with HLA associations occurring only for particular subsets of patients; for example, HLA-B8, DR3 is found to be associated with myasthenia gravis only in patients without a thymoma (111). In such instances the HLA association itself may contribute to a better understanding of the disease process, as will be shown for autoimmune thyroiditis.

The diseases associated with HLA may be divided into two broad categories:

1. Diseases not associated with HLA-D(DR) antigens, for example, hemochromatosis (112), manic-depressive disorders (114a), and psoriasis (2). Mechanisms underlying associations are often unclear, but several of these disorders—hemochromatosis; C2, C4, and 21-hydroxylase deficiencies; spinocerebellar ataxia (reviewed in Ref. 2);

and Paget's disease (115)—are caused by genes linked to HLA.

2. Diseases associated with HLA D/DR alleles and having an autoimmune basis or at least evidence of autoaggression, for example, insulin-dependent diabetes, Graves' disease, and rheumatoid arthritis.

The mechanisms underlying these associations are incompletely understood. Likely possibilities include the following:

1. Associations are in fact with specific Ir genes occuring in linkage disequilibrium with DR antigens. As outlined above, these may be genes for Ia-like antigens, that is, class II molecules restricting immune response in linkage disequilibrium with D/DR loci but not identical with them. Over the last few years, evidence has accumulated suggesting that HLA phenotypes restrict a number of immunologic phenomena (43). In the context of HLA/disease association, it has been demonstrated that antigen-specific T cell proliferative response can be achieved in the presence of M0 which share at least one HLA-D antigen with the responder T cell (43). Studies at the population level find correlations between specific HLA determinants and the level of immune response to autologous and heterologous antigens. Immune response or suppressor gene action is only one of several explanations for such association (116). Recent linkage studies (performed in families), however, strongly suggest that low response is controlled by a dominant gene mapping within the MHC (116). Studies have yet to be done linking Ir genes to HLA, proving that low responsiveness is indeed due to immune suppressor (Is) gene action by demonstrating that this gene determines the generation of suppressor T cells, and documenting the locus of action of the Is or Ir genes. On the basis of the foregoing discussion one might guess at the answers to such questions; however, to experimentally document them is to place MHC-linked Ir genes in the human on a firm basis.

Many organ-specific autoimmune disorders are associated with DR3, which may suggest tightly linked specific Ir genes, or a broad multifunction Ir gene (immunopotentiating gene). We have argued (13, 117) that DR3 is in linkage disequilibrium with a defective immune-suppressor gene possibly acting at the level of the regulatory T cells, and that specific Ir genes on the same or the homologous chromosome add to the genotype to determine MHC-linked liability to particular autoimmune disorders. By analogy with gene complementation findings in the mouse (see Section 4.3), DR3 might for instance be in linkage disequilibrium with a null gene for the equivalent of the α chain of an Eαβ type molecule , the nonfunction of which allowed unrestrained Th function. A second MHC-linked gene would be the "disease-specific" Ir gene. Although suggested, there is no evidence for gene complementation in this sense.

Against these speculations must be set the specificity of Ir and Is gene action, although DR3-positive healthy persons have been found to exhibit less efficient FcR (receptor) function than DR3 negative persons and to express a lower percentage of Tγ cells, (94) consistent with the broad role suggested for DR3. If it is assumed that reduction of suppressor T cell numbers merely reflects FcR expression (and not the genetic program of the particular T cell subset) and that DR expression on immunocompetent cells is tightly linked to that of FcR (80), then the influence of DR3 in modulating FcR expression is, strictly, nonimmunologic. The efficient stimulatory capability of B8 (?DR3) in MLR (118) suggests that the deviation in membrane-associated function may de due to DR3 itself or gene products in linkage disequilibrium (possibly by increased modulability) which affect FcR function in a secondary fashion.

So much for the DR3-associated groups of diseases. The lessons learned from H-2 do not end here, however. Among autoimmune endocrine disorders pernicious anemia and Hashimoto's thyroiditis are associated with DR5, and DR3 reciprocally decreases in fre-quency among affected persons (119, 120). DR5 is structurally dissimilar to other DR antigens*; it has been suggested (121) that synthesis may be controlled by a separate locus or by more than one locus. It is relevant in this context that a specific mutation at H-2^k causes spontaneous autoimmune thyroiditis in the mouse (122), and that the susceptibility to immune thyroiditis was mapped to the K end of H-2 (49).

Notwithstanding all of the above, an association with a DR antigen does not imply an autoimmune background for a disorder; for instance, testicular choriocarcinoma is associated with DR7 (101).

2.   HLA antigens may act as receptors for viruses or ligands. As a result of such hapten interactions HLA antigens may be so altered as to be seen as "nonself," and cytotoxic T cells generated against the combination. This mechanism has been postulated to explain the association of subacute thyroiditis with HLA-B35 (13, 123); B35 itself or tissue-restricted MHC-linked polymorphic markers (see below) may be particularly effective in presenting thyrotropic viruses to T cells. Bacterial products may bind to specific HLA antigens which have a special affinity for these products and thereby influence the immune response; this may be the mechanism for the association of B27 with reactive arthropathies (113). If T cell receptors for nonself (antigens) are cross-reactive with T cell receptor for MHC determinants (52) it is theoretically possible for cross-tolerance and thus nonresponse to certain agents to occur. HLA alleles may also modulate ligand binding or postbinding events (see above).

---

* The conclusion that HLA-DR5 is structurally different from other DR antigens (121) was based on the peptide mapping of synthetically radiolabeled DR antigen obtained from lymphoblastoid lines. It now appears that line 3158 (nominally HLA-DR5) is not of human origin but from marmoset (194). The previous conclusion that the α chain of DR may contribute to the polymorphism of this antigen system is thus invalid. Additionally, Goyret and Silver (194) provide evidence for the human homologues of murine I-E and I-A.

3. HLA antigens may be related to deficiency of certain complement components. An abnormal function of one or more of the complement components coded for by the MHC could result in susceptibility to infection or give rise to autoimmunity. Patients with C2 or C4 deficiencies often present with a lupus erythematosus-like syndrome (24). It is possible that electrophoretically defined complement allotypes may differ in their biological activity, and some alleles of C2 and C4 are in strong linkage disequilibrium with specific HLA-B antigens. The finding that a biologically inactive C4 variant is in strong linkage disequilibrium with HLA-Cw6 and B17 (124) supports this possibility. Most mutations do not change the electric charge of protein; thus it is quite possible that as yet undetected C2, C4, and Bf abnormalities cause immunologic diseases.

Similarly, a gene very close to HLA-B may be involved in regulation of synthesis in the 21β-hydroxylase enzyme system (90).

4. Some disorders may be associated with HLA because MHC gene products influence embryonic differentiation and cell-to-cell interaction. The HLA associations of testicular teratocarcinoma and nonhypertensive hypertrophic cardiomyopathy are recent examples. Hypertrophic cardiomyopathy (HCM) has been found to be inseparably linked to HLA-B, though to different alleles in different families (102). In the absence of observed recombinations (125) between HLA-B and HCM, it is possible that HCM results directly from the influence of the HLA antigen on differentiation. It is possible that the combined immunodeficiency seen in children lacking surface HLA-A and B antigens (70) and the association of IgA and D deficiencies with HLA-B8 may be on this basis (126).

7. INDIVIDUAL DISORDERS

7.1. Insulin-Dependent Diabetes Mellitus

Of endocrine diseases associated with HLA, insulin-dependent diabetes mellitus (IDDM) is by far the most extensively studied. Discussion of IDDM illustrates the information provided by association studies, the insights thus gained into the genetics of autoimmune endocrine disease, and the limitations of present methodology notwithstanding the large amount of information gathered on the disorder.

In Caucasoids, susceptibility to IDDM is increased by possession of HLA-DR3 and HLA-DR4. The risk to double heterozygotes, that is, persons with both DR3 and DR4, is greater than the sum of the risks conferred by the individual alleles, even in homozygous state. The increase in DR3 among IDDM patients is found among Caucasoids, Chinese,

Table 3. HLA antigens and haplotypes relevant to susceptibility and resistance to IDDM

Protective Haplotype	Susceptibility Haplotypes[a]
A3, B7, Bf^s, DR2	A1, Cw-, B8, Bf^s, DR3[b]
	A2, Cw3, B15, Bf^s, DR4
	Aw30, Cw5, B18, Bf^{F1}, DR3[b]
	A-, Cw3, B40, DR4

Reproduced from Farid and Bear (13) with permission of the publishers.
[a] *In order of frequency.*
[b] *It is unclear whether the two DR3 antigens are equivalent. Whereas the genes in linkage disequilibrium with B8/DR3 seem to code for autoimmunity, this relationship has not been established for B18/DR3.*

and probably American blacks; among Japanese, DR8 rather than DR3 seems increased (13, 127, 128). The possible "permissive" role of DR3 in IDDM and other autoimmune endocrine disorders has been alluded to above (Section 6). Since in all populations appropriately typed, an increase in DR4 (or a cross-reacting antigen) has been documented, it is suggested that HLA-DR4, or more likely a gene in linkage disequilibrium with it, specifically predisposes to IDDM (13). It remains a matter for speculation how possession of this particular gene results in immunologic damage to pancreatic islet cells. It might act as an immune response gene specific for determinants expressed on the β cells of the islets. Alternatively or additionally, Ia-like antigens coded for by alleles in linkage disequilibrium with DR4 and restricted in expression to β cells might be particularly immunogenic in the insulin-rich environment of these β cells (129). The suggestion that a specific susceptibility gene for IDDM is universally in linkage disequilibrium with DR4 must be tentative, in that not all findings of characteristic increases of HLA-A, B, and C antigens in IDDM patients of distinct ethnic backgrounds have been supplemented with DR typing (reviewed in Refs. 13, 130). These increased HLA-A, B, and C antigens (with the exception of DR8 in the Japanese) are, however, in linkage disequilibrium with DR3 and DR4.

Linkage disequilibrium extends IDDM associations not only to the HLA antigen alleles, but also to alleles at the complement loci within the HLA region (13, 128). Consequently, certain haplotypes have been identified which confer either resistance or susceptibility to IDDM (Table 3).

In contrast to the susceptibility associated with DR3 and DR4, HLA DR2 (and secondarily by virtue of linkage disequilibrium B7) is extremely rare in patients with IDDM. HLA-Bw52 is rare in IDDM in Japanese; a DR antigen associated with this protective influence has not been documented (13).

Whatever the mode of inheritance proposed for IDDM, the observations reviewed above make it highly probable that genes predisposing to IDDM are part of the MHC.

To determine the genetics of IDDM susceptibility it is obviously necessary to determine whether IDDM is a single disorder or a class of disorders of heterogeneous etiology. That a number of rare genetic syndromes comprise clinical diabetes is clear, and with regard to the bulk of cases it has been proposed that the associations of IDDM with HLA B8 and B15 indicate two forms of the disease: a B8-DR3 form in which islet cell antibodies are frequent and persistent, antipancreatic cell-mediated immunity is increased, and antibodies to exogenous insulin are uncommon; and a B-15-DR4 form with earlier age of onset and increased antibody response to exogenous insulin (131). These age-of-onset relationships have been confirmed in large series of combined data (127), but findings for the association of immunologic features with MHC markers are ambiguous (132). The suggestion that Bf^{F1} occurs predominantly in children with early onset of IDDM (13) has not been sustained by recent work (133). It is, in any event, unclear whether these observations for the bulk of IDDM indicate etiological heterogeneity or rather influences of genetic background on the clinical course of the disease (13, 134). The propensity to develop anti-β cell (islet cell cytoplasm) antibodies or anti-insulin antibodies only demonstrates the possession of appropriate immune response genes which are revealed upon β cell injury or injection of therapeutic insulin; the role of these Ir genes in the pathogenesis of IDDM is not clear. It should be remembered that a variety of antibodies directed against the β cell have been described (see Ref. 135 for review). Some, such as the complement-fixing immunofluorescence assay which is closely related to the early onset of IDDM, and the killing of cultured β cells by islet cell surface antibody, are likely to be of pathogenetic significance. The association of these antibodies with HLA antigens has yet to be demonstrated, although preliminary studies indicate that positivity in immunofluorescence assay correlates with HLA identity to an index sib with IDDM (136).

As an aside, islet cell cytoplasmic antibodies (137) have an unusual IgG subclass restriction and certain heavy chain allotypic markers have been described as predominating among patients who develop high titers against therapeutic insulins compared to those who do not (138), suggesting that immunoglobulin genes may be intimately associated with at least two of the immunologic phenomena observed in patients with IDDM. An increased prevalence of IgA deficiency among B8/DR3 positive patients with early onset of IDDM has been found (139, 140); this may in part reflect the increased incidence of IgA deficiency among the HLA-B8/DR3 background population; there is some indication that IgA levels are generally reduced in IDDM patients (140).

That IDDM is a familial disorder is clear; sibs and offspring of affected persons are more than 20 times more likely than other persons to develop the disease (141, 142). The nature of its genetic background remains obscure, however.

Formal genetic analysis of diseases and traits of obscure inheritance (segregation analysis) is traditionally based on collections of pedigree of large numbers (preferably hundreds) of consecutively ascertained index cases. Such samples can be considered representative of the total population of affected persons. From such data can be estimated the probability of dominant, recessive, or more complex inheritance, with adjustment, at the mathematical level, for genetic and environmental variation influencing gene expression and disease liability (for a recent review see Ref. 143). Among these adjustments, *penetrance* denotes the proportion of times genes are expressed compared to Mendelian expectation. Although an unsatisfactory concept to human geneticists as well as other observers (144), penetrance conveniently expresses the

fact that single genes are not always expressed even though the genetic or environmental background to these failures is not known. The concept of *phenocopies* makes allowance for the fact that indistinguishable clinical conditions can reflect in one case unusual environmental insult and in other cases genetic susceptibility; for instance, the ingestion of Vacour can precipitate IDDM indistinguishable from that which occurs spontaneously (145), but such cases are very infrequent. If single gene inheritance seems unlikely, the arbitrary assumption of an underlying normal distribution of disease liability resulting from multiple, additively acting genes and environmental effects may allow a reasonable description of familial clustering of cases, and the calculation of the *heritability* of liability can give an estimate of the upper limit of the proportion of liability due to additive gene effects. If results from such analyses are inconclusive it is at least possible to infer that none of the models of inheritance tested adequately describes susceptibility, or that within the limitations of the data available the models tested are indistinguishable. Attempts can follow to delineate etiological heterogeneity, collect more data, or find limits to the number of possibilities compatible with available data.

Most of the large series of diabetes pedigrees subjected to formal segregation analysis were collected without reference to the distinction between IDDM and insulin-independent diabetes (146–148), and are thus not very informative regarding the inheritance of either condition. In a Mexican series of 175 IDDM patients (149) both recessive and polygenic hypotheses of inheritance were found to explain familial occurrence equally well.

Recent investigation of the inheritance of IDDM, as related to its association with genetic markers in the MHC, has been based on three different sorts of data. Increased RR conferred by certain antigens and the ''overdominance'' for risk of the double heterozygote B8/B15 (DR3/DR4) were observed in series of patients and controls. To the extent that patients and controls in these series are representative, these associations and the genetic liability they imply are characteristic of IDDM in the general population. Given the association of IDDM with MHC markers, studies of MHC markers in families of IDDM patients are of obvious interest. However, whereas collection of pedigrees of patients is logistically relatively easy, collection of MHC data on relatives, particularly healthy ones, is not. Thus numerous reports describe the distribution of MHC markers in small numbers of families, generally selected by virtue of including two or more affected sibs. For this reason alone, even were the results of such studies open to simple interpretation—which they are not— the relevance of the specific findings in these selected families to the susceptibility to IDDM in general would be unclear. Finally, genetic linkage analyses have been undertaken in families with several diabetics; genetic liability in such families may be very different from that in the general population.

The basic revelation of family studies of MHC markers in IDDM is that pairs of affected sibs are more similar in their genotypes than would be expected by chance. Two recent, relatively large studies illustrate this. Pairs of sibs are expected to have in common, two, one, and no parental MHC haplotypes 25, 50, and 25% of the time, respectively. A study of 120 IDDM sib pairs in the UK found 57, 37, and 6% to have two, one, and no haplotypes in common, working with HLA A, B, and C alleles (142); a series of 134 sib pairs pooled from several centers, with DR data, gave closely similar results (127). Thus factors coded for in the MHC must be influencing liability within families, as well as at the population level. The UK study mentioned (142) and a comprehensive investigation in Denmark (150) found the distribution of HLA alleles associated with IDDM liability to be the same in cases with and without affected sibs; this suggests familial cases are indeed similar to nonfamilial cases in MHC-associated liability.

Observed proportions of affected sibs having two, one, and no haplotypes in common

may be compared with those expected if susceptibility were conditioned by an HLA-linked dominant or recessive allele, and the frequency and penetrance of such an allele estimated (151). The excess of affected sib pairs sharing two as opposed to one haplotype is incompatible with dominant inheritance. On the other hand, were the distribution of haplotypes in affected sib pairs the result of a recessive allele, the allele would have to have a frequency of 0.23 (127) to 0.35 (142) and a penetrance of only 0.01 to 0.02. This is incompatible with other observations: some 5 to 10% of sibs of index cases are affected, which suggests a penetrance of about 20% on a hypothesis of recessive inheritance, and the proportion of monozygous (MZ) twins concordant for IDDM, also an indicator of penetrance assuming single gene action, is also probably about 0.20 rather than the widely quoted value of 0.50 (152). Thus, although a major influence of the MHC on the susceptibility to IDDM seems incontestable, this influence does not take the form of a simple dominant or recessive allele.

Because HLA data from families do not support a simple mode of inheritance, a number of more complex proposals have been made as to the nature of genetic liability to IDDM. These have taken the form of mathematical models, to permit testing whether the proposal is consistent with the observed HLA associations, with the risk of IDDM to relatives of patients (including identical MZ twins), and with the frequency of IDDM in the population. Since available estimates of such basic quantities as the population prevalence of IDDM and recurrence risks for relatives were approximate (152, 153), most such models were consistent with the data and could not be critically rejected. Since they make testable predictions, however, they are subject to further testing and refinement as data accumulate (153). For instance, it can be shown that were IDDM determined by a single locus closely linked to HLA, the incidence of IDDM, the risk to sibs of affected persons, and the concordance of MZ twins would each fall in specified ranges of values (154). Particular attention has been given to the possibility that a disease susceptibility gene at a locus elsewhere in the genome, interacting with an HLA locus (epistasis), could account for observed patterns of HLA haplotype sharing in affected sib pairs and observed risks to relatives (153, 155–157). A model invoking three alleles, two for different forms of IDDM and one normal, at a disease susceptibility locus tightly linked to HLA-B, has been developed to take into account arguments for immunologic heterogeneity of IDDM (158). Finally a model postulating a single locus closely linked to HLA, at which a disease susceptibility locus segregates with a penetrance on the order of 0.06 in single dose and 0.6 to 0.8 in double dose, is also consistent with currently available data on disease frequency, recurrence risks, and haplotype sharing (152).

Of the linkage analyses undertaken to date on IDDM, doubt is cast on the first (159) by the exceptionally high levels of intra-HLA recombination in the parents of the IDDM patients studied (160). Linkage studies by Barbosa and colleagues (161, 162) of families singled out as exhibiting dominant or recessive transmission of IDDM are difficult to interpret because such selected families, though possibly representative of the families of most diabetics, may give misleading results in linkage analysis (163). A more comprehensive study, combining both of Barbosa's sets of families with 28 French families (164) and assuming a recessive IDDM locus, has yielded recombination fractions too large to be reconciled easily with the observed association of IDDM with specific MHC markers, even assuming a penetrance as low as 0.2 (linkage must be very close for linkage disequilibrium to persist) (165). Clerget-Darpoux et al. (164) concluded, and it is evident from observations on sib pair haplotype sharing and modelling of disease liability as well as linkage analysis, that mechanisms more elaborate than a single recessive gene must be considered to explain IDDM liability.

Data are now accumulating which push the genetic analysis of IDDM beyond the confines of its association with MHC markers, but are not as yet specifically illuminating regarding the nature of IDDM liability. There is good evidence (165a) of very tight linkage of IDDM with the Kidd blood group locus, probably on chromosome 2. The families analyzed gave no evidence of falling into groups in which IDDM segregated with HLA on one hand and Kidd on the other; thus the influence of at least two unlinked loci in IDDM liability seems certain. Moreover, the fast phenotype of the acetylator polymorphism (a system determined by a single locus also not linked to HLA, which influences the rate of acetylation of a number of drugs) seems associated with IDDM in data combined from three North European populations; this association may extend to noninsulin-dependent diabetes as well (165b). Weitkamp (165c) has presented findings of an analysis of HLA haplotype sharing among well and affected sibs in families with more than one sib affected with IDDM, and either no or one affected parent. These are consistent with a concentration of non-HLA-linked susceptibility alleles as well as HLA-linked alleles in families with more than two affected members. Schanfield et al. (165d) have reported associations in families of IDDM liability with Ig light and heavy chain markers, as well as expected sex and DR associations. In a multiple cross-classification analysis, liability associated with the Km1 marker was found to be influenced by sex, and restricted to certain Gm phenotypes, and Gm and DR interactions in liability were noted.

The genetic analysis of IDDM is thus rapidly developing at present. Efforts at synthesis are necessary for the full interpretation of results to date. Interactive contributions of alleles labeled by MHC and immunoglobulin markers to autoimmune disease liability are hardly a surprising suggestion in the context of this review (see Section 5). Plausible direct contributions of acetylator and Kidd phenotypes to liability are not immediately obvious; speculation here seems premature.

It seems reasonable to proceed on the assumption that MHC loci themselves directly condition IDDM liability by coding for immune response and suppression anomalies. (DR2-conferred resistance deserves more study in this regard.) Postulating a disease susceptibility locus linked to but at some distance from the MHC seems irrelevant; indications of such a locus are probably analytical artifacts. If gene complementation in immune response is involved, there may well be more than one MHC locus relevant to IDDM susceptibility. Arguments that dominant, recessive, or additive gene action at a single locus makes up the MHC-associated genetic contribution to IDDM liability are probably too simple.

The evidence that other loci not in the MHC interact with MHC loci to condition disease susceptibility, provided by the association of IDDM liability with markers at these loci, must be taken into account (153, 165c). It is therefore necessary to distinguish carefully between postulates about the mode of action of MHC-associated disease susceptibility alleles and postulates concerning the inheritance of liability to IDDM. For instance, it has been vigorously argued (166) that gene and genotype frequencies at the Bf locus in IDDM patients and controls indicate the existence of a recessive allele in linkage disequilibrium with Bf^{F1}, with a penetrance of 0.20, which is sufficient to account for population and familial prevalences of IDDM in North American Caucasoids. These workers dismiss the findings of family investigations and ignore haplotype sharing data for other markers. Regardless of the probability of their postulated Bf-associated allele, penetrance of 0.20 is consistent with considerable additional genetic variation in disease liability (as they also point out).

Epidemiologic studies indicate that the incidence of IDDM is cyclic, consistent with the action of infection as a factor precipitating disease onset (167). Moreover, onset of IDDM in pairs of sibs is not random, but occurs at intervals of less than 1 year more than twice as often as expected (168). Thus conventional analytical assumptions that penetrance is uniform from sib to sib (134) and sibship to sibship may be seriously invalid in studying IDDM.

Similarly the conventional analytical assumptions of the relationships of familial cases to the general population of cases may be invalid, even if the familial cases are representative of all cases. The etiological relationships of IDDM and multiple autoimmune endocrine disease remain to be resolved. But heterogeneity of IDDM should not be invoked in the absence of good evidence to excuse the failure of etiological hypotheses. Immunological or biochemical variations which can be studied in family members, such as carbohydrate intolerance (169), anti-islet cell antibodies (136), or evidence of cell-mediated immunity should extend data. The relevance of the increase in capillary basement width in HLA-DR4-positive non-diabetic parents of children with IDDM (170) is unclear. Given the likely difficulty of applying such biological assays to large numbers of patients and the members of their families, the weakness of genetic analysis at the population level without such data, and the probable complexity of underlying liability, the appropriate and essential role of formal genetic analysis is likely to continue to be intermediary and synthesizing, determining whether findings of laboratory, clinical, and family investigations are sufficient to explain population disease patterns.

7.2. Graves' Disease

Graves' disease is associated with HLA-DR3 in Caucasoids and probably in Chinese, and in the Japanese with HLA-Dw12 (13, 117). Evidence from HLA-B typing suggests a dose effect: B8 homozygote Caucasoids are at greater risk than B8 heterozygotes of developing the disease; HLA-Bw46/B40 or Bw46/B14 heterozygotes among the Chinese are at greater risk than persons possessing

Bw46 alone (Bw46 being the antigen associated with the disease in Chinese) (171).

HLA-DR5 is decreased in patients with Graves' disease, though not significantly so (see also Section 7.3). On the other hand, some studies have suggested that B12 "protects" against Graves' disease in Caucasoids as does Bw52 in Japanese (13, 117).

The same group which reported Dw12 to be increased in Japanese Graves' patients using homozygous cell typing has recently reported DR5 to be increased in a selected group of patients (172). This is a surprising result in terms of tissue typing considerations and inconsistent with indications that DR5 is decreased in frequency in Caucasoid Graves' patients (172a).

It was recently suggested (173) that a subset of patients with diffuse goiter and hyperthyroidism (but no eye signs or TSAb elevation) could be distinguished by possession of DR5, Because, however, thyroid radioiodine uptake was not measured, it is possible that these patients may have had silent thyroiditis, in which DR5 is increased (see Section 7.3).

Proceeding on the assumption that DR3 has a broad immunopotentiating influence and the observation that no other DR antigen has been implicated in Graves' disease susceptibility, we concluded that the HLA-linked susceptibility gene(s) for the disease must be randomly distributed among HLA haplotypes. HLA-Dw12 may have a role similar in Japanese to that of DR3 in Caucasians; alternatively, among Japanese the disease susceptibility gene for Graves' disease may be in linkage disequilibrium with Dw12 (see Ref. 13).

HLA-DR3-positive Graves' patients show a tendency to greater T lymphocyte blast transformation in response to thyroglobulin than do DR3-negative patients, but this may have little to do with liability to Graves' disease, reflecting instead enhanced immune response in that group of patients (13). Likewise, a recent demonstration that HLA-DR3-positive patients with Graves' disease, particularly those previously untreated, have lower C4 levels compared to DR3-negative patients (174), probably reflects defective clearance of immune complexes (94) and their greater deposition in thyroidal tissue with the activation of the classical pathway of complement (175).

Attempts have been made to distinguish subgroups within Graves' disease on the basis of HLA typing. Dramatic increases were noted of specific haplotypes (in addition to the increases of those antigens generally associated with Graves' disease) in patients of Chinese origin suffering from periodic paralysis (176). Other lesser correlations were noted; in some studies it was found that hyperthyroidism occurred at a younger age in patients carrying the HLA antigens associated with the disease than in patients negative for those antigens (13). Though earlier studies based mainly on the results of HLA-A, B, and C typing were equivocal, more recent studies have shown an association of Graves' exophthalmos with HLA-DR3 (13).

Because thyroid-stimulating antibody (TSAb) is causally related to Graves' disease and its presence closely correlated with disease activity, studies to relate the presence of TSAb, the outcome of various types of treatment, and HLA antigens have been undertaken. Although neither the presence nor the "titer" of TSAb could be related to HLA antigens, HLA-B8/DR3-positive patients were found much more likely to relapse following a course of antithyroid drugs; in general, they needed a larger dose of radioiodine to render them euthyroid than did patients who lacked B8/DR3 (reviewed in Ref. 13). The association between relapse and possession of DR3 was not universally found; duration of treatment or follow-up are unlikely to be reasons for discrepancies among these studies (177–180). Regardless of these discrepancies, data of MacGregor et al. (179) clearly suggest that the mechanism whereby DR3 contributes to relapse is separate from TSAb, in that immediately after discontinuing antithyroid medication, TSAb levels were *higher* in DR3 negative than in DR3 positive patients.

Because loci not linked to HLA seem important in liability to Graves' disease, its inconsistent relationship with HLA antigens is not completely surprising. In particular a strong association is found between specific heavy chain markers of IgG (Gm) and Graves' disease susceptibility. Genes in linkage disequilibrium with these Gm allotypes could ensure that IgG antibodies capable of combining with TSH receptor are synthesized. An immunologic network independent of the MHC but interactive with it thus seems to contribute to Graves' disease liability (104, 117). It is likely that interactions between idiotype (TSAb in this instance) and anti-idiotype may be important in inducing disease remission (See Ref. 117 for details). The influence of sex on the susceptibility to Graves' disease is well known. The interaction of these and other genetic markers in the simple mathematical models employed to date appears to be complex (13, 117).

The studies of association of HLA and Graves' disease at the population level suggest that two parental haplotypes may participate in conferring disease susceptibility (171, 181). Analysis of the distribution of HLA haplotypes among sib pairs affected with Graves' disease in a small series (28 pairs) showed 68, 25, and 7%, respectively, sharing two, one, and no haplotypes. At the reported levels of prevalence of Graves' disease neither dominant nor recessive inheritance could be excluded in so few data. In families where the disease appeared to be vertically transmitted the haplotypes segregating with disease susceptibility included fewer DR3-positive haplotypes than expected. These findings are in keeping with the suggestion that susceptibility genes for Graves' disease are randomly distributed among HLA haplotypes, supplementation of the phenotype by DR3 positive haplotypes having an immunopotentiating effect increasing the probability of their expression (13).

7.3. Autoimmune Thyroiditis

Studies of HLA association demonstrate the genetic heterogeneity of chronic lympho-cytic thyroiditis along broad, clinically relevant lines. Atrophic thyroiditis, whether or not associated with thyroid failure, is associated with HLA-DR3 (and secondarily B8) whereas goitrous autoimmune (Hashimoto's) thyroiditis is associated with HLA-DR5, without important deviations in the occurrence of HLA-A, B, and C. Pernicious anemia is also associated with HLA-DR5 (120), implying a common immunogenetic basis for thyrogastric autoimmunity (reviewed in Refs. 13, 119, and 182).

Drexhage et al. (183) have recently provided some evidence that goitrogenesis in the context of both autoimmune thyroiditis and Graves' disease may be related to the presence of circulating thyroid growth antibodies. There are no data at present relating such antibodies to DR5; such a relationship would not be simple, because DR5 seems reduced in patients with Graves' disease irrespective of the presence of goiter. If we ascribe to DR3 in thyroiditis as we have in other autoimmune diseases a broad facilitatory role, we must conclude that the disease susceptibility gene for atrophic thyroiditis is not associated with any specific MHC haplotype; that is, it does not maintain linkage disequilibrium. If HLA-DR5 identifies an immune response gene it is necessary to postulate the existence of more than one type of thyroid growth antibody, only one variety of which is related to HLA-DR5. We have previously postulated (see Section 5) that tissue restriction for MHC factors in linkage disequilibrium with DR5 does not necessarily have to be identical in each tissue. Thus a particularly immunogenic combination of tissue-specific antigens and HLA-DR5-related specificity could stimulate cell growth in thyroid tissue and destruction of parietal cells. This schema could embrace the observation that suppressor T cells predominate in the Hashimoto's thyroiditis gland as compared to the Graves' disease gland; suppressor cells are known to produce prostaglandins which have been shown to stimulate thyroid cells in monolayer cultures (13); this hypothesis does not preclude the action of DR5 as an immune response gene for a subset of thyroid growth antibodies.

The subject of postpartum thyroiditis is dealt with at length in Chapter 13. A syndrome of transient hyperthyroidism associated with thyroiditis can occur not only postpartum but also unrelated to pregnancy. Although these two syndromes have features in common, they are distinguishable in several respects. In postpartum cases detectable circulating thyroid autoantibodies, goiter, and subsequent thyroid failure are more common. On the other hand, several authors have noted patients suffering from both syndromes to have relatives suffering from autoimmune endocrine disorders (184, 185; N. R. Farid, unpublished); it is possible that this tendency is more pronounced in transient hyperthyroidism unrelated to pregnancy, although the number of patients studied is limited. HLA studies provide further grounds for separating these two syndromes; postpartum thyroiditis is associated with DR5, and transient hyperthyroidism with thyroiditis unrelated to pregnancy with HLA-DR3 (and secondarily with B8). Women with recurrent postpartum thyroiditis are more likely to be DR5 than those whose postpartum thyroiditis does not recur. Although no striking deviations in the incidence of HLA-A, B, and C antigens have been documented, B35 appears to be somewhat increased in the patients with postpartum thyroiditis. It should be recalled that B35 is strongly associated with subacute thyroiditis, without a significant DR antigen association. Interestingly, HLA-B35 is also associated with subacute thyroiditis in the Chinese (186).

7.4.   Idiopathic Addison's Disease

Adrenal failure, presumably of autoimmune origin, is associated with HLA-B8 and HLA-DR3 (reviewed in Ref. 13). Interestingly, serum adrenocorticoid antibodies are very strongly related to Dw3 (187). Since adrenal-specific cytoplasmic antigens are also expressed on plasma membranes (187a), the association of these antibodies with DR3 sug-

gests the involvement of an HLA-linked Ir gene conditioning response to adrenal antigens and thus in immune injury. No information is available concerning HLA association with Addison's disease in non-Caucasoids. It has been suggested that the rarity of this disorder in the Japanese is due to the virtual absence of B8 and DR3 in that population (187). If so, the disease liability may be conferred by an Ir gene in linkage disequilibrium with DR3, to be distinguished from the broad facilitatory role of DR3 that we have outlined above.

7.5.   Hypergonadotropic Hypogonadism

It has been suggested that primary gonadal failure is associated with B8 (188); in this report it was unclear whether the oophoritis underlying gonadal failure was an isolated disorder or part of the polyglandular failure syndrome. The dearth of information on the association of this disorder with HLA stems from the fact that it is rare and heterogeneous; autoimmune dysfunction of the gonad is only one cause of apparent hypergonadotropic hypogonadism and, short of biopsy, difficult to diagnose conclusively. In a group of 25 patients studied from several centers, increases in HLA-DR3 and HLA-B35 were found in what appeared to be two nonoverlapping subgroups. This finding is in keeping with the probable etiological heterogeneity of the disorder (P. G. Walfish and N. R. Farid, unpublished).

7.6.   Polyglandular Autoimmune Syndrome

This subject is discussed in detail in Chapter 10. We would like to stress the contribution made by HLA typing to the understanding of this syndrome and its single constituent disorders (13). Two types of syndromes comprising Addison's disease have been distinguished: Type 1 syndrome associated with mucocutaneous candidiasis or hypoparathyroidism and Type II syndrome associated with IDDM and thyroid autoimmune diseases (189). HLA-B8 seems increased in patient series with the type II syndrome but not the type I syndrome. HLA-DR data are insufficient to assess at present whether type I syndrome is associated with MHC markers (190, 191).

We have stressed elsewhere (13) that not all the individual components of polyglandular autoimmune syndrome type II are individually associated with HLA-B8/DR3; for example, in goitrous thyroiditis and pernicious anemia, DR5 is significantly increased. Because the syndrome is unusual, the method of ascertainment could influence the combinations of disorders exhibited by patients, although possibly not the magnitude of association with HLA-DR3. Two population studies (192, 193) suggest that susceptibility to disease combinations is determined by separate genes, even though each of the individual disorders is associated with DR3. Study of a limited number of families with multiple cases of polyglandular autoimmune disease strongly suggests that disease susceptibility to different autoimmune diseases is due to closely linked genes on the *same* chromosome. It is quite possible that with the study of more multiplex families, the effects of individual genes may be inferred. Unusual haplotypic arrangements have been noted in some of these families; it is unclear whether this is a characteristic of the polyglandular autoimmune syndromes (192).

REFERENCES

1. Anon., *Time* **116**, 46 (1980).

2. A. Svejgaard, M. Hauge, C. Jersild, P. Platz, L. P. Ryder, L. Staub Nielsen, and M. Thomsen, Eds., *Monographs in Human Genetics*, Vol. 7, Karger, Basel, 1979.

3. L. U. Lamm and G. B. Petersen, *Transplant. Proc.* **11**, 1692 (1979).

4. B. Larsen, in N. R. Farid, Ed., *HLA in Endocrine and Metabolic Disease*, Academic Press, New York, 1981, p. 11.

5. H. Balner, *Transplant. Proc.* **11**, 657 (1979).

6. D. L. Mann, S. Abelson, S. Harris, and D. B. Amos, *Nature* **259**, 145 (1976).

7. J. J. van Rood, A. van Leeuwen, J. J. Keuning, and A. Termijtelen, *Scand. J. Immunol.* **6**, 373 (1977).

8. L. M. Nadler, P. Stashenko, R. Hardy, K. H. Tomaselli, E. J. Yunis, S. F. Schlossman, and J. N. Pesando, *Nature* **290**, 591 (1981).

9. E. Gazit, C. Terhorst, and E. J. Yunis, *Nature* **284**, 275 (1980).

10. T. Cotner, H. Hashimo, P. C. Kung, G. Goldstein, and J. L. Strominger, *Proc. Natl. Acad. Sci. USA* **78**, 3858 (1981).

11. J. Klein, A. Juretic, C. N. Baxevanis, and Z. A. Nagy, *Nature* **291**, 455 (1981).

12. J. Klein, *Science* **203**, 516 (1979).

13. N. R. Farid and J. C. Bear, *Endocr. Rev.*, **2**, 50 (1981).

14. A. Arnaiz-Vellena and H. Festenstein, *Lancet* **2**, 207 (1976).

15. G. Stingl, K. Tamaki, and S. I. Katz, *Immunol. Rev.* **53**, 149 (1980).

16. S. M. Fu, N. Chiorizzi, C. U. Wang, G. Montazeri, H. G. Kunkel, H. S. Ko, and A. B. Gottlieb, *J. Exp. Med.* **148**, 1423 (1978).

17. R. Alejandro, A. Rabinovitch, W. Eeveryn, S. Hajek, J. Miller, and D. H. Mintz, *Diabetes* **30**, 65A (1981) (Abstract).

18. H. L. Ploegh, H. L. Orr and J. L. Strominger, *Cell* **24**, 287 (1981).

19. B. Benacerraf, *Science* **203**, 1229 (1981).

20. C. J. Barnstable, E. A. Jones, and M. J. Crumpton, *Br. Med. Bull.* **34**, 241 (1978).

21. B. A. Cunningham and I. Berggård, *Transplant. Rev.* **21**, 3 (1974).

22. L. Trägårh, K. Wiman, L. Rask, and P. A. Peterson, *Scand. J. Immunol.* **8**, 563 (1978).

23. H. T. Orr, D. Lancet, R. J. Robb, J. A. Lopex de Castro, and J. L. Strominger, *Nature* **282**, 266 (1979).

24. P. J. Lachmann and M. J. Hobart, *Br. Med. Bull.* **34**, 247 (1978).

25. W. F. Bodmer, *Nature* **237**, 139 (1972).

26. G. J. O'Neill, S. Y. Yang, J. Tegoli, R. Berger, and B. Dupont, *Nature* **273**, 668 (1978).

27. W. F. Bodmer and J. G. Bodmer, *Br. Med. Bull.* **34**, 309 (1978).

28. N. K. Jerne, *Ann. Immunol. (Inst. Pasteur)* **125c**, 373 (1974).

29. R. M. Zinkernagel and P. C. Doherty, *Cold Spring Harbor Symp. Quant. Biol.* **41**, 505 (1977).

30. B. Sredni and R. H. Schwartz, *Immunol. Rev.* **54**, 187 (1981).

31. G. Thomson, W. F. Bodmer, and J. Bodmer, in S. Karlin and E. Nevo, Eds., *Population Genetics*

and Ecology, Academic Press, New York, 1976, p. 465.

32. B. Woolf, *Ann. Hum. Genet. Lond.* **19**, 251 (1955).

33. A. Svejgaard, C. Jersild, L. S. Nielsen, and W. F. Bodmer, *Tissue Antigens* **4**, 95 (1974).

34. A. E. H. Emery, *Methodology in Medical Genetics*, Churchill Livingston, New York, 1976.

35. A. Svejgaard and L. P. Ryder, in J. Dausset and A. Svejgaard, Eds., *HLA and Disease*, Munksgaard, Copenhagen, 1977, p. 46.

36. Y. Bishop, S. Fienberg, and P. Holland, *Discrete Multivariate Analysis. Theory and Practice*, MIT Press, Cambridge, Mass., 1971.

37. J. Barbosa, M. M. Chern, N. Reinsmoen, H. Noreen, R. Ramsey, and L. Greenberg, *Tissue Antigens* **14**, 426 (1979).

38. R. S. Spielman, L. Baker, and C. M. Zmijewski, in N. R. Farid, Ed., *HLA in Endocrine and Metabolic Disorders*, Academic Press, New York, 1981, p. 37.

39. K. I. Welsh, P. Pimlot, and J. R. Batchelor, *Tissue Antigens* **17**, 91 (1981).

40. B. Benacerraf and H. O. McDevitt, *Science* **175**, 273 (1972).

41. A. S. Rosenthal, *N. Engl. J. Med.* **303**, 1153 (1980).

42. P. B. Hausman, D. P. Sites, and J. D. Stobo, *J. Exp. Med.* **153**, 476 (1981).

43. E. Thorsby, B. Bergholtz, E. Berle, L. Braathen, and H. Hirschberg, *Transplant. Proc.*, **13**, 903 (1981).

44. D. W. Thomas, K-H. Hsieh, J. L. Schauster, and G. D. Wilner, *J. Exp. Med.* **153**, 583 (1981).

45. T. Tada and K. Okumura, *Adv. Immunol.* **28**, 1 (1979).

46. L. J. Rosenwasser and B. T. Huber, *J. Exp. Med.* **153**, 1113 (1981).

47. C. G. Fathman, M. Kimoto, R. Melvold, and C. S. David, *Proc. Natl. Acad. Sci. USA* **78**, 1853 (1981).

48. P. P. Jones, D. B. Murphy, and H. O. McDevitt, *Immunogenetics* **12**, 321 (1981).

49. N. R. Rose, Y-C. M. Kong, I. Okayasu, A. A. Giraldo, K. Beisel, and R. S. Sundick, *Immunol. Rev.* **55**, 299 (1981).

50. B. Benacerraf, *J. Immunol.* **120**, 1809 (1978).

51. U. R. Kees, *J. Exp. Med.* **153**, 1562 (1981).

52. C. Janeway, B. Jones, H. Binz, M. Frischknecht, and H. Wigzell, *Scand. J. Immunol.* **12**, 83 (1980).

53. J. W. Kappler, B. Skidmore, J. White, and P. Marrack, *J. Exp. Med.* **153**, 1198 (1981).

54. H. Cantor and R. K. Gershon, *Fed. Proc.* **38**, 2058 (1979).

55. B. Benacerraf and R. N. Germain, *Fed. Proc.* **38**, 2053 (1979).

56. R. K. Gershon, D. D. Eardley, S. Durum, D. R. Green, F-W. Shen, K. Yamauchi, H. Cantor, and D. B. Murphy, *J. Exp. Med.* **153**, 1533 (1981).

57. E. L. Reinherz and S. F. Schlossman, *Immunol. Today* **2**, 69 (1981).

58. T. W. Chang, P. C. Kung, S. P. Gingras, and G. Goldstein, *Proc. Natl. Acad. Sci. USA* **78**, 1805 (1981).

59. R. Jackson, M. Bowring, M. Morris, B. Haynes, and G. S. Eisenbarth, *Program of the 63rd Annual Meeting of the Endocrine Society, Cincinnati, June 17–19th, 1981*, p. 195 (Abstract).

60. D. D. Eardley, F. W. Shen, H. Cantor, and R. F. Gershon, *J. Exp. Med.* **150**, 44 (1979).

61. R. H. Zubler, B. Benacerraf, and R. N. Germain, *J. Exp. Med.* **151**, 681 (1980).

62. F. L. Owen, R. Riblet, and B. A. Taylor, *J. Exp. Med.* **153**, 801 (1981).

63. C. A. Janeway, R. A. Murgita, F. J. Weinbaum, R. Asofsky, and H. Wigzell, *Proc. Natl. Acad. Sci. USA* **74**, 4582 (1977).

64. L. A. Herzenberg, K. Okumura, H. Cantor, V. L. Sato, F. W. Shen, E. A. Boyse, and L. A. Herzenberg, *J. Exp. Med.* **144**, 330 (1976).

65. Y. J. Rosenberg and J. M. Chiller, *J. Exp. Med.* **150**, 517 (1979).

66. K. Eichman, *Adv. Immunol.* **26**, 195 (1978).

67. A. D. Steinberg, D. P. Huston, J. D. Taurog, J. S. Cowdery, and E. S. Raveche, *Immunol. Rev.* **55**, 121 (1981).

68. B. F. Haynes, R. S. Metzgar, J. D. Minna, and P. A. Bunn, *N. Engl. J. Med.* **304**, 1319 (1981).

69. S. Broder, T. Uchiyama, L. M. Muul, C. Goldman, S. Sharrow, D. G. Poplack, and T. A. Waldman, *N. Engl. J. Med.* **304**, 1382 (1981).

70. J. L. Touraine, H. Beruel, G. Souillet, and M. Jeune, *J. Pediatr.* **93**, 47 (1978).

71. E. L. Reinherz, L. Moretta, M. Roper, J. Breard, M. Mingari, M. Cooper, and S. Schlossman, *J. Exp. Med.* **151**, 969 (1980).

72. L. Moretta, M. C. Mingari, and A. Moretta, *Immunol. Rev.* **45**, 163 (1979).

73. H. M. Dosch and E. W. Gelfand, *Immunol. Rev.* **45**, 243 (1979).

74. R. F. Fox, L. F. Thompson, and J. R. Huddlestone, *J. Immunol.* **126**, 2062 (1981).

75. R. E. Rocklin, *Adv. Immunol.* **29**, 55 (1980).

76. M. Fresno, G. Nabel, L. McVay-Boudreau, H. Furthmayer, and H. Cantor, *J. Exp. Med.* **153**, 1246 (1981).

77. R. E. Ballieux, C. J. Heijnen, F. Uytdehaag, and B. J. M. Zegers, *Immunol. Rev.* **45**, 3 (1979).

78. H. Y. Tse, J. J. Mond, and W. E. Paul, *J. Exp. Med.* **153**, 871 (1981).

79. D. H. Katz, *Lymphocyte Differentiation, Recognition and Regulation*, Academic Press, New York, 1977.

80. G. Sarmay, J. Ivanyi, and J. Gergely, *Cell Immunol.* **56**, 452 (1980).

81. R. W. Chestnut and H. M. Grey, *J. Immunol.* **126**, 1075 (1981).

82. O. Ringden, B. Rynnel-Dagoo, T. Kunori, C. I. E. Smith, L. Hammar Ström, A. Frejd, and E. Möller, *Transplant. Rev.* **45**, 195 (1979).

83. R. F. Geha, *Immunol. Rev.* **45**, 275 (1979).

84. F. D. Finkelman and P. E. Lipsky, *Immunol. Rev.* **45**, 117 (1979).

85. H. O. McDevitt, T. L. Delovitch, J. L. Press, and D. B. Murphy, *Transplant. Rev.* **30**, 197 (1976).

86. J. L'Age-Stehr, *J. Exp. Med.* **153**, 1236 (1981).

87. N. Nutt, J. Haber, and H. H. Wortis, *J. Exp. Med.* **153**, 1225 (1981).

88. D. Bennett, *Cell* **6**, 441 (1975).

89. D. Owerbach, W. J. Rutter, N. E. Cooke, J. A. Martial, and T. B. Shows, *Science* **212**, 814 (1981).

90. M. I. New, B. Dupont, and L. S. Levine, in N. R. Farid, Ed., *HLA in Endocrine and Metabolic Disorders*, Academic Press, New York, 1981, p. 177.

91. W. Lafuse and M. Edidin, *Biochemistry* **19**, 49 (1980).

92. J. E. Womack, D. L. S. Yan, and M. Potier, *Science* **212**, 63 (1981).

93. C. Staszak, J. S. Goodwin, G. M. Troup, D. R. Pathak, and R. C. Williams, Jr., *J. Immunol.* **125**, 181 (1980).

94. T. J. Lawley, R. P. Hall, A. S. Fauci, S. I. Katz, M. I. Hamburger, and M. J. Frank, *N. Engl. J. Med.* **304**, 185 (1981).

95. A. Helenius, B. Morein, F. Fries, K. Simmons, P. Robinson, V. Schirrmacher, C. Terhorst, and J. L. Strominger, *Proc. Natl. Acad. Sci. USA* **75**, 3846 (1978).

96. D. L. Mann, S. I. Katz, D. L. Melsen, L. D. Abelson, and W. Strober, *Lancet* **1**, 110 (1976).

97. C. F. Bryan, K. Nishiya, M. S. Pollack, B. Dupont, and M. De Sousa, *J. Immunogenet.* **12**, 129 (1981).

98. M. H. Dorner, A. Silverstone, K. Nishiya, A. De Sostoa, G. Munn, and M. De Sousa, *Science* **209**, 1019 (1980).

99. J. Dausset and L. Contu, *Human Immunol.* **1**, 5 (1980).

100. P. C. Doherty and J. R. Bennink, *Fed. Proc.* **40**, 218 (1981).

101. W. C. de Wolf, P. H. Lange, M. Einarson, and E. J. Yunis, *Nature* **277**, 216 (1979).

102. J. R. Darsee, S. B. Heymsfield, and D. O. Nutter, *N. Engl. J. Med.* **300**, 877 (1979).

103. N. Isakov and S. Segal, *Transplant. Proc.* **13**, 963 (1981).

104. N. R. Farid, R. M. Newton, E. P. Noel, and W. H. Marshall, *Tissue Antigens* **12**, 205 (1978).

105. S. Whittingham, J. D. Mathews, M. S. Schanfield, B. D. Tait, and I. R. MacKay, *Clin. Exp. Immunol.* **43**, 80 (1981).

106. A. S. Kadish, F. A. Tansey, G. S. Yu, A. T. Doyle, and B. R. Bloom, *J. Exp. Med.* **151**, 637 (1980).

107. J-W Yoon, M. Austin, T. Onodera, and A. L. Notkins, *J. Exp. Med.* **152**, 1173 (1980).

108. P. K. Süteri, L. A. Jones, J. Roubinian, and N. Talal, *J. Steroid Biochem.* **12**, 425 (1980).

109. Y. Weinstein and Z. Berkovich, *J. Immunol.* **126**, 998 (1981).

110. J. Dausset and A. Svejgaard, Eds., *HLA and Disease*, Munksgaard, Copenhagen, 1977.

111. R. L. Dawkins, in P. I. Terasaki, Ed., *Histocompatibility Testing 1980*, UCLA Tissue Typing Laboratory, Los Angeles, 1980, p. 662.

112. M. Simon, R. Fauchet, H-P Hespel, P. Brissot, B. Genetet, and M Bourel, in N. R. Farid, Ed., *HLA in Endocrine and Metabolic Disorders*, Academic Press, New York, 1981, p. 291.

113. A. F. Geczy, K. Alexander, H. V. Bashir, and J. Edmonds, *Nature* **283**, 782 (1980).

114. E. D. Schwartz, L. R. Luehrman, and G. E. Rodey, *J. Clin. Invest.* **64**, 938 (1979).

114a. L. R. Weitkemp, H. C. Stancer, E. Persed, C. Flood, and S. Guttorman, *N. Engl. J. Med.* **305**, 1301 (1981).

115. A. Haymovits and M. Fotino in N. R. Farid, Ed., *HLA in Endocrine and Metabolic Disorders*, Academic Press, New York, 1981, p. 265.

116. E. G. Engleman, Ed., "Genetic control of the human immune response," *J. Exp. Med.* **152**, August 1980, Part 2 (supplement).

117. N. R. Farid, in N. R. Farid, Ed., *HLA in Endocrine and Metabolic Disorders*, Academic Press, New York, 1981, p. 85.

118. D. Osoba and J. Falk, *Immunogenetics* **6**, 425 (1978).

119. N. R. Farid, L. Sampson, H. Moens, and J. M. Barnard, *Tissue Antigens* **17**, 265 (1981).

120. M. Thomsen, F. Jørgensen, M. Brandsborg, P. Gimsing, J. Lang Nielsen, L. P. Ryder, and A. Svejgaard, *Tissue Antigens* **17**, 97 (1981).

121. S. M. Goyert, J. J. Hubert, R. A. Curry, and J. Silver, *Human. Immunol.* **1**, 161 (1980).

122. R. Maron and I. R. Cohen, *J. Exp. Med.* **152**, 1115 (1980).

123. S. Nyulassy, P. Hnilica, P. Gorman, V. Hirschova, and J. Stefanovic, *J. Clin. Endocrinol. Metab.* **45**, 270 (1977).

124. G. J. O'Neill, in *Symposium on HLA-Linked Complement Loci*, Program of the 23rd Annual Meeting of the Canadian Federation for Biological Societies, St. John's, Newfoundland, June 8–13, 1980.

125. S. E. Hodge, M. A. Spence, and S. D. Cederbaum, *N. Engl. J. Med.* **301**, 442 (1979) (letter).

126. P. A. Fraser and P. H. Sehur, *Clin. Immunol. Immunopathol.* **19**, 67 (1981).

127. A. Svejgaard, P. Platz, and L. P. Ryder, in P. I. Terasaki, Ed., *Histocompatibility Testing 1980*, UCLA Tissue Typing Laboratory, Los Angeles, 1980, p. 638.

128. J. Nerup and M. Christy, in N. R. Farid, Ed., *HLA in Endocrine and Metabolic Disorders*, Academic Press, New York, 1981, p. 69.

129. T. B. Strom, R. A. Bear, and C. B. Carpenter, *Science* **187**, 1206 (1975).

130. S. Srikanta, M. M. S. Ahuja, A. N. Malaviya, N. K. Mehra, and M. C. Vaidya, *N. Engl. J. Med.* **304**, 1175 (1981) (letter).

131. J. I. Rotter and D. L. Rimoin, *Am. J. Med.* **70**, 116 (1981).

132. M. Christy, A. Green, B. Christau, H. Kromann, J. Nerup, P. Platz, M. Thomsen, L. P. Ryder, and A. Svejgaard, *Diabetes Care* **2**, 209 (1979).

133. E. Wolf, J. R. Markwick, L. Wells, and A. G. Cudworth, *Diabetologia* **21**, 80 (Abstract) (1981).

134. M. Curie-Cohen, *Tissue Antigens* **17**, 136 (1981).

135. G. F. Cahill, Jr. and H. O. McDevitt, *N. Engl. J. Med.* **304**, 1454 (1981).

136. A. G. Cudworth, G. F. Bottazzo, and D. Doniach, in W. J. Irvine, Ed., *Immunology of Diabetes*, Teviot Scientific Publications, Edinburgh, 1980, p. 67.

137. B. M. Dean, J. M. McNally, and D. Doniach, *Diabetologia* **19**, 268 (Abstract) (1980).

138. Y. Nakao, H. Matsumoto, T. Miyazaki, N. Mizuno, N. Arima, A, Wakisaka, K. Okomoto, Y. Akazawa, K. Tsuji, and T. Fujita, *N. Engl. J. Med.* **304**, 407 (1981).

139. W. I. Smith, B. S. Rabin, A. Huellmantel, D. H. van Thiel, and A. Drash, *Diabetes* **27**, 1092 (1978).

140. S. Hoddinot, J. Dornan, J. C. Bear, and N. R. Farid, *Diabetologia* (in press).

141. B. Degnbol and A. Green, *Ann. Hum. Genet.* **42**, 25 (1978).

142. A. Walker and A. G. Cudworth, *Diabetes* **29**, 1036 (1980).

143. R. C. Elston, in H. Harris and K. Hirschhorn, Eds., *Advances in Human Genetics*, Vol. 11, Plenum, New York, 1981, p. 63.

144. J. M. Opitz, *Am. J. Med. Genet.* **8**, 265 (1981).

145. J. E. Craighead, *N. Engl. J. Med.* **299**, 1439 (1978).

146. D. S. Falconer, *Ann. Hum. Genet. Lond.* **31**, 1 (1967).

147. C. Smith, D. S. Falconer, and L. V. P. Duncan, *Ann. Hum. Genet.* **35**, 281 (1972).

148. M. J. Goodman and C. S. Chung, *Clin. Genet.* **8**, 66 (1975).

149. C. Zavala, N. E. Morton, D. C. Rao, J. M. Lalouel, I. A. Gamboa, A. Tejeda, and R. Lisker, *Hum. Hered.* **29**, 325 (1979).

150. P. Platz, B. K. Jakobsen, N. Morling, L. P. Ryder, A. Svejgaard, M. Thomsen, M. Christy, H. Kromann, J. Benn, J. Nerup, A. Green, and M. Hauge, *Diabetologia* **21**, 108 (1981).

151. G. Thomson and W. Bodmer, in J. Dausset and A. Svejgaard, Eds., *HLA and Disease*, Munksgaard, Copenhagen, 1977, p. 84.

152. R. S. Spielman, L. Baker, and C. M. Zmijewski, *Ann. Hum. Genet. Lond.* **44**, 135 (1980).

153. G. Thomson, *Ann. Hum. Genet. Lond.* **43**, 383 (1980).

154. B. Suarez, S. E. Hodge, and T. Reich, *Diabetes* **28**, 527 (1979).

155. F. Clerget-Darpoux and C. Bonaiti-Pellie, *Ann. Hum. Genet. Lond.* **44**, 195 (1980).

156. F. Clerget-Darpoux, C. Bonaiti-Pellie, I. Deschamps, J. Hors, and N. Feingold, *Ann. Hum. Genet. Lond.* **45**, 199 (1981).

157. S. E. Hodge, *Am. J. Hum. Genet.* **33**, 381 (1981).

158. S. E. Hodge, J. I. Rotter, and K. L. Lange, *Ann. Hum. Genet. Lond.* **43**, 399 (1980).

159. P. Rubenstein, N. Suciu-Foca, and J. F. Nicholson, *N. Engl. J. Med.* **297**, 1036 (1977).

160. J. V. Neel, *N. Engl. J. Med.* **297**, 1062 (1977).

161. J. Barbosa, M. M. Chern, H. Noreen, V. E. Anderson, and E. J. Yunis, *J. Clin. Invest.* **62**, 492 (1978).

162. J. Barbosa, M. Chern, V. E. Anderson, H. Noreen, S. Johnson, N. Reinsmoen, R. McCarthy, R. King, and L. Greenberg, *J. Clin. Invest.* **65**, 592 (1980).

163. B. K. Suarez and P. Van Eerdewegh, *Diabetologia* **20**, 524 (1981).

164. F. Clerget-Darpoux, C. Bonaiti-Pellie, J. Hors, I. Deschamps, and N. Feingold, *Clin. Genet.* **18**, 51 (1980).

165. L. L. Cavalli-Sforza and W. F. Bodmer, *The Genetics of Human Populations*, W. H. Freeman, San Francisco, 1971.

165a. S. E. Hodge, C. E. Anderson, K. Neiswanger, L. L. Field, M. A. Spence, R. S. Sparkes, M. C. Sparkes, M. Crist, P. I. Terasaki, D. L. Rimoin, and J. L. Rotter, *Lancet* **2**, 893 (1981).

165b. H. J. Bodansky, P. L. Drury, A. G. Cudworth, and D. A. Price Evans, *Diabetes* **30**, 907 (1981).

165c. L. R. Weitkamp, *Am. J. Hum. Genet.* **33**, 776 (1981).

165d. M. S. Schanfield, R. Brown, S. Sarjeantson, and R. L. Kirk, *Am. J. Hum. Genet.* **33**, 133A (Abstract) (1981).

166. D. Raum, Z. Awdeh, and C. T. Alper, *Immunogenetics* **12**, 59 (1981).

167. D. R. Gamble, *Epidemiol. Rev.* **2**, 49 (1980).

168. D. R. Gamble, *Diabetologia* **19**, 341 (1980).

169. R. S. Speilman, L. Baker, and C. M. Zmijewski, in C. F. Sing and M. Skolnick, Eds., *Genetic Analysis of Common Disease: Applications to Predictive Factors in Coronary Disease*, Alan R. Liss Inc., New York, 1979, p. 567.

170. J. F. Marks, P. Raskin, and P. Stastny, *Diabetes* **30**, 475 (1981).

171. S. H. Chan, P. P. B. Yeo, K. F. Lui, G. B. Wee, K. T. Woo, P. Lim, and J. S. Cheah, *Tissue Antigens* **12**, 109 (1978).

172. H. Uno, T. Sasazuki, H. Tamai, and H. Matsumoto, *Nature* **292**, 768 (1981).

172a. N. R. Farid and J. C. Bear, *Nature*, **295**, 629 (1982) (letter).

173. H. Schleusener, G. Schernthaner, W. Mayr, P. Kotulla, U. Bogner, K. Wenzel, R. Finke, and H. Meinhold, *Program of the 12th Annual Meeting European Thyroid Association, Pisa, 1981*, p. 14a, Abstract.

174. W. Tom and N. R. Farid, *Hum. Hered.* **31**, 227 (1981).

175. H. Fujiwara, M. Torisu, Y. Koitabashi, T. Baba, and M. Esaki, *Clin. Immunol. Immunopathol.* **19**, 98 (1981).

176. P. P. B. Yeo, S. H. Chan, K. F. Lui, G. B. Wee, P. Lim, and J. S. Cheah, *Br. Med. J.* **2**, 930 (1978).

177. W. J. Irvine, R. S. Gray, P. J. Morris, and A. Ting, *Lancet* **2**, 898 (1977).

178. K. Bech, B. Lumholtz, J. Nerup, M. Thomsen, P. Platz, L. P. Ryder, A. Svejgaard, K. Siersboek-Nielsen, J. Møholn Hansen, and J. H. Larsen, *Acta Endocrinol.* **86**, 510 (1977).

179. A. M. McGregor, B. Rees Smith, R. Hall, M. M. Peterson, M. Miller, and P. J. Dewar, *Lancet* **2**, 1101 (1980).

180. P. A. Dahlberg, G. Holmlund, F. A. Karlsson, and J. Safwenberg, *Acta Endocrinol.* **97**, 42 (1981).

181. N. R. Farid, J. M. Barnard, and W. H. Marshall, *Tissue Antigens* **8**, 181 (1976).

182. M. Weissel, R. Höfer, H. Zasmeta, and W. R. Mayr, *Tissue Antigens* **16**, 256 (1980).

183. H. A. Drexhage, G. F. Bottazzo, L. Bitensky, J. Chayen, and D. Doniach, *Lancet* **2**, 287 (1980).

184. H. G. Fein, J. M. Goldman, and B. D. Weintraub, *Am. J. Obstet. Gynecol.* **138**, 504 (1980).

185. T. F. Nikolai, J. Brosseau, M. A. Kettrick, R. Roberts, and E. Beltaos, *Arch. Intern. Med.* **140**, 478 (1980).

186. P. P. B. Yeo, S. H. Chan, T. C. Aw, K. F. Lui, A. Rauff, T. Mathew, C. H. Chang, S. Doraisingham, P. Lim, and J. S. Cheah, *Tissue Antigens* **17**, 249 (1981).

187. A. Svejgaard, M. Christy, J. Nerup, P. Platz, L. P. Ryder, and M. Thomsen, in N. R. Rose, P. E. Bigazzi, and N. L. Warren, Eds., *Genetic Control of Autoimmune Disease*. Elsevier/North Holland, New York, 1978, p. 101.

187a. E. L. Khoury, L. Hammond, G. F. Bottazzo, and D. Doniach, *Clin. Exp. Immunol.* **45**, 48 (1981).

188. J. Nerup, C. L. Cathilenenu, J. Seignalet, and M. Thompson, in J. Dausset and A. Svejgaard, Eds., *HLA and Disease*, Munksgaard, Copenhagen, 1977, p. 149.

189. M. Neufeld, R. M. Blizzard, and N. McLaren, *Clin. Res.* **27**, 812A (Abstract) (1980).

190. K. Arulanathan, J. M. Dwyer, and M. Genel, *N. Engl. J. Med.* **300**, 164 (1979).

191. M. J. Brueton, H. M. Chapel, and L. P. Mackintosh, *Tissue Antigens* **15**, 101 (1980).

192. N. R. Farid, B. Larsen, R. Payne, E. P. Noel, and L. Sampson, *Tissue Antigens* **16**, 23 (1980).

193. G. F. Bottazzo, A. G. Cudworth, D. H. Moul, D. Doniach, and H. Festenstein, *Br. Med. J.* **2**, 1253 (1978).

194. S. M. Goyret and J. Silver, *Nature* **294**, 266 (1981).

4

Prevalence of Autoimmune Endocrine Disease

W. M. G. Tunbridge

Newcastle General Hospital and
University of Newcastle upon Tyne
Newcastle upon Tyne, United Kingdom

Contents

1. EPIDEMIOLOGIC PROBLEMS

Determination of the prevalence of any disease depends on accurate diagnosis and the method of selection employed in the population under consideration. The recognition of the autoimmune origin of many endocrine diseases depends on the demonstration of autoantibodies to the relevant target organ, characteristic histology, and association with other autoimmune diseases. Many endocrine diseases which are believed to be autoimmune in origin may also have other causes. Thus hypothyroidism may be the end result of autoimmune thyroiditis but may also be due to iodine deficiency or previous destructive therapy to the thyroid. Studies of the prevalence of hypothyroidism must therefore distinguish these different causes before the frequency of autoimmune hypothyroidism can be expressed. Furthermore, the degree of damage caused by the destructive processes involved in autoimmune thyroiditis can be variable. Thyroid antibodies can be detected without any biochemical evidence of deterioration of thyroid function or can be associated with an atrophic gland and gross clinical myxedema. Accurate definition is therefore essential before any discussion of the prevalence of a condition can take place. This is particularly important with regard to endocrine disorders such as diabetes, for even diabetologists cannot agree on criteria for its definition which have worldwide acceptance. Gross cases of symptomatic diabetes with high blood sugars may be universally recognized, but the definition of impaired glucose tolerance is still under debate. Furthermore, only a proportion of insulin-dependent diabetics can be shown to have evidence of an autoimmune process, even at the time of diagnosis. The frequency of demonstrable pancreatic islet cell antibodies declines rapidly with time after diagnosis, making it extremely difficult to define which cases may have been due to an autoimmune process. Epidemiologic studies of the prevalence of autoimmune endocrine diseases depend heavily on techniques for the demonstration of circulating antibodies. Techniques for the demonstration of pancreatic islet cell antibodies or adrenal antibodies are more complicated and less readily available than those for detection of, say, thyroid antibodies and may result in an underestimation of the true frequency of the underlying autoimmune processes.

As well as problems of definition, varying etiology and technical limitations in the detection of autoantibodies, environmental factors, and population characteristics may also influence the prevalence of endocrine diseases. Hospital clinics specializing in a particular field of medicine are unlikely to reflect the disease pattern in the surrounding community. Patient referral is highly selective and may well depend on the special interests of the doctors concerned. Prevalence data based on hospital inpatient records are even more limited owing to changing patterns of hospital practice, particularly in endocrinology where most patients are dealt with on an outpatient basis. Nevertheless, hospital studies may provide useful information on the natural history of the disease and the influence of treatment. The true prevalence of a condition in the community depends on studies of cross sections of that community which reasonably reflect its socioeconomic structure and age

and sex distribution. Such studies are costly in time, money, and personnel and are thus relatively scarce, but are important if consideration is to be given to detection of the earliest stages of disease processes and their prevention. The pattern of diseases in the community may also change with time. Addison's disease was largely attributable to tuberculosis earlier this century when the latter was rife and autoimmunity unrecognized. The decline in tuberculosis may have resulted in a decreased frequency of Addison's disease but a higher proportion is recognized as idiopathic, probably autoimmune in origin. Evidence to support this changing pattern is provided by a study of death certificates, but the latter have limitations owing to incomplete or inaccurate documentation. Evidence from postmortem material is more accurate but postmortems are now performed less frequently and are usually highly selective.

Given the above problems, it is perhaps not surprising that data on the prevalence of autoimmune diseases are relatively imprecise. Autoimmune thyroid disease and diabetes mellitus are relatively common, whereas Addison's disease, primary ovarian failure, and hypoparathyroidism are relatively rare. The prevalence of these conditions is now considered in more detail and their associations examined.

2.   AUTOIMMUNE THYROID DISEASES

The spectrum of autoimmune thyroid diseases ranges from Graves' disease at one end to overt myxedema at the other. Both conditions present extreme forms of disordered thyroid function that may occur in a subsection of the population which is believed to have a genetic predisposition to autoimmune thyroid disease.

2.1.   Hyperthyroidism

A United Kingdom survey covering 106 general practices suggested a prevalence of hyperthyroidism of 25 to 30 cases per 10,000 females and a hospital in-patient study calculated 3 cases per 10,000 hospital discharges, but in neither series were diagnostic criteria specified (1). In the United States, an annual incidence of 3 cases per 10,000 females was suggested by a retrospective study of hospital referrals in Olmsted County, Minnesota (2), but this is complicated by the change in diagnostic procedures during the 30 years under review. Where all cases are referred to a few hospitals in a limited area, the hospital records may provide a valid reflection of certain disorders in that area. The annual incidence of hyperthyroidism in Tasmania was found to be 12 per 100,000 population prior to the introduction of iodized bread. Subsequently it rose to 80 per 100,000 and later fell again, presumably as the majority of susceptible individuals previously protected by iodine deficiency from exhibiting the full clinical syndrome declared themselves (3). In a more recent survey of a cross section of the population in Whickham, a noniodine-deficient area in Northeast England, Tunbridge et al. determined the prevalence of the whole spectrum of thyroid disorders in that community (4). Overt hyperthyroidism was diagnosed on the basis of clinical features and laboratory tests which included serum thyroxine and triiodothyronine levels. The overall prevalence of previously treated and new cases of thyrotoxicosis was 20 per 1000 females, rising to 27 per 1000 females when previously treated "possible" cases (whose original records were not available) were included, compared with 1.5 to 2.5 per 1000 males. It was not always possible from the analysis of case records to determine how many of these cases of thyrotoxicosis were originally due to Graves' disease and how many to autonomous thyroid nodules, but the majority appeared to be associated with diffuse goiter, favoring the former. Studies of a cross section of a population, such as the Whickham survey, allow the determination of prevalence data but give little indication of incidence. Nevertheless, it was estimated on the basis of knowledge of the age at onset of the illness that the incidence

of hyperthyroidism in this community was between 2 and 3 per 1000 females per year.

2.2. Overt Hypothyroidism

Iodine deficiency is by far the major cause of hypothyroidism worldwide, but in non-iodine-deficient areas, autoimmune processes are believed to be the major cause. In the Whickham survey, overt hypothyroidism defined by clinical criteria and confirmed by low levels of thyroxine with raised thyroid-stimulating hormone (TSH) levels was established to have occurred in 14 per 1000 females and in 19 per 1000 females when previously treated "possible" cases were included, compared with less than 1 per 1000 males (4). Previous destructive therapy to the thyroid by surgery or radioiodine accounted for a third of the cases and, when iatrogenic diseases were excluded, the prevalence of spontaneous overt hypothyroidism was 10 per 1000 females or 15 per 1000 females including "possible" cases. All these cases had evidence of thyroglobulin or microsomal antibodies. Spontaneous hypothyroidism was previously undiagnosed in 3 per 1000 females. This compares with 2 per 1000 of a sample of approximately 3000 people from two populations in Finland surveyed by Gordin et al.

2.3. Autoimmune Thyroiditis

There is considerable variation in the reported frequency of thyroid antibodies due to differences in techniques used for their estimation, definitions of significant titers, and inherent differences in the populations selected for screening. Early studies of thyroglobulin antibodies were made on selected hospital patients, excluding those with clinical thyroid diseases, or on sera sent to laboratories for other purposes such as blood transfusion or routine Wassermann testing (6, 7). The reported frequency of thyroglobulin antibodies regarded as positive at titers varying from 1:10 to 1:125 or more in the different studies ranged from 7 to 27% of females and 2 to 10% of males. A community study based on a 1 in 10 sample of people registered in a general practice in England, which avoided the selection bias of hospital studies, reported thyroglobulin antibodies at titers of 1:25 or more in 16% females and 4% males (8). A survey in New Zealand reported a low prevalence of thyroglobulin antibody (titers ranging from 1:10 to 1:30) in males with no age trend and in females a prevalence of 2% at age 25, rising to 15% at age 75 (9). In Finland Gordin et al. (5) found thyroglobulin antibody titers of 1:10 or more in 8 and 11%, respectively, of the two populations examined. In the Whickham survey, only 2% of the sample had thyroglobulin antibody titers of 1:20 or more, whereas cytoplasmic antibodies detected by immunofluorescence in serum diluted 1:10 were demonstrated in 10%, with a female to male ratio of 4:1 (4). Although the differences in techniques used to measure thyroid antibodies make strict comparison between these surveys impossible, all consistently show an increased frequency of thyroid antibodies with age in females and at least fourfold increase of antibodies in women compared with men of all ages.

The majority of people with thyroid autoantibodies detected by screening procedures do not have any clinical evidence of disordered thyroid function. Furthermore, many people with histological evidence of autoimmune thyroiditis reach the end of their lives without developing clinical evidence of thyroid disease (10, 11). Nevertheless, biochemical evidence of impaired thyroid function can be detected in a proportion of people with thyroid antibodies. Between 1.5 and 3% of samples of two Finnish communities were shown to have thyroglobulin antibodies and raised TSH levels (5), and 3% of the sample of the Whickham population (5% women and 1% men) were found to have thyroid cytoplasmic antibodies and raised TSH levels (4). Tunbridge et al. (4) found that half the subjects with thyroid antibodies had a high TSH and defined the approximate mean relative risk of having a high TSH with respect to thyroid antibodies as 20:1 for males and 13:1 for females, in-

dependent of age. People with circulating thyroid autoantibodies and raised TSH levels may be deemed to have a minor degree of hypothyroidism.

It is postulated that thyroid failure develops progressively in people with a genetic predisposition to autoimmune thyroiditis. The first markers to appear are thyroid antibodies and with advancing destruction of the thyroid gland there is an increased TSH drive in an attempt to compensate for the decline in circulating hormone levels which eventually results in overt hypothyroidism. Gordin and Lamberg (12) reported that 5 out of 18 subjects with symptomless autoimmune thyroiditis developed overt hypothyroidism during a mean follow-up of 3 years; however, four of their five overtly hypothyroid subjects had had markedly elevated TSH levels when initially assessed. Tunbridge et al. (13) followed 163 asymptomatic people with thyroid antibodies or raised serum thyrotrophin concentrations or both, and 209 age- and sex-matched controls without either marker of thyroid disorder. After 4 years, it was found that mildly raised TSH concentrations alone and the presence of thyroid antibodies alone did not significantly increase the risk of developing overt hypothyroidism during this period but overt hypothyroidism developed at the rate of 5% per year in women who initially had both raised TSH and thyroid antibodies.

2.4. Goiter

Visible diffuse goiter is much commoner in younger women, in contrast to the distribution of thyroid antibodies which increase with age. On the other hand, nodular goiter is commoner in older women. In nonendemic areas, the evidence of association between goiter and thyroid antibodies is very weak. The goiter of puberty and pregnancy probably does not have an autoimmune basis but nodular goiter is more likely to be associated with antibodies in the older age group. The use of the term "Hashimoto's thyroiditis" to embrace not only the large multinodular goiter associated with lymphocytic infiltration and thyroid antibodies but also asymptomatic autoimmune thyroiditis associated with antibodies in the absence of a goiter has tended to confuse the subject. The etiology of sporadic goiter remains unknown in the majority of cases.

3.   DIABETES MELLITUS

The prevalence of diabetes mellitus in Caucasian communities in the Western world is between 1 and 2% of the population, depending on the precise criteria used. This embraces the whole spectrum of diabetes from the acute onset insulin-dependent type usually found in young people to the much commoner noninsulin-dependent type found in older adults. The annual incidence rises with age from less than 2 per 1000 children, with a slight increase around the age of 12 to 15 years, increasing to about 8 per 1000 in middle age and 2% by the seventh decade (14).

There is a seasonal variation in the onset of insulin-dependent diabetes in childhood, with an increased prevalence over the winter or early autumn (15). It has been suggested that these trends may relate to the prevalence of viral infections in the community. An association with Coxsackie B4 virus has been demonstrated in isolated cases and diabetes may follow an episode of mumps but evidence of a precipitating viral infection is lacking in the majority of cases of insulin-dependent diabetes.

There is a well-recognized association between insulin-dependent diabetes and other autoimmune endocrine diseases at all ages (see later). Development of techniques for the detection of pancreatic islet cell antibodies by Bottazzo et al. (16) provided further evidence of an autoimmune basis in some insulin-dependent diabetics. Lendrum et al. (17) found islet cell antibodies in 85% of young insulin-dependent diabetics at the time of diagnosis, but this fell to 50% within a month of diagnosis, and after 3 years less than 20% were found to be antibody positive. In a few patients positive antibodies persist for years. Similar data were also found by Irvine et al. (18). Prevalence of islet cell antibodies in the normal population varied between 1.7% (17) and 0.5% (18) in nondiabetic controls. It has been postulated that insulin-dependent diabetes may be divided into two types: in the first, possibly viral in origin, islet cell antibodies are transient, being secondary to virus-induced beta cell destruction; the second type, truly autoimmune, is associated with other endocrine diseases and persistent islet cell antibodies.

Noninsulin-dependent diabetes is found in an older age group and is often associated with obesity and insulin resistance. Pancreatic islet cell antibodies have been found in about 5% of such patients (17). The presence of pancreatic islet cell antibodies, even in insulin-dependent diabetes, does not prove that they have a pathogenic role. The antibodies are directed against several components in the islets and not just the beta cell which is selectively destroyed. It is not possible in our present state of knowledge to determine the proportion of insulin-dependent diabetes that may be attributed to an autoimmune process.

4.   ADDISON'S DISEASE

In a study of hospital cases in the Northeast region of London related to the population in the area in the 1960s, Mason et al. (19) identified 39 cases of Addison's disease per million population. Evidence was obtained from attending physicians and also from death certificates. The prevalence of tuberculous Addison's disease in the age range 25 to 69 was about 12 per million and of nontuberculous disease about 27 per million. Adrenal failure due to tuberculosis was more common in men and nontuberculous disease more common in women. Analysis of follow-up of these patients together with those certified to have died of Addison's disease in the same period in the three other metropolitan regions of London indicated an annual death rate of 1.4 per million. Approximately half the deaths were due to tuberculosis and the other half associated with adrenal atrophy. It is presumed that cases associated with adrenal atrophy were suffering from end-stage autoimmune adrenal failure.

Techniques for detection of adrenal antibodies are less widely available than those for detecting thyrogastric antibodies. They can be found in some cases of idiopathic Addison's disease but there is a very low prevalence of adrenal cortical antibodies in the general population. There is a slight increase of prevalence of adrenal antibodies in patients with other organ-specific autoimmune disorders but without clinical Addison's disease. The association of idiopathic Addison's disease with other organ-specific autoimmune diseases is considered below.

5. PREMATURE OVARIAN FAILURE

The frequency of this condition in the female population of reproductive years is not established. Etiology is multiple and may be associated with chromosome abnormalities or be secondary to pituitary or hypothalamic disorders. Autoantibodies to ovarian tissue are not found in these conditions. Autoantibodies to ovarian tissue may be found in patients with premature ovarian failure who also have evidence of other autoimmune diseases such as Addison's disease (20). They may develop an immune reaction against antigens that are shared between the adrenal cortex and steroid-producing cells in the gonads. There is a correlation between the age at diagnosis of premature ovarian failure and autoimmune Addison's disease, whereas amenorrhea is relatively uncommon in Addison's disease of tuberculous origin (21).

6. IDIOPATHIC HYPOPARATHYROIDISM

This condition is rare but is believed to fit into the constellation of autoimmune endocrine diseases by virtue of its association with other endocrine disorders and demonstration of immunofluorescent antibodies in a proportion of cases (22). Hypoparathyroidism in children is usually associated with mucocutaneous candidiasis and such patients may also develop autoimmune adrenal failure and later hypogonadism (23).

7. ASSOCIATIONS BETWEEN AUTOIMMUNE ENDOCRINE DISEASES

Before the development of techniques for the detection of autoimmune antibodies, clinical association between certain endocrine diseases had been recognized. Thyroid disorders were recognized to be more common in patients attending diabetic clinics than in the population at large. Schmidt described his syndrome of associated adrenal and thyroid failure in 1926. The development of serologic tests for detection of autoimmune antibodies broadened the concept of these associations. It is, however, necessary to recognize that the coexistence of clinical manifestations of two or more endocrine diseases in the same patient is relatively uncommon. Serologic evidence of other coexistent autoimmune processes is more frequent but such patients do not necessarily go on to develop clinical manifestations of the disorders. Only thyroid antibodies have so far been shown to have some value in the prediction of development of hypothyroidism (12, 13). There is a strong association between thyroid antibodies and gastric parietal cell antibodies which may permit the early diagnosis of mild hypothyroidism in patients with pernicious anemia and vice versa. The distribution by age and sex of gastric parietal cell antibodies is very similar to that of thyroid microsomal antibodies.

Autoimmune Addison's disease shows a strong association with other organ-specific autoimmune diseases. In a series of 294 patients with Addison's disease reported from the Middlesex Hospital (23, 24), 40% had associated disorders including primary ovarian failure (8%), thyroid diseases (ranging from myxedema to thyrotoxicosis) (19%), insulin-dependent diabetes (15%), and idiopathic parathyroid deficiency (4%). In a similar series of 289 patients reported from Edinburgh (21, 25), 37% had associated disorders including primary ovarian failure (8%), thyroid disease (16%), insulin-dependent diabetes (9%), and idiopathic parathyroid deficiency (5%). In each series, a proportion of patients had more than two disorders. It is thus clearly worth looking for other endocrine diseases in patients with Addison's disease. The proportion of patients with positive serology is considerably higher than the number of patients with biochemical or clinical manifestations of other target organ failure. The polyendocrine syndromes are considered in more detail in Chapter 10.

Pancreatic islet cell antibodies were first reported in patients with multiendocrine deficiencies associated with organ-specific autoimmunity (16). Subsequent studies showed that islet cell antibodies declined rapidly after diagnosis in most insulin-dependent diabetics, but in the small proportion whose antibodies persisted there was a strong association with other autoimmune endocrine diseases (17, 26). Even among children who did not have persisting islet cell antibodies, 11% had organ-specific antibodies, which is fivefold more common than would be expected in normal children of the same age, although clinical evidence of other endocrine disease was rare (26). Islet cell antibodies were also detected in a few healthy first-degree relatives of children with insulin-dependent diabetes. Thus it may be possible to identify people with an increased risk of developing diabetes in families with a history of autoimmune endocrine disease.

It is well known that diabetes mellitus and thyroid diseases tend to run in families. The genetic aspects of the autoimmune endocrine diseases are considered in Chapters 2 and 3. Clearly, screening first-degree relatives is more

Table 1.   Prevalence of autoimmune endocrine diseases and circulating antibodies in the community

Disease	Prevalence in the community[a]	Antibodies to
Thyrotoxicosis	F 2.0–2.7% M 1–2/1000	TSH receptors
Myxedema	F 1.4–1.9% M 1/1000	Thyroid microsome
Asymptomatic A.I. Thyroiditis	F < 45 years 8% F > 45 years 12% M all ages 2%	Thyroid microsome
Endocrine exophthalmos	NK	Extraocular muscle Retro-orbital tissue
Pernicious anemia	F > M 0.3%	Intrinsic factor
Parietal cell antibodies	F < 35 years 2.5% F > 35 years 10% M all ages 5%	Gastric parietal cell
Addison's disease	F > M 0.027/1000	Adrenal cortex
Premature menopause with adrenalitis	NK (rare)	Adrenal cortex Steroid cells in gonad
Diabetes mellitus (insulin dependent)	0.5%	Pancreatic islet cells
Idiopathic hypoparathyroidism	NK (rare)	Parathyroid chief cell

[a] (F = female, M = male, NK = prevalence not known.)

likely to detect an increased number of individuals affected by variants of these or other autoimmune disorders than would be found in the general population. Screening such families and long-term follow-up will add to our knowledge of the genetic and natural history of autoimmune endocrine diseases. However, in our present state of knowledge and inability to prevent diabetes, identification of possibly susceptible individuals may well engender unnecessary anxiety.

8. SUMMARY

The prevelance of autoimmune endocrine diseases based on community studies is summarized in Table 1. These data may serve to put the diseases into perspective. It is important to note that the prevalences of overt diseases other than those affecting the thyroid and diabetes mellitus are low. Furthermore, overt endocrine disease occurs in only a small proportion of people with circulating antibodies. The presence of such antibodies may serve as a marker of an autoimmune process but their pathogenic role and prognostic significance remain to be established in many instances. Epidemiologic studies reveal associations between diseases and between autoantibodies but do not provide proof of cause and effect. More long-term studies are needed to determine the practical significance of autoantibodies found in asymptomatic individuals and to reveal the natural history of autoimmune disorders.

REFERENCES

1.   R. Hoffenberg, *Brit. Med. J.* iii, 452 (1974).

2.   J. Furszyfer, L. T. Kurland, et al., *Mayo Clin. Proc.* 45, 636 (1970).

3.   R. J. Connolly, G. I. Vidor, and J. L. Stewart, *Lancet* 1, 500 (1970).

4.   W. M. G. Tunbridge, D. C. Evered, R. Hall, et al., *Clin. Endocrinol.* 7, 481 (1977).

5.   A. Gordin, O. P. Heinonen, P. Saarinen, and B. A. Lamberg, *Lancet* 1, 551 (1972).

6.   E. Hackett, M. Beech, and I. J. Forbes, *Lancet* 2, 402 (1960).

7.   O. W. Hill, *Brit. Med. J.* 1, 1793 (1961).

8.   P. R. Dingle, A. Ferguson, D. B. Horn, J. Tubmen, and R. Hall, *Clin. Exp. Immunol.* 1, 277 (1966).

9.   K. G. Couchman, R. D. Wigley, and I. A. M. Prior, *J. Chronic Dis.* 23, 45 (1970).

10.   E. D. Williams and I. Doniach, *J. Pathol. Bacteriol.* 83, 255 (1962).

11.   P. A. Bastenie, P. Neve, M. Bonnyns, L. Vanhaelst, and M. Chailly, *Lancet* 1, 915 (1967).

12.   A. Gordin and B. A. Lamberg, *Lancet* 2, 1234 (1975).

13.   W. M. G. Tunbridge, M. Brewis, J. French, et al., *Brit. Med. J.* 282, 258 (1981).

14.   D. S. Falconer, L. J. P. Duncan, and C. Smith, *Ann. Hum. Genet.* 34, 347 (1971).

15.   A. Bloom, T. M. Hayes, and D. R. Gamble, *Brit. Med. J.* 3, 580 (1975).

16.   G. F. Bottazzo, A. Florin-Christensen, and D. Doniach, *Lancet* 2, 1279 (1974).

17.   R. Lendrum, G. Walker, A. G. Cudworth, et al., *Lancet* 2, 1273 (1976).

18.   W. J. Irvine, C. J. McCallum, R. S. Gray, et al., *Diabetes* 26, 138 (1977).

19.   A. S. Mason, T. W. Meade, J. A. H. Lee, and J. N. Morris, *Lancet* 2, 744 (1968).

20.   W. J. Irvine, M. M. W. Chan, L. Scarth, et al., *Lancet* 2, 883 (1968).

21.   W. J. Irvine, in G. M. Besser, Ed., *Advanced Medicine*, Vol. 13, Pitman Medicine, Tunbridge Wells, United Kingdom, 1977, p. 115.

22.   R. M. Blizzard, D. Chee, and W. Davis, *Clin. Exp. Immunol.* 1, 119 (1966).

23.   D. Doniach and G. F. Bottazzo, in E. C. Franklin, Ed., *Clinical Immunology Update*, Elsevier/North Holland, Amsterdam, 1981, p. 95.

24.   F. Sotsiou, G. F. Bottazzo, and D. Doniach, *Clin. Exp. Immunol.* 39, 97 (1979).

25.   W. J. Irvine and E. W. Barnes, *Clin. Endocrinol. Metab.* 4, 379 (1975).

26.   G. F. Bottazzo, J. I. Mann, M. Thorogood, J. D. Baum, and D. Doniach, *Brit. Med. J.*, ii, 165 (1978).

5

The Receptor Antibody Diseases

Leonard C. Harrison
Paula Heyma

The Endocrine Laboratory and Department of Medicine
The Royal Melbourne Hospital
Victoria, Australia

Contents

1. INTRODUCTION

Hormones and neurotransmitters initiate their actions by binding to specific cellular receptors on the cell surface (peptide hormones, catecholamines, and neurotransmitters), in the cytoplasm (steroid and sterol hormones), or in the nucleus (thyroid hormones).

The primary function of a receptor is selective recognition of its ligand, as evidenced by stereospecific and high affinity binding. Conformational and/or covalent modifications in the receptor then lead to activation of postreceptor pathways and bioeffects characteristic of the ligand. The ligand has no function without its receptor, which shares at least an equal role in effecting the biological responses traditionally ascribed to the ligand.

Cell surface receptors are generally large glycoproteins with molecular weights in the range 10^5 to 10^6 daltons, that is, orders of magnitude greater than their ligands. They have a complex subunit structure with hydrophobic regions buried in the membrane and require detergents for their solubilization and isolation. Their concentrations range from 10^3 to 10^5 per cell and reflect a dynamic equilibrium which can be altered by many factors controlling their rates of synthesis, degradation, or membrane insertion. The receptors for some peptide hormones and neurotransmitters are coupled via a guanosine triphosphate (GTP) binding protein to the enzyme adenylate cyclase, which hydrolyzes adenosine triphosphate (ATP) to the cyclic nucleotide adenosine-3′,5′-monophosphate (cAMP). Increases in cAMP ("second messenger") lead to activation of protein kinases which phosphorylate and thereby activate or inactivate intracellular enzymes. Unfortunately, the postreceptor mechanisms involved in the actions of metabolic and growth peptides such as insulin, growth hormone, prolactin, and the insulin-like growth factors (IGFs), are less well defined.

A large body of literature has accumulated during the past decade on the characterization, dynamics, and structure of receptors, and the principles derived from studies of hormone receptor systems have been extensively reviewed (1–9). This chapter deals with one facet of the pathophysiology of receptors, namely, autoimmune reactions to cell surface membrane receptors. Studies of receptor autoimmunity have not only provided new insights into the molecular mechanisms of disease states but have led to the availability of highly specific autoantibodies for probing receptor structure and function.

2. EHRLICH REVISITED

Paul Ehrlich (1854–1915) made a monumental contribution to the science of immunochemisty and, in addition, laid the foundations for our present-day concepts of cell surface receptors. His work on bacterial toxin-antitoxin reactions led him to introduce the notion that cells possess "side chains" or receptors)10, 11; Fig. 1). He believed that antitoxins made by cells normally reside on the cell surface as "side chains." Circulating antitoxin results from excessive production of "side chains" triggered by toxin. It is noteworthy that Ehrlich believed "side

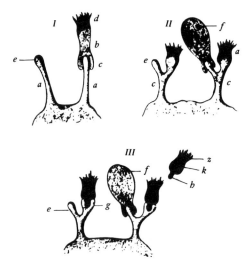

Figure 1. Ehrlich's "side-chain theory" published in connection with the "Anemia" of Ehrlich and Lazarus in Nothnagel's *Special Pathology and Therapy*, Vol. 8, 1898–1901, as an appendix to Ehrlich's *Schlussbetrachtungen*, pp. 163–185. I. Receptor of first order. (*e*) Haptophore complex; (*b*) absorbed toxin molecule with (*c*) haptophore group; (*d*) toxophore group. II. Receptor of second order with (*e*) haptophore group, (*d*) zymophore group, and (*f*)absorbed nutritive molecule. III. Receptor of the third order. (*e*) Haptophore, (*g*) complementophile group, (*k*) complement with (*h*) haptophore, (*z*) zymotoxic group, (*f*) nutritive molecule.

chains'' exist as ''Normalantikorper'' or natural antibodies prior to exposure to toxin. This view was opposed by his contemporary Karl Landsteiner, who held that antibody production was a new event, ''Andersleistung,'' that only followed exposure to toxin. Ehrlich nevertheless was very much concerned with ''side-chain'' specificity. He saw the analogy with Emile Fischer's ''lock-and-key'' principle for enzyme-substrate interactions and hypothesized that ''side-chain'' specificity might be based on steric complementarity. Furthermore, he distinguished between toxin and toxoid, the latter being pharmacologically inactive but still antigenic. He proposed that toxin molecules contain two separate chemical groups: a ''haptophore'' responsible for binding and a ''toxophore'' responsible for pharmacological activity. Toxoid molecules contained only the ''haptophore.'' Thus Ehrlich addressed the question of agonism versus antagonism, and its molecular basis, which for many systems remains unknown. His view of bacterial toxins as bifunctional molecules has proved to be essentially correct and could perhaps even be applied to ligands such as peptide hormones.

We now appreciate that Ehrlich's receptors are the antibodies on the surface of B lymphocytes whose secretion can be provoked by antigen, but progress in defining the chemistry and biology of immunocyte receptors has been relatively slow. The evolution of the receptor concept and its validation have in fact occurred predominantly in other areas, notably pharmacology and endocrinology, disciplines that were founded on the basis of ligands rather than receptors! Indeed, it is from the studies of nonantibody receptors for drugs, hormones, neurotransmitters, and lipoproteins that immunology now derives its paradigms. A further irony is that the refinement of techniques for identifying hormone receptors has revealed the presence of naturally occurring (auto)antibodies against cell surface receptors of nonimmune cells—the ''horror autotoxicus'' that Ehrlich believed would never be a reality. Ehrlich had been unable to generate autoantibodies by immunizing animals with their own red cells, yet several years later Donath and Landsteiner (12) found the first autoantibody, one which lysed red cells after binding with complement to a surface blood group antigen.

Autoimmunity is of course now recognized as an important cause of human disease. However, the molecular specificities and mechanisms of autoimmune reactions have really only been elucidated with autoantibodies to ''nonimmune'' cell surface receptors. From the following descriptions it will be appreciated that, depending on the cell type, autoantibodies to receptors can lead to either activation or inhibition of a diversity of cellular functions, ranging from membrane transport to protein synthesis. These findings have enormous implications for understanding the regulation of the immune system itself, and with it the disorder of self-tolerance in autoimmunity and the role of immune mechanisms in conditions such as cancer and aging. In accord with Ehrlich's original notions Jerne (13) has developed the concept of the immune system as a network of autoantibodies (''complementary idiotypes''), either circulating or bound as immunocyte receptors. Ultimately, we may come full circle to find that the immunopathology of membrane receptors is again concerned primarily with the regulation of receptors on immune cells.

Currently, the disease states associated with receptor autoantibodies are Graves' disease with antibodies to the thyrotropin (TSH) receptor (Chapter 6), myasthenia gravis with antibodies to the acetylcholine (ACh) receptor, severe insulin-resistant diabetes with antibodies to the insulin receptor, and asthma and related disorders with antibodies to the β_2-adrenergic receptor. In this chapter we attempt to focus on the mechanisms of receptor dysfunction in some of these diseases and to highlight aspects which elucidate receptor structure-function relationships. Despite the complexity of receptor structure and the diversity of immune reactions certain common features can be discerned.

Cell surface receptors are obvious targets for immune reactions (14, 15) and their derangement by autoantibodies may underlie many diseases whose pathogenesis is obscure.

3. ACETYLCHOLINE RECEPTORS AND MYASTHENIA GRAVIS

Myasthenia gravis is a disorder of neurotransmission causing weakness and easy fatigability, especially of the facial, ocular, pharyngeal, laryngeal, and respiratory muscles. A characteristic feature in myasthenia is a decremental electromyographic response to successive low-frequency stimuli (2 to 3 Hz), probably representing the electrophysiological counterpart of muscle fatigability. This phenomenon, although not completely understood, can be produced by several mechanisms including the simple functional blockade of ACh receptors with specific antagonists. It is reversed by the use of anticholinesterase drugs, which prolong the action of ACh (see Refs. 16 and 17 for clinical reviews).

3.1. Neuromuscular Transmission

Striated muscle fibers are innervated by myelinated nerve axons extending from motor neuron cell bodies in the spinal cord; the synapse between the motor neuron and the muscle fiber is known as an end plate. The bioelectrical processes subserving muscle activation have been reviewed in detail by Gage (18) and Rang (19). In the nerve ending acetylcholine (ACh) is stored in 500 Å vesicles, each containing up to 10,000 ACh molecules. Depolarization of the normally negative membrane potential at the nerve terminal by a descending action potential wave causes exocytosis of 50 to 200 ACh vesicles into a 900 Å synaptic gap, opposite the postsynaptic membrane where Ach receptors are concentrated on folds at ~20,000 binding sites per square micrometer. Binding of ACh to these receptors triggers the opening of a cation channel through which sodium, calcium, and potassium ions flow according to their concentration gradients. The summation of potential changes from these channel openings generates the end plate potential. When this exceeds a certain threshold level, an action potential is generated and propagated to activate the contractile process. Normally, the amount of ACh released and the occupancy of receptors greatly exceed the minimum necessary for activation (''safety factor''), but the potential decays rapidly as ACh levels fall due to destruction by acetylcholinesterase and to diffusion out of the synapse. Even in the resting state miniature end plate potentials (MEPPs) of about 1 mV are recordable owing to the spontaneous release of the contents of single synaptic vesicles. The early observation by Elmqvist and co-workers (20) that MEPPs were deficient in myasthenic patients led many investigators to conclude, incorrectly, that the defect was an insufficiency of ACh itself. The structure of the presynaptic membrane and the amount of ACh released in the myasthenic are normal, however. The abnormality is due to a decrease in sensitivity to ACh because of reduced numbers of ACh receptors and to an altered structure of the postsynaptic membrane, induced by antibodies to the ACh receptor (21–23).

The ACh receptor is the prototype for studies of receptor structure and function, largely because of the intense effort directed toward understanding the pathogenesis of myasthenia gravis and because ACh receptors are readily available in a concentrated form in the electric organs of *Electrophorus electricus*, the electric eel, and various species of *Torpedo*, the electric ray. The ACh receptor is an integral transmembrane glycoprotein, and in *T. californica* consists of four initimately associated peptide chains of molecular weights 40,000 (α), 50,000 (β), 60,000 (γ), and 65,000 (δ) present in a mole ratio of 2:1:1:1, forming a macromolecular complex with a molecular weight of 250,000 (24). The ACh receptor from *Torpedo* (but not eel or mammalian muscle) exists in the postsynaptic membrane predominantly as a dimer, linked through disulfide bonds in the 65,000 chains (25). The monomer contains the ion channel and two ACh binding sites, the latter formed at least in part by the 40,000 chains, since these chains are affinity labeled by ACh analogues (26). As shown by Raftery and co-workers (24) the four subunits have distinct but homologous sequences, suggesting that they descended from a single ancestral coding gene. Electron microscopy of freeze fractured and negatively stained synaptic membranes containing ACh receptors has shown structures approximately 85 Å in diameter with a central "pit" approximatey 25 Å in diameter. The relationship of the ion channel to these structures and to the central "pit" is still unclear.

3.2. Autoimmunity in Myasthenia Gravis

A number of lines of evidence, including the presence of thymic hyperplasia and antibodies to striated muscle, changes in serum complement, and the occurrence of transient weakness in the newborn of some myasthenic mothers led to suggestions by Simpson (28) and Nastuk and co-workers (29) in 1960 that myasthenia gravis was an autoimmune disease, possibly mediated by autoantibodies to the ACh receptor. The snake toxin α-bungarotoxin, a specific blocker of the ACh binding site at the neuromuscular junction, was discovered shortly after by Chang and Lee (30), but despite the availability of this unique probe of the ACh receptor the mechanisms of impaired neurotransmission in myasthenia remained controversial for another decade. By 1971, however, ultrastructural studies by Engel and Santa (31) had convincingly demonstrated that the basic lesion in myasthenia was in the postsynaptic membrane. The missing link in the pathogenesis was then provided with the fortuitous observation by Patrick and Lindstrom (32) that rabbits immunized by ACh receptors purified from the electric organs of *Electrophorus* developed muscular weakness similar to that seen in humans with myasthenia

gravis (MG). This experimental model, now called experimental autoimmune myasthenia gravis (EAMG), was associated with autoantibodies to the ACh receptor and provided the clue to the identification of such antibodies in the human syndrome (33–39). Most studies have demonstrated that autoantibodies to the ACh receptor do not mainly behave as competitive antagonists of ACh binding, but lead to receptor loss by (1) accelerating internalization and degradation of the receptor (40–42) and (2) complement-mediated focal lysis. Antibody-induced receptor degradation is called "antigenic modulation" and is analogous to the "down-regulation" of receptors induced by exposure to homologous ligands (3). Actually Engel has recently demonstrated (personal communication) that receptor degradation and synthesis are both increased, but that the insertion of newly synthesized receptors into the end plate is impaired. The ability of ACh receptor antibodies to induce receptor loss requires antibody bivalency and therefore may depend on cross-linking of receptor subunits (43). Studies with EAMG in animals also show that neurotransmission is affected to a lesser extent by direct antibody binding than by loss of ACh receptor (17). Comprehensive descriptions of the immunopathology of ACh receptors in MG and EAMG may be found in recent reviews by Lindstom (44) and Vincent (27).

Although EAMG has been an invaluable model it is not altogether identical to human MG. Animals immunized with purified ACh receptor together with Freund's and *B. pertussis* adjuvants develop an acute myasthenic syndrome after 8 to 12 days. This is associated with measurable levels of ACh receptor antibody but, most strikingly, with intense phagocytic infiltration of the end place, complement fixation, and membrane lysis leading to rapid denervation. This acute phase may be an artifact or an enhanced reaction due to the *B. pertussis* since it is not usually seen in animals immunized without this adjuvant. The chronic phase of EAMG occurs after 30 to 40 days and is associated with high titers of ACh receptor antibody, loss of receptors, "simplification" of the postsynaptic membrane folds, and complement-dependent lysis, but no phagocytic infiltration. This pathology resembles that seen in human myasthenia. In both situations the amount of ACh receptor, bound antibody, and bound C3 complement is greatest in the least severely affected subjects, consistent with the evidence that loss of ACh receptor causes impaired transmission.

EAMG can be passively transferred by globulins from an affected to a normal rat (45). Transfer is rapid and within a day or two there is an intense phagocytic infiltration resembling EAMG. This indicates that antibodies alone (with complement) are capable of inducing a cellular response at the end plate. Passive transfer from man to mouse has also been accomplished (46). Passive transfer and acute EAMG do not occur if C3 complement is depleted by treatment with cobra venom factor, even though antibodies are bound (47). This indicates the importance of complement fixation in opsonizing the membrane for destruction by phagocytes. "Antigenic modulation" does not appear to require complement, but simply the presence of bivalent antibodies. The human counterpart of the passive transfer experiment is the transplacental transfer of antibodies from some myasthenic mothers to their offspring, where weakness in the neonate declines over 4 to 6 weeks with the disappearance of antibodies.

3.3.   Properties of ACh Receptor Antibodies

The antibodies in experimental animals with chronic EAMG or in humans with MG are 7S IgG, the major subclass being IgG3 (44). Production of ACh receptor antibodies is T-lymphocyte dependent and is not seen in rats subjected to neonatal thymectomy and X-irradiation (48). The responses to immunization in these animals can be reconstituted by B plus T lymphocytes, but not by B lymphocytes alone. Thymectomy of adult immunized rats does not, however, prevent EAMG.

Antisera against each of the four subunits of the *Torpedo californica* receptor cross-react with receptors in human muscle and with the same subunits from other species (49), suggesting conservation of some common determinants exposed on the extracellular surface. However, species specificity is also present as indicated by the limited cross-reactivity of MG patient sera with ACh receptors from rat muscle or electric organs. Thus antibodies in MG sera did not react with eel ACh receptor, although antibodies to eel receptor do cross-react with human muscle ACh receptor (50). In both EAMG and MG most antibodies are against a "main immunogenic region" on the 40,000 (α) subunit, but in both cases antibodies to many antigenic determinants are produced (51).

Lindstrom and co-workers (44) have demonstrated that EAMG in rats develops after immunization with any single receptor subunit, suggesting that there is no single myasthenogenic determinant. This is in keeping with the evidence that the myasthenic state is due to the accelerated degradation of receptors triggered by antibody cross-linking, rather than by antibody interference with the function of a specific determinant. Most of the antibodies are directed at determinants other than the ACh binding site. The binding of α-bungarotoxin to human ACh receptor is inhibited by only about one-third of MG sera (52). Furthermore, Lindstrom and colleagues have shown that antibody-ACh receptor complexes extracted from affected muscle can still bind toxin. It makes little difference also whether antibodies are measured by using [^{125}I]-toxin ACh receptor as antigen, or [^{3}H]-acetyl ACh receptor in which the toxin binding sites are free.

A further interesting finding concerns the differences between "junctional" receptors concentrated at the end plate and "extrajunctional" receptors found at lower densities over the entire surface of embryonic or denervated adult muscle fibers. Although both forms of the receptor have the same gross subunit structure they differ in several respects, including immunoreactivity. Weinberg and Hall (53) found in the rat that extrajunctional receptors have determinants not present on junctional receptors, which are recognized by some human myasthenic antibodies but not by several antisera to purified ACh receptors. One interpretation, therefore, might be that the autoimmune reaction in MG is against an embryonic receptor antigen, perhaps resembling the ACh receptor on myoid cells of the thymus (54).

Tzartos and Lindstrom (55) and Lennon and Lambert (56) raised monoclonal antibodies against purified ACh receptors and found that their infusion into normal rats produced myasthenia. This indicates that myasthenia can result from a defect in a single clone of immunocytes, producing an antibody presumably against a single determinant on the receptor. Lindstrom and colleagues have also used the monoclonal antibodies to map the receptor structure (51); approximately 50% are species nonspecific and many react with a "main immunogenic region" on the 40,000 (α) subunit outside the ACh binding site. They suggest that these antibodies may be directed against a highly conserved immunogenic region important in receptor function, which could be the prime target of the autoimmune response in MG. Delineation of the antibody specificities at the monoclonal level could lead to specific forms of immunotherapy for MG as discussed below.

3.4. Humoral versus Cellular Immunity

Humoral and cellular immune responses can both be demonstrated in myasthenia, but the chief effector mechanism appears to be humoral. The humoral response is T cell-dependent and EAMG animals demonstrate delayed-type hypersensitivity to the ACh receptor. Lymph node cells can transfer myasthenia, but the result is not as dramatic as after passive transfer with antibodies (48). It is also much more delayed and probably results from antibody production in the recipient.

Purified ACh receptor stimulates ^{3}H-thymidine uptake in peripheral blood lymphocytes from MG patients, but this is not a universal finding (57). Furthermore, cellular responses to the ACh receptor have also been observed in some cases of polymyositis without the clinical features of MG (58). ACh receptor antibodies have not been found in polymyositis and are present in less than 1% of patients with other autoimmune and neurological disorders (37). The evidence for a primary pathogenetic role for ACh receptor antibodies in myasthenia has already been discussed. In summary, (1) antibodies, not cells, are found at the end plates in MG and chronic EAMG (17); (2) EAMG can be induced by passive transfer of antibodies from man to mouse (46) or from rat to rat (45), or by infusion into normal rats of monoclonal antibodies against ACh receptor (55, 56); and (3) removal of antibodies by plasmapheresis results in clinical and electrophysiological improvement (59).

3.5. Measurement of ACh Receptor Antibodies

The frequency of antibody detection in MG patients depends on the assay employed and the source of ACh receptor. The most sensitive assay is the so-called radioimmunoassay, the indirect immunoprecipitation of solubilized receptor from human muscle labeled with [^{125}I]-bungarotoxin (36–39). The immunoprecipitation assay is positive in greater than 90% of patients. It does not detect antibodies directed against the binding site, but this is not a major problem since most antibodies are against other determinants. In fact, receptor-antibody complexes can be extracted from muscle, labeled with [^{125}I]-toxin, and then precipitated with antihuman IgG (60).

Although the titer of antibodies is generally low in patients with localized, for example, ocular, MG, the correlation between titer and the severity of generalized MG is poor (37), and patients in remission have been reported to have titers within the range seen in active disease (52). Thus the abilities of the antibodies to immunoprecipitate solubilized receptors do not always match their functional effects. Given the evidence for the pathogenic role of antibodies in MG this lack of correlation must indicate considerable heterogeneity between patients' antibodies. Sera could contain additional antibodies to solubilized receptors not recognized by the receptors in situ, especially if the autoimmune response was maintained by the shedding of postsynaptic membrane. Additional factors possibly responsible for the discrepancy between antibody titers and clinical status could include the degradation upon storage of specific antibody subclasses (e.g., IgG$_3$) responsible for functional effects, the function of the complement system in individual patients, and the ability to repair end plate damage.

3.6.   Factors Bearing on the Etiology and Treatment of Myasthenia Gravis

Rational therapy for myasthenia gravis, and for other autoimmune diseases, would aim to eradicate the autoantigen for the clones producing autoantibodies, or restore immunoregulation to normal. Unfortunately, because of our ignorance of the precipitating and sustaining factors in autoimmunity, and the lack of detailed knowledge of the molecular specificity of autoimmune phenomena that we observe, therapy remains largely empirical. There is no evidence for an intrinsic receptor defect in myasthenia gravis or the other autoimmune receptor diseases. However, there is evidence for impaired immunoregulation.

Caucasians with MG fall into two general classes: (1) the majority are young females with a peak age of onset in the third decade; approximately 65% have thymic hyperplasia and tissue typing reveals a significantly higher frequency of the HLA antigens A1, B8, and DR3, (2) A minority are older males, thymoma is common, and there are a high frequency of antibodies to striated muscle and an increased frequency of HLA antigens A2 and

A3. In Japanese, thymic hyperplasia is associated with HLA B12 and thymoma with HLA B5 (61). Thymectomy, particularly in young females, is generally associated with clinical improvement but the mechanism is unknown and this procedure is not usually associated with a dramatic fall in receptor antibody titers. The role of the thymus in MG is still poorly understood. Since the thymus contains ACh receptors on myoid cells (54) it has been postulated that MG may be initiated in the thymus. Thymectomy is not always beneficial, which suggests that the thymus is not the sole source of autoantigenic stimulation. However, it is possible that in established MG the shedding of ACh receptors from damaged end plates could maintain the autoimmune process.

Penicillamine treatment of rheumatoid arthritis has been associated with the reversible development of MG (62) and ACh receptor antibodies (63). Penicillamine treatment has also been associated with autoimmune responses to other antigens, suggesting that this drug induces a defect in immunoregulation (64).

Corticosteroids and other immunosuppressive agents given to patients with MG result in clinical improvement and a decrease of antibody titer (17, 27, 44). Antibody concentration can be decreased and a temporary clinical improvement observed after plasmapheresis (exchange of the patient's plasma with normal plasma) (59). Drainage of the thoracic duct which removes lymphocytes as well as antibodies is also effective (65), but such procedures which physically remove the autoimmune effectors must be combined with immunosuppressive drug treatment to prevent rebound synthesis of new receptor antibodies.

Autoimmune myasthenia can result from a monoclonal antibody against one determinant on the ACh receptor (55, 56). Thus loss of regulation of a single antibody-producing clone could result in autoimmune disease. The corollary is that it may be possible to actively or passively immunize against such clones. Indeed, antibodies (anti-idiotypic antibodies) reactive against antibodies to the ACh receptor have been raised in mice by immunization with sensitized spleen cells or purified antibodies to the ACh receptor (66).

4. INSULIN RECEPTORS AND DIABETES MELLITUS

Diabetes mellitus is the syndrome characterized by chronic hyperglycemia, defects in insulin secretion and/or action, and in most cases, chronic complications involving small and large blood vessels. Clinically, diabetes is classified into two major types: type I or insulin-dependent diabetes (20% of cases) occurs predominantly in young persons and is ascribed to an absolute lack of pancreatic insulin-producing beta cells; type II or non-insulin-dependent diabetes (80% of cases) occurs predominantly in middle-aged persons who tend to be obese, and is associated with a relative lack of insulin secretion in the face of tissue resistance to the action of insulin. These are convenient but oversimplified distinctions that belie our knowledge of the basic pathogenetic processes involved. Even so, considerable progress has been made recently in defining possible immunopathological mechanisms in diabetes. A large body of evidence indicates that Type 1 diabetes, whatever the precipitating cause, involves autoimmune destruction of the pancreatic beta cells (67), but neither the effector mechanisms nor the autoantigens have been clearly defined.

Under the mantle of type II diabetes are an increasing number of genetic and acquired diseases with "secondary diabetes," where tissue resistance to insulin is the characteristic and common feature (68). In this section we describe one such form of diabetes, an autoimmune syndrome of insulin resistance associated with autoantibodies to the insulin receptor. Although apparently uncommon this syndrome has been studied in considerable detail and insulin receptor autoantibodies have been unique probes of receptor structure and function.

4.1. The Insulin Receptor

The structure of the receptor has been elucidated by labeling the binding sites with photoreactive ^{125}I-insulins (69–71) or chemically cross-linked ^{125}I-insulin (72, 73) or by autoantibody precipitation of receptors surface-labeled with ^{125}I (74, 75) or biosynthetically labeled with ^{35}S (76). In addition, the receptor protein has been analyzed after sequential chromatographic purification on columns of immobilized lectins and insulin (77) or receptor antibodies (78). The consensus from these studies is that the insulin receptor in several human and rat tissues is a multivalent oligomer of molecular weight 300,000 to 350,000, composed of disulfide-linked 130,000 and 90,000 subunits. Both subunits are surface glycoproteins (75, 76, 79), but whether one or both are transmembranous is unknown. The Stokes radius of the native, Triton-solubilized receptor is approximately 72 Å, corresponding to a molecular weight of approximately 300,000 (80–82), similar to that of the nonreduced labeled receptor isolated in SDS-polyacrylamide gels. The stoichiometry of the disulfide-linked oligomer has not been determined directly but analysis of graded reduction products after chemically cross-linking ^{125}I-insulin suggests a combination of two pairs of 130 and 90K subunits (72, 83). The 130 and 90K subunits appear to be distinct peptides although homology could be present and indeed would be expected if the subunits arose by gene duplication (cf. ACh receptor).

A number of smaller receptor-specific peptides have been isolated in these studies and probably represent degradation products of the major subunits (74, 84). There is some evidence that the 90K subunit is composed of two 45K "domains" (78, 84). The subunit structure of the receptor appears to be the same in rat adipocytes and hepatocytes and in human lymphocytes and placental tissues, but in rat brain Yip and co-workers (85), using photoreactive ^{125}I-insulin labeling, could not identify the 90K subunit. Since the brain appears to bind insulin, this raises the possibility that the 90K subunit could be an effector or regulator subunit. Indeed, not all investigators have been able to identify the 90K subunit in other tissues (71, 72) using covalent ^{125}I-insulin labeling methods, although it is specifically recognized by polyclonal receptor autoantibodies that recognize the 130K subunit (73, 75, 76). Insulin binding is coupled to a variety of postreceptor events in different tissues and although the gross structure of the receptor may be the same in most tissues, it seems likely that fine differences must exist to subserve different postbinding functions. This is suggested because solubilized receptors from different species, and from different tissues within the same species, exhibit different reactivities with polyclonal antisera in a receptor radioimmunoassay (86).

The specific functions of the 130,000 and 90,000 subunits remain to be elucidated. It has been proposed that they each contribute to a single binding site, analogous to the heavy and light chains of an immunoglobulin molecule (72, 83). However, the inconstant covalent labeling of the 90,000 subunit with ^{125}I-insulin does not support this notion, but rather that the 130,000 subunit is a "high affinity" site and the 90,000 subunit a "low affinity" site. On the other hand, a "two-site" model would require a high ratio of low to high affinity sites for which there seems to be, in fact, contrary evidence. Any model must ultimately account for the nonlinear concave Scatchard plot of insulin binding to both membrane-bound and solubilized receptors, attributed by De Meyts (87) to "negative cooperativity."

An alternative model might be a multivalent receptor of 130K recognition-binding subunits, with the 90K subunit being an associated protein, for example, an affinity regulator, effector-coupler, or transport/channel. Recent studies in lymphocytes have demonstrated that the binding of ^{125}I-insulin under physiological conditions leads to covalent labeling of the receptor (88). This finding has been confirmed in an insulin-sensitive tissue, the adipocyte,

and shown to involve a disulfide exchange between insulin and the 130K subunits (89). Disulfide exchange occurs on the membrane before internalization and appears to be a necessary requirement for insulin action (89). We have proposed that this mechanism of receptor activation, which amounts to "insulin bridging" of receptor subunits, provides an explanation for the known insulin-like effects of oxidants (e.g., H_2O_2, vanadate) and cross-linking agents (receptor antibodies and lectins).

4.2. Insulin Receptors and Insulin Resistance

The first direct evidence for the role of receptors in disease came from the studies on insulin receptor function in states of "insulin resistance." A host of physiological and pathological causes of insulin resistance are associated with changes in the concentration and/or affinity of insulin receptors (reviewed in Refs. 1, 3, 4, and 6). The prototype for insulin resistance is obesity. In obesity there is an increased frequency of glucose intolerance despite the presence of increased plasma insulin levels, and the response to exogenous insulin is diminished (90). In the studies of Kahn and co-workers (91) on obese mice it was demonstrated that insulin resistance was associated with a decrease in the concentration of insulin receptors on various target cells, and that this decrease was inversely proportional to the ambient insulin concentration. This finding was subsequently confirmed in obese humans (92–94). The decreased receptor concentration was found to correlate with indexes of insulin resistance (93) and a reduction in caloric intake was shown to decrease insulin concentration and restore receptor concentrations toward normal (92).

In addition to obesity, insulin levels may be elevated with type 2 diabetes, acromegaly (growth hormone excess), chronic liver or kidney disease, and insulinoma. Hyperinsulinemia in these conditions is also associated with a reciprocal decrease in receptor concentration and with insulin resistance (3, 4, 6). These findings support the idea that a major factor regulating receptor expression is insulin itself. Gavin and co-workers (95) demonstrated that insulin could induce specific "down-regulation" of its receptors in cultured human lymphocytes, and this process was subsequently shown to involve accelerated internalization and intracellular degradation of receptors rather than inactivation of their binding function or internalization with a block in recycling (76, 86, 96). Nevertheless, in many insulin-resistant states insulin is not the prime effector, despite the fact that it is usually the common denominator. Insulin action is part of a complex homeostatic system, and defects at any level from the brain to the peripheral tissues can produce the same steady-state disturbance. For example, insulin resistance may occur with a defect intrinsic to the receptor, leading to higher levels of circulating glucose and amino acids, pancreatic stimulation, and secondary hyperinsulinemia.

The maximum bioactivity of insulin requires that only a fraction of the total cellular receptors be occupied by hormone at any one time (97). Therefore, the effect of reducing receptor concentration is to decrease sensitivity to insulin, that is, to shift the dose response to the right without altering the maximum possible response (98). Decreased sensitivity also results if receptor affinity is reduced, as for example in acidosis or Cushing's syndrome (glucocorticoid excess). Thus a reduction in either the concentration or the affinity of insulin receptors leads to impaired tissue sensitivity to insulin. In many situations, however, including type 2 diabetes with fasting hyperglycemia, the predominant type of insulin resistance is an impairment of the maximum response, indicating the presence of a defect distal to receptor binding (99).

4.3.   Autoantibodies and Insulin Resistance

Autoantibodies to the insulin receptor were discovered by Flier and co-workers in 1975 in the sera of three nonobese women with severe insulin resistance and the skin disorder acanthosis nigricans (100). These patients had evidence of generalized autoimmune disease and were classified as having the type B syndrome of insulin resistance and acanthosis nigricans, to distinguish them from type A patients with insulin resistance and acanthosis nigricans who also had hirsutism and polycystic ovarian disease but who lacked receptor autoantibodies (101). A total of only 18 patients with insulin receptor autoantibodies has been documented thus far, making this disorder probably the least common of the known receptor antibody diseases.

Insulin receptor antibodies are polyclonal and predominantly of the IgG class (102). They inhibit insulin binding (100, 102, 103), acutely mimic the actions of insulin (104–106), and immunoprecipitate solubilized insulin receptors (107). The clinical features of the patients have been recently reviewed (108, 109) and are summarized in Table 1. Most patients have presented with symptomatic diabetes resistant to extremely high doses of insulin (up to 24,000 units per day). As with other autoimmune diseases females predominate, but there are notably few Caucasians. Nearly all patients have had acanthosis nigricans, a thickening of the skin with pigmentation over the extensor surfaces of the neck and joints, frequently extending over the trunk and face and associated with multiple skin tags. The significance of acanthosis is uncertain but the severity of the lesions seems to mirror the degree of insulin resistance and of hyperinsulinemia. One possibility, therefore, is that acanthosis represents a "growth effect" of supraphysiological concentrations of insulin. Most patients have evidence of generalized autoimmune disease usually manifest by nonspecific serologic markers, although five patients have had the classic features of systemic lupus erythematosus. In contrast, insulin receptor antibodies were not detected in screening more than 80 sera from patients with other autoimmune diseases (Harrison and Flier, unpublished).

Table 1.   Features of patients with insulin receptor antibodies

Total number of patients documented	18
Females/males	14/4
Age range: 15–62 years	
Race: 12 black, 3 Caucasian, 2 Japanese, 1 Mexican-American	
Presenting feature	
Symptomatic diabetes	11
"Reactive" hypoglycemia	1
Lupus erythematosus	1
Sjogren's syndrome	2
Polyarthralgia	1
Asymptomatic associated with ataxia-telangiectasia	2
Acanthosis nigricans	13
Severe glucose intolerance	15
Tendency to ketosis	8
Severe insulin resistance	17
Generalized autoimmune features at some time (e.g., vitiligo, alopecia, submandibular gland enlargement, thyroiditis, glomeruloneprhritis, hemolytic anemia, arthralgias, splenomegaly, antinuclear antibodies)	16
Development of hypoglycemia	3
Improvement or remission (with or without therapy)	9

The clinical course has been variable, although the tendency has been for insulin resistance to improve and antibody titers to fall, with or without therapy (110–113). At least half of the patients have been given immunosuppressive drugs, usually glucocorticoids with or without cyclophosphamide, but in only two cases could a remission be reasonably attributed to treatment (110, 113). Two patients have been serially plasma exchanged and in one case this procedure resulted in a progressive decrease in antibody titer and a concomitant increase in insulin binding to the patient's cells in vitro (114). These changes were accompanied by disappearance of ketosis and by a slight increase in insulin sensitivity in vivo, but the results were short-lived and the antibody levels rebounded within several days of the last exchange. To be of practical benefit plasma exchange should be combined with immunosuppressive treatment to inhibit antibody synthesis.

Three patients have developed hypoglycemia, in one case severe and intractable and leading to death (113). The insulin receptor antibodies do have insulin-like actions acutely in vitro but are usually associated with clinical insulin resistance consistent with their ability to desensitize cells chronically in vitro (115, 116). The evolution of hypoglycemia in the female who died was not accompanied by any apparent change in the properties of her antibodies on normal cells and could not be attributed to excessive levels of insulin or insulin-like growth factors. There was, however, a major increase in insulin binding to her own cells owing to a marked increase in low affinity binding sites. Insulin binding to her cells was not blocked by her receptor antibodies in vitro. These findings could be explained by massive proliferation of receptors maximally blocked by antibodies, since the effect of her antibodies on normal receptors in vitro was to abolish high affinity binding. It seems likely that this receptor proliferation was responsible for hypoglycemia, but whether insulin or antibodies were required for activation is unknown. It is reasonable to speculate that the receptor antibodies failed to downregulate or desensitize her receptors and continued to act as agonists, in an analogous fashion to thyroid-stimulating antibodies in

Graves' thyrotoxicosis. We have also studied another patient not included here (Harrison and Underhill, unpublished) with an abdominal malignancy and acanthosis nigricans, who presented with hypoglycemia and was found to have insulin receptor autoantibodies. This suggests that these antibodies might sometimes behave as agonists in vivo.

Antibodies to the insulin receptor have also been discovered in the New Zealand obese (NZO) mouse, an animal model of obesity and insulin-resistant diabetes (117). NZO mice were inbred from a stock colony which had originally given rise to the NZB and NZB/W models of autoimmune hemolytic anemia and systemic lupus erythematosus. The latter strains have been the subject of extensive immunologic investigations. When Marion Bielschowsky first characterized the metabolic syndrome in NZO mice she suggested that the insulin resistance might be due to an antagonist of insulin action (118), but the possibility that the antagonist could be an autoantibody does not seem to have been entertained until recently. In contrast to the human antibodies those in the sera from NZO mice are of low titer and are IgM. These IgM antibodies are labile and their activity deteriorates quickly during storage or with freezing and thawing. They only partially inhibit insulin binding to human receptors but can be detected by their ability to immunoprecipitate solubilized receptors (117). However, more evidence is required to establish that the insulin receptor antibodies in NZO mice have a pathogenetic role as "insulin antagonists." Further evidence for the immune basis of the NZO syndrome is the finding of autoantibodies to single- and double-stranded DNA in NZO sera and the demonstration that NZO kidneys contain dense glomerular deposits of IgM (119).

4.4. Autoantibodies and Insulin Receptor Function

Binding of insulin to receptors on fresh circulating monocytes from type B patients is markedly impaired. Analysis of the defect may be difficult because of the low level of binding and this itself suggests a loss of receptors. However, in the few patients studied a decrease in receptor affinity has been the predominant feature; that is, the antibodies behave as "competitive antagonists." Thus greater concentrations of unlabeled insulin are required to decrease tracer ^{125}I-insulin binding, and the Scatchard plot of binding shows a loss of curvilinearity owing to absence of high affinity binding at low insulin concentrations (Fig. 2) (120, 121). Total binding capacity (receptor concentration) is not usually reduced in these analyses. An "average affinity profile" shows that the receptors are "locked" in a low affinity state (Fig. 2). Similar binding defects can be reproduced in vitro by incubating normal cells with antireceptor serum or globulins at 22°C, and are partially reversed by an acid wash of cells designed to elute surface immunoglobulins (103, 120, 121).

The lack of any major change in apparent receptor concentration in these studies is somewhat surprising since the antibodies are themselves rapidly internalized (122) and might be expected to "down-regulate" receptors. It is assumed that insulin receptors on monocytes are sensitive to regulation (e.g., by insulin) because their concentration usually mirrors that on classical target tissues such as liver and fat under various conditions in vivo (4), but direct studies in vitro to confirm this point are lacking. Incubation of human lymphocytes (IM-9 line) for 60 minutes at 22°C with antireceptor sera causes a decrease in receptor affinity (103). However, when these experiments are performed for 3 hours at 37°C antireceptor sera cause a marked decrease in receptor concentration (Harrison and Itin, unpublished). It has also been shown that an affinity defect induced by brief exposure of lymphocytes to an antireceptor serum progressed to an apparent defect in receptor concentration with further exposure at 37°C (Kasuga and Harrison, unpublished). These findings suggest that insulin receptor autoantibodies do indeed down-regulate the re-

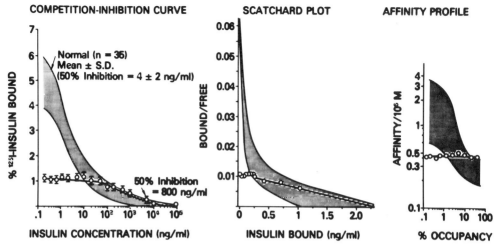

Figure 2. ^{125}I-insulin binding to circulating monocytes in a patient (B-6) with the type B syndrome of insulin resistance and acanthosis nigricans (mean ± SEM of four studies). The impairment of insulin binding to the patient's cells (0-0) is due to a decrease in receptor affinity, indicated by the high concentration of unlabeled insulin required to inhibit ^{125}I-insulin binding by 50% (left panel), by the decrease in curvilinearity of the Scatchard plot (center panel), and by the flat affinity profile (right panel).

ceptor under physiological conditions, via an effect on receptor affinity. In fact, down-regulation has been demonstrated in hepatocytes exposed to rabbit antiserum against partially purified insulin receptors (123). The observation that binding to monocytes shows predominantly an affinity defect (120, 121) (Fig. 2) is hard to reconcile with these in vitro results. Monocyte receptors may not be modulated by antibodies in similar fashion to those on other cells, but this seems unlikely. Alternatively the methods of data analysis may be misleading since several assumptions underlying Scatchard analysis are not met in receptor binding studies, and the "negative cooperativity" model of insulin binding requires further proof. An explanation for the results shown in Figure 2 might be that patients' monocytes do have a loss of high affinity receptors, with a residual population of low affinity receptors whose binding function is not altered by antibodies.

Any generalization about the mechanisms underlying the effects of receptor antibodies must account for the fact that they are polyclonal and functionally heterospecific. Flier (103) found that inhibition of insulin binding to lymphocytes after short-term exposure to

antireceptor sera was due to several mechanisms. These included competitive occupancy of binding sites, decreased rates of association, increased rates of dissociation, and negatively cooperative effects, which depended not only on the particular antiserum but also on its concentration. The molecular basis of each of these effects is unknown but two observations suggest that they may largely be due to allosteric mechanisms with changes in binding site conformation, rather than to direct "competitive" effects on the binding site. First, one antireceptor serum was shown to reduce receptor affinity in particulate placental membranes, but to decrease apparent receptor number in solubilized placental membranes (107). Second, acute exposure of lymphocytes in vitro to certain antireceptor sera produces a right shift in the binding competition curve without a decrease in binding of tracer ^{125}I-insulin (124). This is consistent with an increase in low affinity receptors presumably due to conformational change and exposure of cryptic binding sites. Irrespective of these acute effects, as outlined above, chronic occupancy of receptors by insulin receptor autoantibodies probably induces receptor loss.

4.5. Specificity of Insulin Receptor Autoantibodies

Antireceptor sera are approximately equipotent in inhibiting binding to a variety of human and other mammalian tissues, but are less potent against nonmammalian receptors (100). There is no apparent preferential effect of the patients' sera on binding to their own receptors, and patients' fibroblasts in culture have normal binding properties (120). This suggests that the underlying binding site in affected patients is grossly normal, but does not exclude the possibility that it is autoantigenic.

Insulin receptor autoantibodies are specific for the insulin receptor. They do not inhibit the binding of other hormones, nor do they immunoprecipitate receptors for other hormones including insulin-related growth factor peptides (107). The interaction of the antibodies with the receptor has been studied directly. Purified antireceptor IgG was labeled with ^{125}I and then receptor-purified by binding and elution from cultured IM-9 lymphocytes. The eluted [^{125}I]-IgG, enriched for [^{125}I]-antireceptor IgG, bound to a variety of cells in direct proportion to their insulin receptor concentration, and a major part of the binding was specifically competed for by insulin and insulin analogues (125). This indicated that a subpopulation of the antibodies, at least, bound at or very close to the binding site for insulin. Consistent with this is the ability of insulin to impair immunoprecipitation of the receptor (75, 107). Recent studies have clearly demonstrated that a major proportion of the IgG antibodies in several antireceptor sera recognize the insulin binding subunits (probably the 130K subunit) in an oligomeric receptor (75). On the other hand, it is likely that some antibodies bind to determinants away from the insulin binding site (but perhaps on the same subunit) because antireceptor sera will still recognize the solubilized receptor (86) and mimic insulin's actions (104) after destruction of insulin binding activity by trypsin.

Blockade of insulin binding by autoantibodies has no effect on insulin degradation (126) and binding and degrading activity are not copurified during affinity purification of placental insulin receptors (78). We would therefore conclude that insulin-degrading activity is physically distinct from the receptor, although it has been reported (127) that one antireceptor serum inhibits both binding and degradation.

4.6. Autoantibodies and Insulin Action

The clinical state associated with insulin receptor autoantibodies has generally been one of insulin resistance, consonant with the ability of the antibodies to impair insulin binding. However, the acute effect of the antibodies in most systems in vitro is to mimic the actions of insulin (Table 2). The spectrum of antibody bioactivity covers all of insulin's actions except the direct growth effect of high concentration of insulin. It includes effects that are both dependent and nondependent on glucose transport, effects on both membrane and cytoplasmic systems, and chronic effects that require protein synthesis. The titer of most antisera with respect to stimulation of glucose uptake in fat cells is higher than that determined by binding inhibition and approaches the titer for immunoprecipitation (108, 109), confirming the presence of some populations of antibodies directed against determinants outside of the insulin binding site.

The studies on antibody bioactivity have led to several important insights into the nature of insulin action. Antibody bioactivity, unlike inhibition of insulin binding, requires bivalency (105). Purified IgG or F(ab)$_2$ fragments are equally effective in their ability to inhibit insulin binding and mimic insulin's actions; monovalent Fab fragments inhibit binding but have no intrinsic bioactivity. The bioactivity of Fab fragments on cells, however, is restored by the addition of anti(Fab)$_2$ IgG. These findings indicate that bioactivity not only depends on receptor occupancy, but also requires bivalent binding or cross-linking of receptor

Table 2.   Insulin-like effects of insulin receptor autoantibodies

Adipocytes

Stimulation of glucose transport, incorporation into lipid and glycogen, and oxidation to CO_2
Stimulation of amino acid transport and incorporation into protein
Inhibition of lipolysis
Activation of glycogen synthase
Inhibition of phosphorylase
Activation of pyruvate dehydrogenase and acetyl CoA carboxylase

3T3-L1 Fatty Fibroblasts

Stimulation of glucose transport and oxidation to CO_2
Activation of lipoprotein lipase

Muscle

Stimulation of glucose transport and incorporation into glycogen
Activation of glycogen synthase

Liver

Stimulation of amino acid transport
Activation of glycogen synthase
Down-regulation of receptors

IM9-Lymphocytes

Down-regulation of receptors

---

subunits. The importance of this requirement for the modulation of acetylcholine receptors by antibodies has already been discussed. A further example is the IgE-mediated degranulation of mast cells leading to histamine release. This event requires cross-linking of the IgE receptor with either IgE and second antibody, antibodies to the receptor itself, or chemically cross-linked IgE dimers (128).

The suggestion was made by Kahn (105) that cross-linking might be involved in activation by insulin. They showed that antibodies to insulin sometimes enhanced the effect of suboptimal concentrations of insulin prebound to its receptors. In addition, fluorescence microscopy reveals that insulin, like receptor autoantibodies, can induce "patching" and "capping" on the cell surface (129). Anticytoskeletal agents, however, have no effect on the bioactivity of either receptor antibodies or insulin, and cell surface events such as macroscopic aggregation and internalization (of fluorescent-labeled ligands) do not appear to be necessary for cellular activation. Also, it is important to note that the rates of internalization of bivalent and monovalent receptor antibodies are identical, although only the

former possess bioactivity (Kasuga and Harrison, unpublished). None of the evidence cited appears to be directly relevant to cross-linking at a molecular level. Insulin circulates as a monomer, but the possibility that it could dimerize on a multivalent receptor is not unreasonable. Alternatively, there is now direct evidence for a disulfide exchange between the A and B chains of insulin and its binding subunits. This process could provide an "insulin bridge" to cross-link the receptor at the molecular level (89).

The ability of cross-linking ligands other than insulin (receptor antibodies and certain lectins) as well as oxidizing agents (H_2O_2, spermine, vitamin K_5, vanadate) to mimic the actions of insulin indicates that the receptor is the chief effector molecule. Thus the "information" for insulin action is contained within the receptor. This implies also that insulin degradation, or a product thereof, is not required (e.g., as a "second messenger") for insulin action. The only effect of insulin not mimicked by receptor autoantibodies is growth stimulation (^{3}H-thymidine incorporation into fibroblast DNA). King and coworkers (130) have shown that this effect of insulin (usually seen only at supraphysiological concentrations) is mediated through receptors for insulin-like growth factors (IGFs) rather than through the insulin receptor.

The paradox of insulin-like receptor antibodies in vitro and donor patients who are insulin resistant and hyperglycemic is not explained by species differences, since the antibodies are bioactive in both human and rodent adipocytes (106). The explanation appears to be that the bioactivity is only short-lived, as shown by Karlsson and co-workers (115) in studies using cultured 3T3-L1 fatty fibroblasts. In these cells receptor antibodies inhibit insulin binding and stimulate glucose uptake and oxidation, as in freshly isolated adipocytes. The insulin-like effects are transient, however, reaching the maximum by 1 hour and then decreasing. After several hours basal activity returns to normal and is resistant to stimulation by insulin, concanavalin A, and further addition of receptor antibodies. Insulin binding remains inhibited. Although continued occupancy of receptors by antibodies shifts the dose response for insulin action to the right, there is also a decrease in maximum responsiveness. This desensitization requires antibody bivalence but its mechanism has not been clearly defined. The locus of the desensitization is probably close to the binding site since the insulin-like actions of spermine and vitamin K_5 are unaltered (131). Desensitization is not affected by anticytoskeletal and antilysosomal agents, but requires that the cells have a source of energy such as glucose or pyruvate or a glucose derivative capable of being phosphorylated (131).

5. β-ADRENERGIC RECEPTORS AND ATOPY

Atopy (Greek: "strange disease"), a term introduced by Coca and Cooke in 1923 (132), now denotes a state characterized by (1) familial predisposition to asthma, allergic rhinitis ("hay fever"), eczema, and urticaria (skin wheals); (2) increased levels of serum IgE;

and (3) abnormal autonomic reactivity. The latter encompasses decreased sensitivity to β-adrenergic agonists and increased sensitivity to α-adrenergic and cholinergic agonists (133).

Coca and Cooke (132) reported the clinical and familial association between the above-mentioned diseases and suspected a common immunopathological basis. Consistent with this notion was the fact that the "immediate hypersensitivity" of (atropic) individuals to extrinsic "allergens" could be passively transferred by blood or serum (134). However, the effector role of the immune system in atopy has not been specifically defined, beyond the demonstration that certain antigens can provoke IgE-mediated release of smooth muscle constrictors such as histamine from mast cells. What of the autonomic abnormalities in atopy, and their relationship to immune function? A possible connection between allergy and immunity is the discovery of autoantibodies to the β_2-adrenergic receptor in atopic subjects (135) and the subsequent demonstration that these antibodies are related to autonomic dysfunction (136).

5.1. Atopy and Autonomic Function

Studies performed in vivo, beginning two decades ago, have documented that asthmatic subjects have an impaired response to β-adrenergic agonists. The effect of epinephrine or isoproterenol on plasma levels of glucose, free fatty acids, and cAMP, or on pulse pressure is less in asthmatics, and moreover is inversely correlated with an enhanced effect of acetylcholine or histamine on bronchial constriction (137–143). In 1968, Andor Szentivanyi (144) proposed the β-adrenergic theory of the pathogenesis of asthma—an imbalance in autonomic control due to decreased β-adrenergic sensitivity of bronchial smooth muscle, mucous glands, and mucosal vessels. During the next several years this hypothesis gained further support from studies showing impaired cAMP responses specifically to β-adrenergic agonists in leukocytes from asthmatics (145–148; for discussion see Ref. 133).

This raised the question whether there was an intrinsic defect in the putative β-adrenergic receptor, hitherto defined only indirectly by pharmacological criteria.

Initially, attempts to study β-adrenergic receptors by binding the natural agonist [³H]-epinephrine were fraught with technical problems, but with the advent of the high affinity antagonists, [³H]-dihydroalprenolol and [¹²⁵I]-hydroxybenzylpindolol (IHYP), it became possible in the mid-1970s to identify directly sites that fulfilled the criteria for specific β-adrenergic receptors (for review see Ref. 7). In keeping with the previous bioresponse studies it was soon shown that cells from asthmatics did indeed exhibit a reduction in the apparent number of β-receptors (149–151), but for several years this observation was attributed solely to down-regulation of receptors, induced by exposure to pharmacological concentrations of β-adrenergic drugs administered for the treatment of asthma. Although drug-induced down-regulation (and desensitization) clearly occurs there is now sufficient evidence from studies in untreated and asymptomatic subjects to indicate that a defect in β-receptor binding is a basic feature of asthma (see Ref. 133). Similar conclusions apply also to subjects with atopic eczema confirming earlier reports of impaired catecholamine responses in lymphocytes from such subjects (152). The decrease in β-receptor binding in atopic subjects has recently been linked with an increase in α-adrenergic receptor binding and Szentivanyi has now extended his concept to a "dual receptor" hypothesis (145).

5.2. Atopy, Autonomic Function, and Autoimmunity

In 1978 one of us (L. H.) began a search for autoantibodies which might stimulate the parathyroid glands in patients with primary hyperparathyroidism, analogous to the thyroid-stimulating antibodies in patients with Graves' disease. Isolated bovine parathyroid cells (from Dr. Edward Brown of The National Institutes of Health) were incubated with dilutions of patient or control serum. After washing, the cells were exposed to an excess of ¹²⁵I-protein A and specific uptake of radioactivity was used to indicate the presence of residual surface-bound IgG. Two of the sera tested were positive in that they contained IgG to a component of bovine parathyroid cell membrane, but neither was from a patient with hyperparathyroidism. One was from a control subject suffering from asthma. The parathyroid cells were known to possess β-adrenergic receptors and these findings, coupled with our interest in autoimmune receptor disease, led us to speculate that asthmatics might produce autoantibodies to the β-adrenergic receptor. Subsequently, the ¹²⁵I-protein A assay using human placental membranes was applied to the screening of coded sera from atopic patients under the care of Dr. M. Kaliner at The National Institutes of Health. Three sera positive in the protein A assay, seven negative sera, and four control sera were coded and assayed by Drs. C. Fraser and J. C. Venter of Buffalo, New York, for the presence of antibodies which might specifically immunoprecipitate solubilized lung β-receptors. Three of the 14 samples contained IgGs which indirectly immunoprecipitated Triton-solubilized canine lung β-receptors prelabeled with IHYP (135). These three samples, one from a patient with allergic rhinitis and two from patients with asthma, were those that had been positive in the protein A assay (human placental membranes used for the protein A screening assay were shown to contain 30 femtomoles of IHYP binding sites per milligram of protein).

In the initial report of these findings (136) IgG from the patient with allergic rhinitis also inhibited the binding of IHYP to lung and placenta but not cardiac membranes (Fig. 3), indicating that at least some of the antibodies recognized determinants on β₂-receptors in situ, at or near the ligand binding site. The inability to totally immunoprecipitate all available IHYP-labeled receptors, as well as the lower titer with immunoprecipitation versus binding inhibition, suggested that the anti-

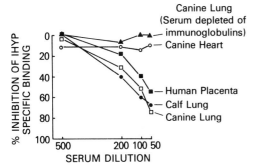

Canine Lung
(Serum depleted of
immunoglobulins)
— Canine Heart

— Human Placenta
— Calf Lung
— Canine Lung

Figure 3. Effect of serum from a patient with allergic rhinitis (No. 10) on ^{125}I-hydroxybenzylpindolol binding to membrane-bound B-adrenergic receptors.

bodies in this one serum were predominantly directed at the IHYP binding site in the solubilized receptor.

In a follow-up study IgG antibodies were detected in 9 of 60 coded sera: 3/19 control, 1/9 pre-allergic, 4/17 asthma, 0/8 allergic rhinitis, 1/7 cystic fibrosis (153). Most importantly, the presence of antibodies was associated with autonomic abnormalities (153, 136). Subjects with antibodies required higher doses of infused isoproterenol to elevate their pulse pressure or plasma cyclic AMP. Moreover, this evidence for β-adrenergic resistance was accompanied by increased sensitivity to the effects of the α-adrenergic agonist phenylephrine on pupillary dilation and with increased sensitivity to the effects of the cho-

linergic agent carbachol) on pupillary constriction (Table 3). It is interesting to note that the three control subjects with antibodies required a greater dose of isoproterenol to raise pulse pressure (12 ± 1.73) than the 16 control subjects without antibodies (7.5 ± 0.55).

Further studies on the molecular actions of β-receptor antibodies are consistent with their role as β-receptor antagonists. Thus after preincubation of cultured human lung cells (VA-13 line) with antireceptor IgG there is a marked decrease in sensitivity and responsiveness of cAMP to stimulation by isoproterenol (Fig. 4). It remains to be shown whether this effect is only due to blockade at the receptor level, or whether other mechanisms such as desensitization at a postreceptor step or accelerated receptor loss are also involved.

5.3. Significance of β-Receptor Autoantibodies

These findings would be consistent with a primary role for β-receptor autoantibodies in mediating autonomic dysfunction in at least some atopic subjects. The simplest interpretation is that the antibodies impair β-receptor-mediated relaxation of airways smooth muscle, unmask the opposing influence of α-receptor

Table 3.   Association between β-adrenergic receptor antibody status and autonomic sensitivity

	Antibody		
	Positive	Negative	
Infusion rate of isoproterenol (ng/kg/min) to increase			
Pulse pressure > 22 mm HG	15.0 ± 1.90 (n = 9)	7.7 ± 0.40 (n = 20)	p < .001
Plasma cAMP > 50%	12.4 ± 1.80 (n = 9)	8.1 ± 0.62 (n = 13)	p < .02
Phenylephrine (%) to dilate pupils > 0.5 mm	2.06 ± 0.30 (n = 9)	2.55 ± 0.08 (n = 57)	p < .05
Carbachol (%) to constrict pupils > 0.5 mm	0.61 ± 0.08 (n = 9)	0.78 ± 0.03 (n = 57)	p < .05

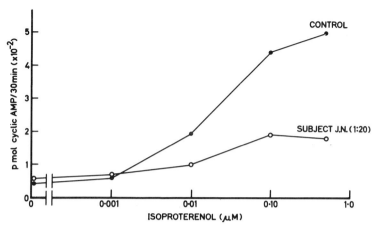

Figure 4. Inhibition of cAMP response to isoproterenol in human lung fibroblasts (Va-13 line) exposed to serum globulins from asthma subject J. N.

agonists and acetylcholine, and lower the threshold for release of mediators such as histamine, prostaglandins, and leukotrienes. It will be important to delineate the influence of β-adrenergic dysfunction on these biochemical pathways and on the classical effector mechanism of mast cell histamine release triggered by IgE, as well as to determine whether other receptor autoantibodies are present. Furthermore, an explanation is required for the anatomical localization of atopic manifestations to the lower airways in asthma, the upper airways in allergic rhinitis, and the skin in urticaria and atopic eczema.

Atopy must now be considered within the spectrum of autoimmune disorders, and this concept is supported by studies demonstrating a defect in suppressor T lymphocyte function in atopic subjects (154). Clearly, "forbidden clones" that recognize self-antigens may be more pervasive than hitherto suspected. On the other hand, if autoimmunity was a naturally regulated state perhaps it could be viewed as a continuum: from a normal state of regulated autoimmunity, through the emergence of (?) nonpathogenic autoantibodies with advancing age or after exposure to certain drugs, to the emergence of pathogenic autoantibodies in classic autoimmune states. In the latter there is usually tissue destruction by cells or complement, but there may be other pathological situations exemplified by atopy where the

manifestations are due solely to the specific functional effects of autoantibodies. The implications for the treatment of atopic diseases are the same as discussed for the other receptor antibody diseases. Corticosteroids and immunosuppressive drugs used occasionally for intractable asthma or atopic eczema might act to impair autoantibody production. Plasmapheresis, reported to be effective in a single case of severe asthma (155), warrants further appraisal.

6. EXPANDING THE SPECTRUM OF RECEPTOR ANTIBODIES

Antibodies to several partially purified receptors have been produced by experimental immunization of animals. Their application to the study of receptor function reinforces the concepts already outlined. Thus rabbit antibodies to insulin receptors purified from rat liver membranes do not compete with [125I]-insulin for binding, but do precipitate solubilized receptors and mimic insulin's actions (156). This is consistent with the notion that there is no single insulinomimetic determinant of the receptor. Guinea pig antibodies to prolactin receptors purified from pregnant rabbit mammary glands inhibit the binding of [125I]-prolactin to several tissues and species, suggesting that the structural determinants of binding in prolactin receptors are phylogenetically conserved (157). The same antibodies also block the biological action of prolactin, thereby demonstrating that binding sites for prolactin are authentic receptors (158). A rabbit antiserum with specific antagonist properties against dopamine receptors has been raised against the TCX11 line of mouse neural cells. Globulins in this antiserum inhibit ^{3}H-dopamine binding and dopamine stimulation of adenylcyclase in rat caudate tissue, and inhibit the depolarization of TCX11 cells in response to dopamine (159).

The occurrence of species-specific IgG autoantibodies to parathyroid hormone (PTH) receptors has been reported in patients with chronic renal failure (160). PTH receptor autoantibodies would provide a novel explanation for the secondary hyperparathyroidism of chronic renal failure usually attributed to hypocalcemia secondary to impaired phosphate clearance and vitamin D action. However, a major problem with all PTH binding studies has been the difficulty of preparing biologically active [^{125}I]-PTH by conventional iodination methods. This report of PTH receptor autoantibodies requires confirmation using [^{125}I]-PTH that has demonstrably normal receptor binding properties.

It seems likely that antibodies to receptors will be found in a larger number of diseases. The obvious candidates are the "organ-specific" or "polyglandular" autoimmune diseases: Hashimoto's thyroiditis (hypothyroidism), idiopathic primary hypoparathyroidism, Addison's disease (hypoadrenalism), type I (insulin-dependent) diabetes, pernicious anemia (atrophy of gastric parietal cells), and some cases of impaired fertility associated with autoantibodies to ovaries and sperm (161, 162). In most of these diseases there is hypofunction and (ultimately) destruction of specific cell types. Traditionally, these diseases have been classified according to the presence of "organ-specific" autoantibodies, usually detected by relatively insensitive immunofluoresence methods using fixed tissue sections. The molecular specificities and functional effects of such antibodies require

definition. Most "organ-specific" autoantibodies are directed at cytoplasmic components and are probably a secondary feature, distinct from the autoimmune process(es) that initiates cellular dysfunction and membrane lysis. The coexistence of multiple autoantibodies with specificities for both surface membrane and intracellular sites is clearly exemplified by autoimmune thyroid disease.

Investigators have begun to reappraise these examples of "organ-specific" autoimmunity, and two are worthy of note. Using sera from type I diabetics Lemmark and co-workers have provided elegant immunofluorescence pictures of autoantibodies to the surface of isolated pancreatic islet cells (see Chapter 8) (163). Most important, these antibodies specifically impair insulin release, and the majority are associated with binding of complement (164). The identification of the relevant membrane "autoantigens" is crucial to our understanding of diabetes. Loveridge and co-workers have found that sera from patients with pernicious anemia contain antibodies to the surface of gastric parietal cells, and that these sera inhibit acid production by parietal cells (165). Therefore, is the loss of parietal cells and their 'intrinsic factor' (responsible for vitamin B$_{12}$ absorption) initiated by autoantibodies to the surface gastrin receptors that regulate acid secretion?

The paradigms established for studying receptor autoimmunity, especially for the acetylcholine and insulin receptors, demonstrate the extent to which immune mechanisms can be explored, as well as the utility of autoantibodies in probing receptor structure and function. Undoubtedly the application of receptor methodology will lead to redefinition of organ-specific autoimmunity in terms of receptor-specific autoimmunity, and will provide insights into disease states whose mechanisms are currently obscure.

ACKNOWLEDGMENTS

Our thanks to Drs. Jon Lindstrom, Andrew Engel, and Roger Dawkins for their comments on the section on acetylcholine receptors. Expert secretarial assistance was provided by Mrs. Linda Stafford. We are indebted to the Victor Hurley Medical Research Fund of the Royal Melbourne Hospital and the Asthma Foundation of Victoria for their financial support.

REFERENCES

1. C. R. Kahn, in E. D. Korn, Ed., *Methods in Membrane Biology*, Vol. 3, Plenum, New York, 1975, pp. 81–146.

2. K. J. Catt and M. L. Dufau, *Annu. Rev. Physiol.* 39, 529–557 (1977).

3. J. Roth, M. A. Lesniak, R. S. Bar, M. Muggeo, K. Megyesi, L. C. Harrison, J. S. Flier, H. Wachslicht-Rodbard, and P. Gordon, *Proc. Soc. Biol. Med.* 169, 191–205 (1979).

4. R. S. Bar, L. C. Harrison, M. Muggeo, P. Gorden, C. R. Kahn, and J. Roth, *Adv. Int. Med.* 24, 23–52 (1979).

5. J. D. Baxter and J. W. Funder, *N. Engl. J. Med.* 301, 1149–1161 (1979).

6. L. C. Harrison and J. Roth, *Aust. N. Z. J. Med.* 10, 78–88 (1980).

7. B. B. Hoffman and R. J. Lefkowitz, *Ann. Rev. Pharmacol. Toxicol.* 20, 581–608 (1980).

8. J. Kaplan, *Science* 212, 14–20 (1981).

9. M. Rodbell, *Nature* 284, 17–22 (1980).

10. *The Collected Papers of Paul Ehrlich*, Vol. 2, Pergamon Press, Oxford, 1957, p. 178.

11. P. Ehrlich, *Studies on Immunity*, 1st ed., Wiley, London, 1906.

12. J. Donath and K. Landsteiner, *Munch. Med. Wochenschr.* 51, 1590–1593 (1904).

13. N. K. Jerne, *Ann. Immunol. (Paris)* 125C, 373–389 (1974).

14. V. A. Lennon and P. R. Carnegie, *Lancet* 1, 630–633 (1971).

15. P. R. Carnegie and I. R. Mackay, *Lancet* 2, 684–686 (1975).

16. D. B. Drachman, *N. Engl. J. Med.* 298, 136–142, 186–193 (1978).

17. A. G. Engel, in P. J. Winken and G. W. Bruyn, Eds., *Handbook of Clinical Neurology*, Vol. 41, Part II, North-Holland, Amsterdam, 1979, pp. 95–145.

18. P. W. Gage, *Physiol. Rev.* 56, 177–247 (1976).

19. H. P. Rang, *Q. Rev. Biophys.* 7, 283–399 (1974).

20. D. Elmqvist, W. W. Hofmann, J. Kugelberg, and D. M. J. Quastel, *J. Physiol. (London)* 174, 417–434 (1964).

21. D. M. Fambrough, D. B. Drachman, and S. Satyamurti, *Science* 182, 293–295 (1973).

22. A. G. Engel, J. Lindstrom, E. H. Lambert, and V. A. Lennon, *Neurology* 27, 307–315 (1977).

23. J. M. Lindstrom and E. H. Lambert, *Neurology* 28, 130–138 (1978).

24. M. A. Raftery, M. W. Hunkapiller, C. D. Strader, and L. E. Hood, *Science* 208, 1454–1456 (1980).

25. S. L. Hamilton, M. McLaughlin, and A. Karlin, *Biochem. Biophys. Res. Commun.* 79, 692–699 (1977).

26. A. Karlin, C. L. Weill, M. G. McNamee, and R. Valderrama, *Cold Spring Harbor Symp. Quant. Biol.* 60, 203–210 (1975).

27. A. Vincent, *Physiol. Rev.* 60, 756–824 (1980).

28. J. A. Simpson, *Scott. Med. J.* 5, 419–436 (1960).

29. W. L. Nastuk, O. J. Plescia, and K. E. Osserman, *Proc. Soc. Exp. Biol. Med.* 105, 177–184 (1960).

30. C. E. Chang and C. Y. Lee, *Arch. Int. Pharmacodyn. Ther.* 144, 241–257 (1962).

31. A. G. Engel and T. Santa, *Ann. N.Y. Acad. Sci.* 183, 46–63 (1971).

32. J. Patrick and J. Lindstrom, *Science* 180, 871–872 (1973).

33. R. R. Almon, C. G. Andrews, and S. H. Appel, *Science* 186, 55–57 (1974).

34. A. N. Bender, S. P. Ringle, W. K. Engel, M. P. Daniels, and Z. Vogel, *Lancet* 1, 607–609 (1975).

35. A. Aharonov, O. Abramsky, R. Tarrab-Hazdei, and S. Fuchs, *Lancet* 2, 340–342 (1975).

36. S. H. Appel, R. R. Almon, and N. Levy, *N. Engl. J. Med.* 293, 760–761 (1975).

37. J. M. Lindstrom, M. E. Seybold, V. A. Lennon, S. Whittingham, and D. D. Duane, *Neurology* 26, 1054–1059 (1976).

38. T. W. Mittag, P. Kornfeld, A. Tormay, and C. Woo, *N. Engl. J. Med.* 294, 691–694 (1976).

39. V. M. Monnier and B. W. Fulpius, *Clin. Exp. Immunol.* 29, 16–22 (1977).

40. S. H. Appel, R. Anwyl, M. W. McAdams, and S. Elias, *Proc. Natl. Acad. Sci. USA* 74, 2130–2134 (1977).

41. I. Kao and D. B. Drachman, *Science* 196, 527–529 (1977).

42. S. Heinemann, S. Bevan, R. Kullberg, J. Lindstrom, and J. Rice, *Proc. Natl. Acad. Sci. USA* 74, 3090–3094 (1977).

43. D. B. Drachman, C. W. Angus, R. N. Adams, J. D. Michelson, and G. J. Hoffman, *N. Engl. J. Med.* 298, 1116–1122 (1978).

44. J. Lindstrom, *Adv. Immunol.* **27**, 1–50 (1979).

45. J. M. Lindstrom, A. G. Engel, M. E. Seybold, V. A. Lennon, and E. H. Lambert, *J. Exp. Med.* **144**, 739–753 (1976).

46. K. V. Toyka, D. B. Drachman, A. Pestronk, and I. Kao, *Science* **190**, 397–399 (1975).

47. V. A. Lennon, M. E. Seybold, J. M. Lindstrom, C. Cochrane, and R. Yulevitch, *J. Exp. Med.* **147**, 973–983 (1978).

48. V. A. Lennon, J. Lindstrom, and M. E. Seybold, *Ann. N.Y. Acad. Sci.* **274**, 283–299 (1976).

49. J. Lindstrom, B. Walter, and B. Einarson, *Biochemistry* **18**, 4470–4480 (1979).

50. J. Lindstrom, M. Campbell, and B. Nave, *Muscle Nerve* **1**, 140–145 (1978).

51. S. J. Tzartos, D. E. Rand, B. L. Einarson, and J. M. Lindstrom, *J. Biol. Chem.* **256**, 8635–8645 (1981).

52. A Vincent and J. Newson-Davis, in B. Cessarelli and F. Clementi, Eds., *Advances in Cytopharmacology. Neurotoxins—Tools in Neurobiology*, Vol. 3, Raven Press, New York, 1979, pp. 267–278.

53. C. B. Weinberg and Z. W. Hall, *Proc. Natl. Acad. Sci. USA* **76**, 504–508 (1979).

54. S. Fuchs, I. Schmidt-Hopfeld, G. Tridente, and R. Tarrab-Hazdai, *Nature* **287**, 162–164 (1980).

55. S. J. Tzartos and J. M. Lindstrom, *Proc. Natl. Acad. Sci. USA* **77**, 755–759 (1980).

56. V. A. Lennon and E. H. Lambert, *Nature* **285**, 238–240 (1980).

57. O. Abramsky, A. Aharanov, C. Webb, and S. Fuchs, *Clin. Exp. Immunol.* **19**, 11–16 (1975).

58. B. Conti-Tronconi, M. Morgutti, M. G. Albizzati, and F. Clementi, *Z. Neurol.* **217**, 281–286 (1978).

59. J. Newsom-Davis, C. D. Ward, S. G. Wilson, A. J. Pinching, and A. Vincent, in P. C. Dau, Ed., *Plasmapheresis and the Immunobiology of Myasthenia Gravis*, Houghton Mifflin, Boston, 1979, pp. 199–208.

60. J. M. Lindstrom, B. L. Einarson, V. A. Lennon, and M. E. Seybold, *J. Exp. Med.* **144**, 726–738 (1976).

61. T. Yoshida, M. Tsuchiya, A. Ono, H. Yoshimatsu, E. Satoyoshi, and K. Tsuji, *J. Neurol. Sci.* **32**, 195–201 (1977).

62. R. C. Bucknall, A. St. J. Dixon, E. N. Glick, J. Woodland, and D. W. Zutshi, *Br. Med. J.* **1**, 600–602 (1975).

63. C. L. Masters, R. L. Dawkins, P. J. Zilko, J. A. Simpson, R. J. Leedman, and J. M. Lindstrom, *Am. J. Med.* **63**, 689–694 (1977).

64. R. L. Dawkins, P. L. Zilko, J. Carrano, M. J. Garlepp, and B. L. McDonald, *J. Rheumatol.* **8**, 56–61 (1981).

65. G. Matell, K. Bergström, C. Frankssen, L. Hammarström, A. K. Lefvent, E. Möller, G. Von Reis, and E. Smith, *Ann. N.Y. Acad. Sci.* **274**, 659–676 (1976).

66. S. Fuchs, in P. C. Dau, Eds., *Immunobiology of Myasthenia Gravis*, Houghton Mifflin, Boston, 1979, pp. 20–31.

67. J. Nerup and A. Lernmark, *Am. J. Med.* **70**, 135–141 (1981).

68. L. C. Harrison and J. S. Flier, in S. Podolsky and M. Viswanahan, Eds., *Secondary Diabetes: The Spectrum of The Diabetic Syndrome*, Raven Press, New York, 1980, pp. 269–286.

69. C. C. Yip, C. W. T. Yeung, and M. L. Moule, *Biochemistry* **19**, 70–76 (1980).

70. S. Jacobs, E. Hazum, Y. Shechter, and P. Cuatrecasas, *Proc. Natl. Acad. Sci USA* **76**, 4918–4921 (1979).

71. M. H. Wisher, M. D. Baron, R. H. Jones, P. H. Sönksen, D. J. Saunders, P. Thamm, and D. Brandenburg, *Biochem. Biophys. Res. Commun.* **92**, 492–498 (1980).

72. P. F. Pilch and M. P. Czech, *J. Biol. Chem.* **255**, 1722–1731 (1980).

73. M. Kasuga, E. Van Obberghen, K. Yamada, and L. C. Harrison, *Diabetes* **30**, 354–357 (1981).

74. U. Lang, C. R. Kahn, and L. C. Harrison, *Biochemistry* **19**, 64–70 (1980).

75. L. C. Harrison and A. Itin, in D. Andreani, R. De Pirro, R. Lauro, J. Olefsky, and J. Roth, Eds., *Current Views on Insulin Receptors*, Academic Press, New York, 45–52 (1981).

76. E. Van Obberghen, M. Kasuga, A. Le Cam, J. Hedo, A. Itin, and L. C. Harrison, *Proc. Natl. Acad. Sci. USA* **78**, 1052–1056 (1981).

77. S. Jacobs, Y. Shechter, K. Bissell, and P. Cuatrecasas, *Biochem. Biophys. Res. Commun.* **77**, 981–988 (1977).

78. L. C. Harrison and A. Itin, *J. Biol. Chem.* **255**, 12066–12072 (1980).

79. J. Hedo, L. C. Harrison, and J. Roth, *Biochemistry* **20**, 3385–3392 (1981).

80. P. Cuatrecasas, *J. Biol. Chem.* **247**, 1980–1991 (1972).

81. B. H. Ginsberg, C. R. Kahn, J. Roth, and P. De Meyts, *Biochem. Biophys. Res. Commun.* **73**, 1068–1074 (1976).

82. L. C. Harrison, T. Billington, I. J. East, R. J. Nichols, and S. Clark, *Endocrinology* **102**, 1485–1495 (1978).

83. J. Massague, P. Pilch, and M. Czech, *Proc. Natl. Acad. Sci. USA* **77**, 7137–7141 (1980).

84. S. Jacobs, E. Hazum, and P. Cuatrecasas, *J. Biol. Chem.* **255**, 6937–6940 (1980).

85. C. C. Yip, M. L. Moule, and C. W. T. Yeung, *Biochem. Biophys. Res. Commun.* **96**, 1671–1678 (1980).

86. L. C. Harrison, J. S. Flier, A. Itin, C. R. Kahn, and J. Roth, *Science* **203**, 544–547 (1979).

87. P. DeMeyts, A. R. Bianco, and J. Roth, *J. Biol. Chem.* **251**, 1877–1888 (1976).

88. G. Saviolakis, L. C. Harrison, and J. Roth, *J. Biol. Chem.* **256**, 4924–4928 (1981).

89. S. Clark and L. C. Harrison, *J. Biol. Chem.* in press.

90. E. A. H. Sims, E. S. Horton, and L. Salans, *Ann. Rev. Med.* **22**, 235–250 (1971).

91. C. R. Kahn, D. M. Neville, and J. Roth, *J. Biol. Chem.* **248**, 244–250 (1973).

92. R. S. Bar, P. Gorden, J. Roth, C. R. Kahn, and P. De Meyts, *J. Clin. Invest.* **58**, 1123–1135 (1976).

93. L. C. Harrison, F. I. R. Martin, and R. A. Melick, *J. Clin. Invest.* **58**, 1435–1441 (1976).

94. J. M. Olefsky, *J. Clin. Invest.* **57**, 1165–1172 (1976).

95. J. R. Gavin, III, J. Roth, D. M. Neville, Jr., P. De Meyts, and D. N. Buell, *Proc. Natl. Acad. Sci. USA* **71**, 84–88 (1974).

96. F. A. Kosmakos and J. Roth, *J. Biol. Chem.* **255**, 9860–9869 (1980).

97. T. Kono and F. W. Barham, *J. Biol. Chem.* **246**, 6210–6216 (1971).

98. C. R. Kahn, *Metabolism* **27**, 1893–1902 (1978).

99. J. M. Olefsky, *Diabetes* **30**, 148–162 (1981).

100. J. S. Flier, C. R. Kahn, J. Roth, and R. S. Bar, *Science* **190**, 63–65 (1975).

101. C. R. Kahn, J. S. Flier, R. S. Bar, J. A. Archer, P. Gorden, M. M. Martin, and J. Roth, *N. Engl. J. Med.* **294**, 739–745 (1976).

102. J. S. Flier, C. R. Kahn, D. B. Jarrett, and J. Roth, *J. Clin. Invest.* **58**, 1442–1449 (1976).

103. J. S. Flier, C. R. Kahn, D. B. Jarrett, and J. Roth, *J. Clin. Invest.* **60**, 784–794 (1977).

104. C. R. Kahn, K. L. Baird, J. S. Flier, and D. B. Jarrett, *J. Clin. Invest.* **60**, 1094–1106 (1977).

105. C. R. Kahn, K. L. Baird, D. B. Jarrett, and J. S. Flier, *Proc. Natl. Acad. Sci. USA* **75**, 4209–4213 (1978).

106. L. C. Harrison, E. Van Obberghen, C. Grunfeld, G. L. King, and C. R. Kahn, in R. Cohn and H. Kohler, Eds., *Membranes, Receptors, and the Immune Response*, Alan R. Liss, New York, 1980, pp. 109–126.

107. L. C. Harrison, J. S. Flier, J. Roth, F. A. Karlsson, and C. R. Kahn, *J. Clin. Endocrinol. Metab.* **48**, 59–65 (1979).

108. L. C. Harrison and C. R. Kahn, *Prog. Clin. Immunol.* **4**, 104–125 (1980).

109. C. R. Kahn and L. C. Harrison, in P. J. Randle, D. F. Steiner, and W. J. Whelan, Eds., *Carbohydrate Metabolism and Its Disorders*, Vol. 3, Academic Press, London, in press.

110. M. Kibata, K. Hiramatsu, Y. Shimizu, T. Fuchimoto, M. Sasaki, M. Shimono, K. Miyake, J. S. Flier, and C. R. Kahn, *Proc. Symp. Chem. Physiol. Pathol. (Japan)* **15**, 58 (1975).

111. K. Kawanishi, K. Kawamura, Y. Nishina, A. Goto, S. Okada, T. Ishida, T. Ofuji, C. R. Kahn, and J. S. Flier, *J. Clin. Endocrinol. Metab.* **44**, 15–21 (1977).

112. W. G. Blackard, J. H. Anderson, and F. Mullinax, *Ann. Int. Med.* **86**, 584–585 (1977).

113. J. S. Flier, R. S. Bar, M. Muggeo, C. R. Kahn, J. Roth, and P. Gorden, *J. Clin. Endocrinol. Metab.* **47**, 985–995 (1978).

114. M. Muggeo, J. S. Flier, R. A. Abrams, L. C. Harrison, A. B. Deisseroth, and C. R. Kahn, *N. Engl. J. Med.* **300**, 477–480 (1979).

115. F. A. Karlsson, E. Van Obberghen, C. Grunfeld, and C. R. Kahn, *Proc. Natl. Acad. Sci. USA* **76**, 809–813 (1979).

116. F. A. Karlsson, C. Grunfeld, C. R. Kahn, and J. Roth, *Endocrinology* **104**, 1383–1392 (1979).

117. L. C. Harrison and A. Itin, *Nature* **279**, 334–336 (1979).

118. M. Bielschowsky and F. Bielschowsky, *J. Exp. Biol.* **34**, 181–198 (1956).

119. K. Melez, L. C. Harrison, J. N. Gilliam, and A. D. Steinberg, *Diabetes* **29**, 835–840 (1980).

120. M. Muggeo, C. R. Kahn, R. S. Bar, M. Rechler, J. S. Flier, and J. Roth, *J. Clin. Endocrinol. Metab.* **49**, 110–119 (1979).

121. R. S. Bar, M. Muggeo, C. R. Kahn, P. Gorden, and J. Roth, *Diabetologia* **18**, 209–216 (1980).

122. J. L. Carpentier, E. Van Obberghen, P. Gorden, and L. Orci, *Diabetes* **28**, 345 (Abstr.) (1979).

123. J. F. Caro and J. M. Amatruda, *Science* **210**, 1029–1031 (1980).

124. L. C. Harrison, M. Muggeo, R. S. Bar, J. S. Flier, T. Waldmaun, and J. Roth, *Clin. Res.* **27**, 252 A (1979).

125. D. B. Jarrett, J. Roth, C. R. Kahn, and J. S. Flier, *Proc. Natl. Acad. Sci. USA* **73**, 4115–4119 (1976).

126. J. S. Flier, E. Maratos-Flier, K. Baird, and C. R. Kahn, *Diabetes* **26**(Suppl. 1), 354 (Abstr. 7) (1977).

127. D. Baldwin, S. Terris, and D. F. Steiner, *J. Biol. Chem.* **255**, 4028–4034 (1980).

128. H. Metzger and M. K. Bach, in M. K. Bach, Ed., *Immediate Hypersensitivity: Modern Concepts and Development*, Marcel Dekker, New York, p. 561.

129. J. Schlessinger, E. Van Obberghen, and C. R. Kahn, *Nature* **286**, 729–731 (1980).

130. G. L. King, C. R. Kahn, M. M. Rechler, and S. P. Nissley, *J. Clin. Invest.* **66**, 130–140 (1980).

131. C. Grunfeld, E. Van Obberghen, F. A. Karlsson, and C. R. Kahn, *The Endocr. Soc. Proc. 61st Ann. Meet., Anaheim, Calif., June 13–15, 1979*, p. 73 (Abstr. 3).

132. A. F. Coca and R. A. Cooke, *J. Immunol.* **8**, 163–168 (1923).

133. A. Szentivanyi, *J. Allergy Clin. Immunol.* **65**, 5–11 (1980).

134. C. Prausnitz and H. Kustner, *Zbl. Bakt. Orig.* **86**, 160–165 (1921).

135. J. C. Venter, C. M. Fraser, and L. C. Harrison, *Science* **207**, 1361–1363 (1980).

136. J. C. Venter, C. M. Fraser, L. C. Harrison, and M. Kaliner, *Fed. Proc.* **40**, 355 (Abstr. 697) (1981).

137. D. U. Cookson and C. E. Reed, *Am. Rev. Respir. Dis.* **88**, 636–643, (1963).

138. E. Middleton and S. R. Finke, *J. Allergy* **42**, 288–299 (1968).

139. S. Makino. J. J. Oulette, C. E. Reed, and C. W. Fishel, *J. Allergy* **46**, 178–189 (1970).

140. C. W. Parker, in K. F. Austen and L. M. Lichtenstein, Eds., *Asthma. Physiology, Immunopharmacology, and Treatment*, Academic Press, New York, 1973, pp. 185–210.

141. C. E. Reed, *J. Allergy Clin. Immunol.* **53**, 34–41 (1974).

142. P. W. Trembath and J. Shaw, *Br. J. Clin. Pharmac.* **3**, 1001–1005 (1976).

143. J. Apold and L. Aksnes, *J. Allergy Clin. Immunol.* **59**, 343–347 (1977).

144. A. Szentivanyi, *J. Allergy* **42**, 203–231 (1968).

145. P. J. Logsdon, E. Middleton, and R. G. Coffey, *J. Allergy Clin. Immunol.* **50**, 45–56 (1972).

146. C. W. Parker and J. W. Smith, *J. Clin. Invest.* **52**, 48–59 (1973).

147. M. E. Conolly and J. K. Greenacre, *J. Clin. Invest.* **58**, 1307–1316 (1976).

148. S. Makino, K. Ikemori, T. Kashima, and T. Fukuda, *J. Allergy Clin. Immunol.* **59**, 348–352 (1977).

149. K. Kariman and R. J. Lefkowitz, *Clin. Res.* **25**, 503 A (1977).

150. S. P. Galant, L. Duriseti, S. Underwood, and P. A. Insel, *N. Engl. J. Med.* **299**, 933–936 (1978).

151. S. M. Brooks, K. McGowan, I. L. Bernstein, P. Altenau, and J. Peagler, *J. Allergy Clin. Immunol.* **63**, 401–406 (1979).

152. W. W. Busse and T. P. Lee, *J. Allergy Clin. Immunol.* **58**, 586–596 (1976).

153. C. M. Fraser, L. C. Harrison, M. C. Kaliner, and J. C. Venter, *Clin. Res.* **28**, 236 A (1980).

154. M. Rola-Pleszczynski and R. Blanchard, *J. Invest. Dermatol.* **76**, 279–283 (1981).

155. J. Gartmann, P. Grob, and M. Frey, *Lancet* **2**, 40 (letter) (1978).

156. S. Jacobs, K-J. Chang, and P. Cuatrecasas, *Science* **200**, 1283–1284 (1978).

157. R. P. C. Shiu and H. G. Friesen, *Biochem. J.* **157**, 619–626 (1976).

158. R. P. C. Shiu and H. G. Friesen, *Science* **192**, 259–261 (1976).

159. P. R. Myers, M. Donlon, K. McCarthy, D. Livengood, and W. Shain, *Biochem. Biophys. Res. Commun.* **72**, 1311–1318 (1976).

160. H. Jüppner, A. A. Bialasiewicz, and R. D. Hesch, *Lancet* **2**, 1222–1224 (1978).

161. I. L. Solomon and R. M. Blizzard, *J. Pediatr.* **63**, 1021–1033 (1963).

162. M. Neufeld, N. Maclaren, and R. Blizzard, *Pediatr. Ann.* **9**, 43–53 (1980).

163. Å. Lernmark, Z. R. Freedman, C. Hofmann, A. H. Rubenstein, D. F. Steiner, R. L. Jackson, R. J. Winter, and H. S. Traisman, *N. Engl. J. Med.* **299**, 375–380 (1978).

164. T. Kanatsuna, Å. Lernmark, A. H. Rubenstein, and D. F. Steiner, *Diabetes* **30**, 231–234 (1981).

165. N. Loveridge, L. Bitensky, J. Chayen, J. U. Hausamen, J. M. Fisher, K. B. Taylor, J. D. Gardener, G. S. Bottazzo, and D. Doniach, *Clin. Exp. Immunol.* **41**, 264–270 (1980).

6

Thyroid Autoantibodies and Disease: An Overview

Terry F. Davies
Erica De Bernardo

Division of Endocrinology
Mount Sinai School of Medicine
New York, New York

Contents

1. THE SPECTRUM OF AUTOIMMUNE THYROID DISEASE

1.1. Background

There have been steady advances in our understanding of the pathological processes involved in human autoimmune thyroid disease since the discovery of human thyroglobulin antibodies by Roitt et al. (1) and thyroid-stimulating antibodies (TSAb) by Adams and Purves (2), both published in 1956. Studies have indicated that the clinical presentation of autoimmune thyroid disease can be strongly correlated with the variety of thyroid auto-antibodies which predominate in the circulation of the individual patient. This is not to say, however, that other important immune abnormalities are not present. Nevertheless, this chapter serves to describe the measurement and relevance of thyroid autoantibodies so that the subsequent discussion of immune function in thyroid disease can be more easily evaluated (Chapter 7).

We now recognize a variety of autoantibodies which can be readily measured in the clinical laboratory but the cause(s) of their secretion remains hypothetical. Much of the evidence, reviewed in Chapters 1–3, suggests that autoimmune thyroid disease is associated with an inherited susceptibility and hence the disease is commonly familial. Recent family studies indicate that autoimmune thyroid disease may be restricted within families to particular combinations of HLA and perhaps Gm types (see Chapter 3). However, not all members of the family with such characteristics become afflicted (3), indicating additional important contributing factors which we do not fully understand.

1.2. Hyperthyroidism (Graves' Disease)

When the circulating thyroid autoantibodies exhibit intrinsic thyroid-stimulating activity the patient presents with clinical signs of thyroid overactivity. Such a presentation may be associated with a number of abnormalities which together constitute the syndrome of Graves' disease (4). Examples of such an association include ophthalmic and skin signs that are unique to the disease and are considered also to be autoimmune in origin (5). On the whole, however, these associations may best be judged as closely linked, genetically independent, autoimmune diseases which may exhibit distinct natural histories from the thyroid abnormality.

1.3. Hypothyroidism (Hashimoto's Disease)

In contrast, when sera exhibit evidence of cytotoxic activity (6), patients present with gross evidence of thyroid failure associated

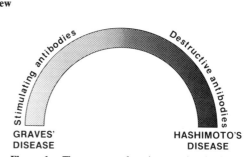

Figure 1.   The spectrum of autoimmune thyroid disease when observed on the basis of autoantibody activity. Preponderance of stimulating antibodies leads to hyperthyroid Graves' disease whereas excess destructive antibodies cause hypothyroid Hashimoto's disease.

either with thyroid atrophy (atrophic autoimmune, or Hashimoto's, thyroiditis) or goiter formation (goitrous autoimmune thyroiditis) most probably depending on the balance between thyroid cell destruction and inflammatory infiltration. Furthermore, patients may initially exhibit Graves' hyperthyroidism, or the associated signs thereof, and progress to thyroid failure. Indeed, claims have been made that thyroid failure is the natural pattern of long-standing Graves' disease. This would seem unlikely but the number of patients expected to demonstrate such "activity shifts" in their autoimmune responses remains uncertain.

1.4. The Spectrum

Although there are considerable differences between Graves' and Hashimoto's diseases, including their HLA associations (see Chapter 3), the thyroidal diathesis of which they form a part can be viewed as a spectrum of disease, dependent on the predominating immune abnormality, and into which almost all patients can be categorized (Fig. 1).

2. AUTOANTIBODIES ASSOCIATED WITH THYROID OVERACTIVITY

2.1. Thyroid-Stimulating Antibodies (TSAb)

History
Serum IgG preparations from hyperthyroid patients with Graves' disease contain TSAb

which can be measured by a wide variety of techniques. The initial observations by Adams and Purves (2) fortuitously followed their use of a guinea pig bioassay for TSH as outlined in Chapter 1. They demonstrated that sera from Graves' patients sometimes exhibit thyroid-stimulating ability quite distinct from TSH insomuch as its stimulating activity is grossly prolonged, hence the name "long acting thyroid stimulator" or LATS. A short time later McKenzie introduced a similar but more practical assay based on mice, which has been widely used in many laboratories (7). LATS was only positive in 15–20% of untreated and unselected patients. However, a binding inhibition assay developed by Adams and Kennedy (8) was subsequently used to detect antibody which interacted with human thyroid in vitro rather than mouse thyroid in vivo, and was termed LATS-Protector (LATS-P) since it inhibited LATS from binding to the human thyroid. LATS-P was found in the great majority of untreated Graves' patients. As with all bioassays that become popular these systems suffered from problems with precision and interassay variation, necessitating the use of large numbers of animals and the search for a simpler in vitro system.

Thyroid Slice Assay

All the most practical techniques now utilize the generation of cyclic AMP by TSH or TSAb as the precise end point. Systems based on thyroid membranes (9), slices (10), and cells (11) have all been utilized. The membrane techniques have proved to be relatively insensitive in most workers' experience and cannot be recommended (11). The thyroid slice assay for thyroid stimulators, however, is simple and sensitive and was first introduced by Onaya et al. (12). In this procedure thyroid slices are incubated with serum or IgG fractions from patients with hyperthyroid Graves' disease or normal controls, and the cyclic AMP accumulated during a 1 to 2 hour incubation period is subsequently measured by homogenizing the tissue and extracting intrathyroidal cyclic AMP. Cyclic AMP radioimmunoassays have improved significantly in recent years

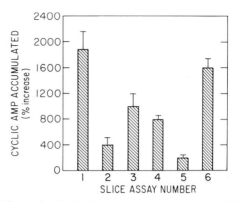

Figure 2. Results from six separate human thyroid slice assays using the same Graves' sera but different thyroid tissue. The sample was positive in each of the assays but the titer of activity was not reliable when using percent increase from basal cyclic AMP.

and, used with an acetylation procedure (13), can detect less than 1 femtomole of cyclic AMP. However, for the slice system such sophistication is not necessary owing to the abundance of the nucleotide in the relatively large amount of tissue used at each point (approximately 15 mg). Thyroid tissue can be conveniently obtained from around thyroid adenoma specimens regularly available in most major medical centers, but such tissue needs to be used immediately. Although sensitive, the slice assay suffers from problems with interassay variation owing to differences in human thyroid reactivity (Fig. 2) (14). Nevertheless, about 60 to 80% (10, 11) of Graves' patients do demonstrate TSAb in the slice system, which remains a cheap but impractical assay.

Human Thyroid Cell Bioassay

In contrast to the slice assay, the use of human thyroid cell monolayers appears to be the basis of a highly reproducible TSAb assay and in our experience is the method of choice (11, 15). Nevertheless, it is not a simple procedure, requiring expertise in cell culture and the use of an acetylated radioimmunoassay for cyclic AMP. Similar tissue is required as for the slice system, but in this technique it is dispersed with collagenase and the cells cultured for 5 to 7 days following which they are frozen in liquid nitrogen. Prior to the bioassay, a vial of cells is thawed, plated in multiwells overnight, and used for the bioassay the following morning (Fig. 3). In this method there are no problems with poorly responding assays since all cultures can be tested prior to a series of bioassays. Such cells are often considerably more sensitive to stimulation than any other easily available system, responding to as little as 10 micro I.U./ml of bTSH standard. The only known system more sensitive is the cytochemical bioassay technique which requires considerable attention, much expense, and has a slow throughput (16).

Recent analysis of 45 unselected and untreated Graves' patients in our own laboratory indicated that 71% of the patients had TSAb activity in the human thyroid cell assay compared to 23% of a small group (n = 13) of treated patients. Significance was assessed by *t*-testing of patients' immunoglobulin-induced responses compared to normal controls in each assay (15).

The clinical application of these bioassay techniques has generated useful but limited information concerning the role of TSAb in the etiology and natural course of Graves' disease (10) and remains to be fully exploited.

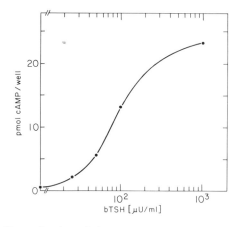

Figure 3. A standard response curve for bTSH in the human thyroid cell bioassay system. Note that the cyclic AMP radioimmunoassay measures femtomoles of cyclic AMP so that a precise standard curve can be constructed from 0 to 100 microunits per milliliter bTSH.

2.2.   TSH Receptor Antibodies (TBI)

The TSH Receptor

The TSH receptor is a surface membrane glycoprotein complex linked to a catalytic subunit responsible for the production of cyclic AMP following interaction with TSH. Such binding sites are present on the surface of thyroid follicular cells (17), adipose (18), and testicular (19) tissue. Although we know that in detergent-solubilized form the TSH receptor has a molecular weight of approximately 50,000 to 150,000 (20) depending on the preparative technique, and has essential disulfide bridges (21), we know little of its precise structure. There is also evidence that gangliosides and phospholipids may form important components of the receptor complex (22).

TSH receptors are present in relatively small amounts when compared with other sites for anterior pituitary hormones. For example, the thyroid cell in vitro is reported to have only 500 to 1000 sites per cell for TSH (23) compared to the Leydig cell, which has 20,000 binding sites for LH (24). Purification of the receptor has been further antagonized by its instability except when frozen below $-70°C$. Analysis of the sites by photoaffinity labeled TSH appears to be the most promising technique for further evaluation of this difficult receptor.

TSH-Binding Inhibition

Many immunoglobulin fractions which exhibit TSAb activity have also been shown to inhibit the binding of ^{125}I-bTSH to intact thyroid cells, membrane preparations, and solubilized TSH receptors (17, 25, 26). This TSH-binding inhibition (TBI) is therefore considered to be secondary to the presence of antibodies to the TSH receptor or a closely located membrane site.

Fractionation of sera from patients with Graves' disease by ion-exchange chromatography, gel filtration, and isoelectric focusing have shown the TBI activity to be associated with a relatively restricted population of IgG (27) and the receptor antibody binding site to be formed by a combination of heavy and light chains in the Fab part of the IgG molecule (28). Hence Graves' disease joins the group of receptor antibody diseases discussed in Chapter 5.

Site of Action of TBI

As solubilized TSH receptors have been subjected to further purification, including affinity techniques, there has been no loss of TBI activity by the Graves' IgG preparations investigated (29). In addition, the nonspecific effects of normal IgG appear to be lessened by examination of TSH receptors in the soluble form. Despite the generation of these consistent data, there has been persisting doubt about the mechanism of this TSH-binding inhibition and whether it represents a direct interaction by the antibody with the TSH receptor binding sites or a secondary effect due to stereospecific changes induced by membrane interactions at a distance from the true receptor. In order to investigate these criticisms we have recently examined such Graves' IgG interaction by its ability to protect the TSH receptor binding sites from inactivation induced by protein modification (30). In control studies, 80% of the binding of ^{125}I-bTSH was inhibited after membrane exposure to the disulfide reducing agent dithiothreitol (DTT). In the presence of TSH-occupied receptor sites there was a dose-related protection of the receptors, with 100% protection following incubation with 30 milli I.U./ml bTSH. In these studies the residual TSH receptors were examined after removal of receptor occupying molecules by 2 M NaCl. Incubation of membranes with 10 mM DTT after prebinding normal IgG caused no TSH receptor protection. However, each of the Graves' IgG examined was able to provide complete protection of the TSH receptor binding sites in proportion to their dissociable fraction following 2 M NaCl. Hence Graves' IgG, but not normal IgG, contain antibodies which are able to protect the TSH receptor binding sites in the same way as TSH. Although these data provided further evidence that Graves' sera contain antibodies to the TSH receptor binding

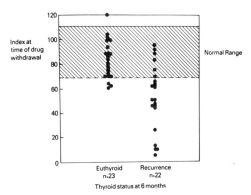

Figure 4. Patients were treated for 6 months with antithyroid drugs following which TBI was measured and the drugs withdrawn. Six months later the patients were divided into relapse and remission groups and are illustrated with their respective TBI results. Data were expressed as an index in relation to normal IgG-induced TBI activity. Inhibition greater than 30% was considered abnormal based on normal controls. Note that all patients with high levels of inhibition were in the relapse group by 6 months after antithyroid drug withdrawal.

site itself, only the availability of purified TSH receptor preparations will finally settle this controversy.

Clinical Application of TBI Assay

When it was realized that Graves' IgG inhibited 125I-bTSH binding, there became available a simple test for Graves' specific autoantibody. The availability of such a rapid, inexpensive, and simple approach to the measurement of an important thyroid autoantibody has generated a large literature on the subject of TBI activity in Graves' disease. TBI activity has been shown to be useful as a relatively specific marker for Graves' disease, for example, in cases of ophthalmic Graves' disease, in the prediction of relapse and remission (Fig. 4) (31, 32), and in the occurrence of neonatal hyperthyroidism (33). These correlations and others are summarized in Table 1.

Comparison of TSAb and TBI in Hyperthyroid Graves' Disease

Once the presence of TSH-receptor antibodies in the circulation of patients with TSAb was demonstrated, it was widely assumed that the two activities were synonymous. This was supported by a good correlation between

Table 1.   TSH binding inhibition (TBI)
in Graves' disease

Prevalence (approximately 70%)	(28, 31, 32, 34, 36, 38)
Positive correlations	
Serum T3	(38, 39)
TRH testing	(34, 38)
Early ^{131}I-uptake	(38)
Thyroid histology	(35)
Response to RAI	(75)
Relapse and remission	(31, 32, 74)
Pretibial myxedema	(38)
Neonatal Graves' disease	(33)
Negative correlations	
Ophthalmic Graves'	(68)
HLA typing	(43, 74, 75)
Antithyroid drug response	(31, 74, 76)

TBI activity and disease status as evidenced by technetium uptake (34), T3 suppressibility (34), thyroid histology (35), and TRH sensitivity. Hence all the in vivo derived parameters of TSAb correlated well with TBI activity. However, when direct correlations between in vitro TSAb by slice assay and TBI by radioreceptor assay were attempted, only poor coefficients were obtained (36). There were many potential reasons for this. In hyperthyroid Graves' disease the patient obviously has TSAb; therefore only TSAb positive patients need be considered. First, the slice assay for TSAb has problems with precision and one would not expect to deliver good correlations with a low precision system. Secondly, different thyroid preparations have been used in the two systems and we know the inherent variability of the TSAb responses (Fig. 2). However, when the bioassay and receptor assay are determined with similar tissue, such as murine thyroid, then somewhat better correlations have been obtained (37).

Comparison of TSAb and TBI in Treated Graves' Disease

In treated Graves' disease, of course, these arguments do not apply since the treatment may indeed affect the immune response and activity of the antibody, as evidenced by declining levels of thyroid autoantibodies in many patients (31, 32, 38). In fact, there is much evidence in such patients for receptor binding antibodies which do not stimulate the thyroid but may inhibit the action of TSH itself (see Section 3.3). The role of the immunosuppresive action of the thionamide group of antithyroid drugs in this phenomenon is a subject of considerable interest (39, 40).

TBI Activity in Non-Graves' Disease

The presence of TBI activity has been reported in some patients with thyroid cancer (38) and subacute thyroiditis (41) but not with multinodular goiters (42). The bioactivity of such receptor antibodies has not been reported but inferred in a case of hyperthyroidism associated with metastatic thyroid carcinoma (43). Presumably, such antibodies are secondary responses to antigenic stimulation in individuals with the inherited ability to produce antibodies with TBI activity.

3.   AUTOANTIBODIES ASSOCIATED WITH THYROIDAL DESTRUCTION

3.1   Thyroglobulin Antibodies (Tg-Ab)

Measurement of Tg-Ab

Antibodies to human thyroglobulin (Tg-Ab) are most commonly detected by the use of Tg-sensitized tanned red blood cells (TRC) which agglutinate in the presence of anti-Tg (48), but can also be measured by radiometric assay (45), enzyme-linked immunoassay (46), plaque-forming cell assay (47), and immunofluorescence. They are not complement fixing.

Prevalence of Tg-Ab

Only 2% of the normal population have Tg-Ab by tanned red cell hemagglutination (TRC) (48), but hTg binding to peripheral mononuclear cells have been observed in most normal individuals and constituted approximately 0.03% of peripheral mononuclear cells (49). However, Tg binding is not synonymous with Tg-Ab secretion, and such binding also appears to be of low affinity and questionable physiological relevance (50). Furthermore, we have recently documented that such secretion is not usually demonstrable in peripheral mononuclear cells (PMC) from normal individuals using a specific plaque-forming cell technique. In contrast, this technique has indicated that approximately 0.5% of peripheral mononuclear cells capable of immunoglobulin secretion have the capacity to secrete hTg-Ab in patients with autoimmune thyroiditis (Fig. 5) (47). The number of Tg-binding and hTg-secreting cells in thyroid infiltrates is also very much greater than found in the peripheral circulation (51), confirming either local antigenic stimulation of appropriate cells or their preferential accumulation within the thyroid gland (see Chapter 7).

Role of Tg-Ab

The pathogenetic role of Tg-Ab in man has been inferred by correlations with lymphocytic infiltration of the thyroid and their high titer in autoimmune thyroiditis (52) compared to lower titers in patients with Graves' disease. Tg-Ab would clearly have access to antigen as it passes through the surface of the thyroid follicular cell and therefore has the potential to initiate thyroiditis as demonstrated in laboratory animals (53). However, not all animal strains serve as good models for thyroiditis, indicating an important

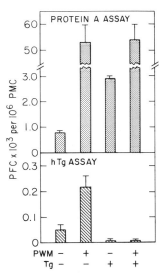

Figure 5. Demonstration of a specific Tg plaque-forming-cell (PFC) assay using peripheral mononuclear cells from a patient with autoimmune thyroiditis and high titers of Tg-Ab. Data obtained with protein A-dependent PFC (upper panel) and hTg-dependent PFC (lower panel) are demonstrated. Cells were incubated for 7 days with or without pokeweed mitogen (PWM, 5 μl/ml) or human Tg (50 μg/ml) as indicated.

genetic component to its susceptibility (see Chapter 2). In a similar way, mothers with high titers of Tg-Ab do not give birth to babies with thyroiditis. Such children may develop autoimmune thyroid disease later in life, indicating that either the genetic susceptibility has a slow penetrance or some external factor(s) are involved.

3.2. Thyroid Microsomal Antibodies (M-Ab)

Measurement of M-Ab

Many patients with autoimmune thyroid disease demonstrate antibodies to an antigen first isolated in a freeze-dried thyroid microsomal preparation (54). A tanned red cell method for such antibodies is now widely available and uses the supernatant from a sonicated 80,000 g fraction of thyroid homogenate (55) and sensitive radioimmunoassays have also been described (56). M-Ab is complement fixing and considered part of the cytotoxic reaction of thyroid cells when confronted with sera from patients with Hashimoto's disease (6).

Prevalence of M-Ab

Up to 7% of the population have thyroid microsomal antibody (M-Ab) by the TRC method (48) and 20% by radioassay. The prevalence of M-Ab, as with most autoantibodies, also increases with age (48, 57). Over 90% of patients with autoimmune thyroiditis and approximately 50% of Graves' patients have easily detectable M-Ab, the titers in thyroiditis being particularly high.

Role of M-Ab

M-Ab show a better correlation with histological thyroiditis than do hTg-Ab and are more often associated with elevated TSH in the general population (58). Of people with M-Ab, 70 to 80% have evidence of thyroid disease.

The precise nature of the microsomal antigen remains uncertain but recent work indicates that labeled M-Ab binds to the surface of thyroid follicular cells (59) as well as to intrathyroidal proteins in cut thyroid tissue. Hence a major component of M-Ab must be a cell surface antigen, which would suggest a primary role for the antibody in thyroid pathology. However, M-Ab titers have not been shown to correlate with TSAb or TBI activity but it is clearly important to distinguish between the intracellular and extracellular antibodies measured by the presently available techniques before reaching a conclusion. It would appear that TSAb is merely one of a number of cell surface antibodies and that the cruder M-Ab assays may measure populations of different molecules.

3.3.   TSH Receptor Blocking Antibodies

Comparison of thyroid-stimulating with ^{125}I-bTSH-binding inhibition has revealed a number of situations where TSAb or TBI may be detected alone (36, 60). In particular, patients with euthyroid Graves' disease presenting with ophthalmopathy, or following treatment, may have TSH receptor-blocking antibodies detected by the TBI assay but in the absence of TSAb (61). Such antibodies have been associated with hypothyroidism in neonates following transplacental passage (62). In vitro they demonstrate blockade of TSH action, which would account for thyroid atrophy and clinical hypothyroidism (14, 60, 62). The prevalence of this category of antibodies is uncertain at present and requires further study but TBI activity is demonstrable in 10 to 15% of patients with autoimmune thyroiditis (28). The physiological role of TBI in patients with thyroid carcinoma remains to be evaluated (38).

3.4   Miscellaneous Thyroid Autoantibodies

The immune diathesis associated with autoimmune thyroid disease is commonly associated with other autoimmune endocrine syndromes and other organ-specific antibodies (see Chapters 5 and 10). In addition there are a variety of thyroid autoantibodies known but on which we have relatively little data:

1.   Antibodies to the thyroid hormones T3 and T4 have been well described but are not directly relevant to the issue of autoimmune thyroid disease (63).

2.   Colloid antibodies cause uniform staining of the colloid in fixed thyroid sections but their pathological significance is unknown (64). They are seen primarily in patients with autoimmune thyroid disease and up to 10% of the normal population.

3.   The patchy staining of the thyroid cell surface described for the antibody of Fagraeus and Jonsson (65) is best considered part of the spectrum of antibodies of which TSAb and TBI activity are another two examples.

4.   Much discussion has been aroused by reports of thyroid growth-stimulating and growth-blocking antibodies in goitrous and atrophic thyroid disease, particularly autoimmune thyroiditis (66, 67). Unfortunately the

data presented have not allowed a clear differential from TSAb and/or TBI activity and await confirmation in other laboratories.

4.   IMMUNE ASPECTS OF GRAVES' OPHTHALMOPATHY

Clinically noticeable retro-orbital inflammation, usually bilateral, occurs in a small proportion of patients with past or present hyperthyroid Graves' disease (68). In addition, the ophthalmic changes may be seen occasionally in autoimmune thyroiditis or without any associated thyroid disease at all (61, 69). Its development bears no correlation with the thyroid autoantibodies we so far recognize except that patients with the most severe disease may be more likely to have significant levels of TSAb and TBI. This suggests that we are dealing with a quite distinct, but closely linked, disorder.

Pathologically there are retro-orbital features of an autoimmune reaction with mononuclear infiltration as well as interstitial accumulation of fat and collagen, particularly in the eye muscle. Sophisticated testing by ultrasound and CAT scans show that many patients with hyperthyroid Graves' disease have some muscle involvement (70).

Specific autoantibodies and autoantigens have not been identified as causative. An association with Tg-Ab–Tg complex trapping in retro-orbital muscle has elegant in vitro experimental support (71) but failure to associate such complexes with eye disease (72) and the rarity of ophthalmic complications in autoimmune thyroiditis suggest that other, more important factors are operating. Similarly, a role for TSH fragments has not found support (73). Clearly we need to identify the specific antigens and antibodies before we can begin to understand this fascinating, but sometimes devastating, disorder.

5.   CONCLUSIONS

The identification of thyroid autoantibodies in the sera of patients with thyroid disease has allowed us to recognize the immune defects in such patients in a simple and precise manner. Evidence has accumulated that certain of these antibodies, such as TSAb and M-Ab, have the potential for primary initiators of disease rather than being simply secondary phenomena. Hence our intellectual curiosity has swung from evaluation of thyroid function and the abnormal thyroid gland to the investigation of the immune system and the mechanisms by which the thyroid becomes so frequently the target. Even if we inherit the potential for thyroid autoantibody secretion there appear to be additional important factors operating for disease development. A multifactorial cause may appear to be an easy way to answer a difficult dilemma but the evidence being generated suggests that this is exactly what we are dealing with.

ACKNOWLEDGMENTS

Supported by NIH grants AM 28243 and AM 07027 and the Irma T. Hirschl Charitable Trust.

REFERENCES

1. I. M. Roitt, D. Doniach, and P. N. Campbell, *Lancet* **2**, 830 (1956).
2. D. D. Adams and H. D. Purves, *Proc. Univ. Otago Med. Sch.* **34**, 11 (1956).
3. H. Uno, T. Sasazuki, H. Tamai, and H. Matsumoto, *Nature* **292**, 768 (1981).
4. R. J. Graves, *London Med. Surg.* **7**, 516 (1835).
5. J. R. Wall, J. Henderson, C. R. Shakosch, and D. M. Joyner, *Can. Med. J.* **124**, 856 (1981).
6. R. J. V. Pulvertaft, D. Doniach, I. M. Roitt, and R. V. Hudson, *Lancet* **2**, 214 (1959).
7. J. M. McKenzie, *J. Clin. Endocrinol. Metab.* **21**, 635 (1961).
8. D. D. Adams and T. H. Kennedy, *J. Clin. Endocrinol.* **27**, 173 (1967).
9. K. Bech and S. Nistrup Madsen, *Clin. Endocrinol.* **11**, 47 (1979).
10. M. Zakarija, J. M. McKenzie, and K. Bonovac, *Ann. Intern. Med.* **93**, 28 (1980).
11. W. E. Hinds, N. Takai, B. Rapoport, S. Filetti, and O. H. Clark, *J. Clin. Endocrinol. Metab.* **52**,

1204 (1981).

12. T. Onaya, M. Kotani, T. Yamada, and Y. Ochi, *J. Clin. Endocrinol. Metab.* **36**, 859 (1973).

13. J. F. Harper and G. Brooker, *J. Cycl. Nucl. Res.* **1**, 207 (1975).

14. M. Platzer, E. Friedman, A. Schwartz, and T. F. Davies, submitted (1983).

15. T. F. Davies and M. Platzer, in preparation (1983).

16. V. B. Petersen, B. R. Smith, and R. Hall, *J Clin Endocrinol. Metab.* **96**, 199 (1975).

17. G. Fayet, B. Vernier, A. Girand, S. Lissitzky, A. Pinchera, J. H. Romaldini, and G. Fenzi, *FEBS Lett.* **32**, 299 (1973).

18. C. S. Teng, B. R. Smith, J. Anderson, and R. Hall, *Biochem. Biophys. Res. Commun.* **66**, 836 (1975).

19. T. F. Davies, B. R. Smith, and R. Hall, *Endocrinology* **503**, 6 (1978).

20. P. J. D. Dawes, V. B. Petersen, B. R. Smith, and R. Hall, *J. Endocrinol.* **78**, 89 (1978).

21. Y. Ozawa, I. J. Chopra, D. H. Solomon, and F. Smith, *Endocrinology* **105**, 1221 (1979).

22. F. Omodeo-Sale, R. O. Brady, and P. H. Fishman, *Proc. Natl. Acad. Sci. USA* **75**, 5301 (1978).

23. P. M. Povey, B. R. Smith, T. F. Davies, and R. Hall, *FEBS Lett.* **72**, 251 (1976).

24. B. Vernier, A. Fayet, and S. Lissitzky, *Eur. J. Biochem.* **42**, 355 (1974).

25. S. W. Manley, J. R. Bourke, and R. W. Hawker, *J. Endocrinol.* **61**, 437 (1974).

26. V. B. Petersen, P. J. D. Dawes, B. R. Smith, and R. Hall, *FEBS Lett.* **83**, 63 (1977).

27. M. Zakarija, *Hormone Res.* **13**, 1 (1980).

28. R. Hall, B. R. Smith, and E. D. Mukhtar, *Clin. Endocrinol.* **4**, 213 (1975).

29. C. Rickards, P. Buckland, B. R. Smith, and R. Hall, *FEBS Lett.* **127**, 17 (1981).

30. T.F. Davies and M. Platzer, *Clin. Endocrinol.*, in press (1983).

31. T. F. Davies, P. P. B. Yeo, D. C. Evered, F. Clark, B. R. Smith, and R. Hall, *Lancet* **2**, 1181 (1977).

32. C. S. Teng and R. T. T. Yeung, *J. Clin. Endocrinol. Metab.* **50**, 144 (1980).

33. D. S. Munro, S. M. Dirmikis, H. Humphries, T. Smith, and G. D. Broadhead, *Br. J. Obstet. Gynaecol.* **85**, 837 (1978).

34. R. Clague, E. D. Mukhtar, G. A. Pyle, J. Nutt, F. Clarke, M. Scott, D. C. Evered, B. R. Smith, and R. Hall, *J. Clin. Endocrinol. Metab.* **43**, 550 (1976).

35. K. Endo, K. Karagi, J. Konishi, K. Ikekubo, T. Okuno, Y. Takeda, T. Mori, and K. Torizuka, *J. Clin. Endocrinol. Metab.* **46**, 734 (1978).

36. A. Sugenoya, A. Kidd, V. V. Row, and R. Volpe, *J. Clin. Endocrinol. Metab.* **48**, 402 (1979).

37. Y. Shishiba, Y. Ozawa, N. Ohtsuki, and T. Shimizu, *J. Clin. Endocrinol. Metab.* **54**, 858 (1982).

38. E. D. Mukhtar, B. R. Smith, G. A. Pyle, R. Hall, and P. Vice, *Lancet* **1**, 713 (1975).

39. A. M. McGregor, M. M. Petersen, S. M. McLachlan, P. Rooke, B. R. Smith, and R. Hall, *N. Engl. J. Med.* **303**, 302 (1980).

40. I. Weiss and T. F. Davies, *J. Clin. Endocrinol. Metab.* **53**, 1223 (1981).

41. C. R. Strakosch, D. Joyner, and J. R. Wall, *J. Clin. Endocrinol. Metab.* **46**, 345 (1978).

42. J. H. Bolk, J. W. F. Elte, J. K. Bussemaker, A. Haak, and O. Van der Heide, *Lancet* **2**, 61 (1979).

43. M. H. Snow, T. F. Davies, B. R. Smith, W. M. Ross, R. G. B. Evans, C. S. Teng, and R. Hall, *Clin. Endocrinol.* **10**, 413 (1979).

44. A. J. Fulthorpe, I. M. Roitt, D. Doniach, and K. Couchman, *J. Clin. Pathol.* **14**, 654, 1961.

45. M. Bayer and J. P. Kriss, *J. Clin. Endocrinol. Metab.* **49**, 557 (1979).

46. Y. Endo, J. Nakano, K. Horinouchi, S. Ohtaki, M. Izumi, and E. Ishikawa, *Clin. Chim. Acta* **103**, 67 (1980).

47. I. Weiss and T. F. Davies, *J. Clin. Endocrinol. Metab.* **54**, 282 (1980).

48. W. M. G. Tunbridge, *Clin. Endocrinol.* **7**, 481 (1977).

49. A. D. Bankhurst, G. Torrigiani, and A. D. Allison, *Lancet* **1**, 236 (1973).

50. I. M. Roberts, S. Whittingham, and I. R. Muckay, *Lancet* **2**, 936 (1973).

51. T. H. Totterman, *Clin. Immunol. Immunopathol.* **10**, 270 (1978).

52. H. Yoshida, N. Amino, K. Yagawa, U. Kunori, M. Satoh, K. Mijai, and Y. Kumahara, *J. Clin. Endocrinol. Metab.* **46**, 859 (1978).

53. J. A. Clagett, B. C. Wilson, and W. O. Weigle, *J. Exp. Med.* **140**, 1439 (1974).

54. W. R. Trotter, G. Belyavin, and A. Waddaus, *Proc. Roy. Soc. Med.* **50**, 961 (1957).

55. T. Bird and J. Stephenson, *J. Clin. Pathol.* **26**, 636 (1973).

56. T. Mori and J. P. Kriss, *J. Clin. Endocrinol.* **33**, 688 (1971).

57. B. B. Taylor, J. A. Thompson, and F. L. Card, *Age Aging* **3**, 122 (1974).

58. W. M. G. Tunbridge, M. Brewis, J. M. French, D. Appleton, T. Bird, F. Clark, D. C. Evered, J. Grimley-Evans, R. Hall, P. Smith, J. Stephenson, and E. Young, *Br. Med. J.* **282**, 258 (1981).

59. G. F. Fenzi, L. Bartalena, E. Macchia, M. Monzana, and A. Pinchera, *Acta Endocrinol.* **225**, 46 (1979).

60. J. Orgiazzi, D. E. Williams, I. J. Chopra, and D. H. Solomon, *J. Clin. Endocrinol. Metab.* **42**, 341 (1976).

61. C. S. Teng, B. R. Smith, B. Clayton, D. C. Evered, F. Clark, and R. Hall, *Clin. Endocrinol.* **6**, 207 (1977).

62. N. Matsoura, Y. Yamada, Y. Nohara, J. Konishi, K. Kasagi, K. Endo, H. Kojima, and K. Wataya, *N. Engl. J. Med.* **303**, 738 (1980).

63. F. Anders Karlson, L. Wibell, and L. Wide, *N. Engl. J. Med.* **296**, 1146 (1977).

64. B. Balfour, D. Doniach, I. M. Roitt, and K. G. Couchman, *J. Exp. Pathol.* **42**, 307 (1961).

65. A. L. Fagraeus and J. P. Jonsson, *Immunology* **28**, 413 (1970).

66. H. A. Drexhage, G. F. Bottazzo, D. Doniach, L. Bitensky, and J. Chayen, *Lancet* **2**, 287 (1980).

67. H. A. Drexhage, G. F. Bottazzo, L. Bitensky, J. Chayen, and D. Doniach, *Nature* **289**, 594 (1981).

68. J. R. Wall, J. Henderson, C. R. Strakosch, and D. M. Joyner, *Can. Med. J.* **124**, 855 (1981).

69. B. J. Ormston, L. Alexander, D. C. Evered, F. Clark, T. Bird, T. Appleton, and R. Hall, *Clin. Endocrinol.* **2**, 369 (1973).

70. S. C. Werner, J. Coleman, and L. A. Franzen, *N. Engl. J. Med.* **290**, 1447 (1974).

71. J. P. Kriss and S. Q. Mehdi, *Proc. Natl. Acad. Sci. USA* **76**, 2003 (1979).

72. S. Ohtaki, Y. Endo, K. Horinouchi, S. Yoshitake, and E. Ishikawa, *J. Clin. Endocrinol. Metab.* **52**, 239 (1981).

73. I. A. Kourides, B. D. Weintraub, E. C. Ridgeway, and F. Maloof, *J. Clin. Endocrinol. Metab.* **40**, 872 (1975).

74. A. M. McGregor, B. R. Smith, R. Hall, M. M. Petersen, M. Miller, and P. J. Dewar, *Lancet* **1**, 1101 (1980).

75. T. F. Davies, M. Platzer, and N. R. Farid, *Clin. Endocrinol.*, **16**, 183 (1982).

76. C. A. Hardisty, L. Hanford, and D. S. Munro, *Clin. Endocrinol.* **14**, 509 (1981).

7

Immune Function in Autoimmune Thyroid Disease

Sandra M. McLachlan

Department of Medicine
Royal Victoria Infirmary
Newcastle upon Tyne, United Kingdom

Bernard Rees Smith

Endocrine Immunology Unit
Welsh National School of Medicine
Cardiff, United Kingdom

Contents

1. INTRODUCTION

Antibodies to a number of components of thyroid tissue appear to be involved in the pathogenesis of autoimmune thyroid disease. Substantial evidence suggests that the hyperthyroidism in patients with Graves' disease is due to antibodies to the TSH receptor which stimulate the thyroid by binding to the receptor and activating adenylate cyclase (1–8). In Hashimoto's thyroiditis, antibodies to thyroglobulin (9) and to thyroid microsomes (10) are associated with the destruction of the thyroid epithelium, although the exact role of these antibodies in the disease process is not yet established. TSH-receptor antibodies have been shown to be of IgG class (11) and this is also true of the majority of antibodies to thyroglobulin and thyroid microsomes; however, low levels of IgA and IgM class antibodies have also been reported (12). Recently some preliminary observations have suggested the existence of another group of thyroid autoantibodies which stimulate thyroid cell growth but do not induce hyperthyroidism (13). In addition to possessing one or more antibodies to thyroid antigens, some patients with autoimmune thyroid disease have other organ-specific autoantibodies, notably gastric parietal cell antibodies (14).

Autoimmune thyroid disease therefore covers a wide spectrum ranging from hypo- to hyperthyroidism and including differences in types of autoantibodies, serum concentrations of autoantibodies, sex, and age of onset of disease. Hence it is to be anticipated that the general immune function in such patients will vary, encompassing at least the variations arising from age differences (15, 16). However, the essential feature common to all such patients is the *specific* response to thyroid antigens and in general this appears to be superimposed on an otherwise relatively normal immune response. This is seen perhaps most clearly by comparing the immune response of patients with autoimmune thyroid disease and those with nonorgan-specific autoimmune diseases such as systemic lupus erythematosus (SLE) and rheumatoid arthritis (Table 1). Patients with SLE frequently have gross immune defects such as low numbers of circulating T cells (17), decreased responses to mitogens (18, 19) and cytotoxic antibodies present in serum to T cell subsets involved in regulating immune responses in vitro and probably in vivo (20–24). In contrast, most studies have shown that patients with Hashimoto's thyroiditis and Graves' disease have normal numbers of T and B cells, normal

responses to mitogens and allogeneic cells (30–38) and lymphocytoxic antibodies have not been reported in the serum of such patients. Cells spontaneously secreting immunoglobulin may be present in the peripheral blood of SLE patients (20, 46, 47, 50, 51), and the ability of their peripheral blood lymphocytes to synthesize immunoglobulin in culture over a 6 to 7 day interval is higher than in control donors; conversely the addition of pokeweed mitogen to such cultures did not result in increased immunoglobulin production as has been observed for lymphocytes from normal individuals (47–51) and as is described below for patients with autoimmune thyroid disease (Sections 3.1 and 3.2). The in vivo response by Hashimoto's patients to other antigens, for example, tetanus toxoid, does not appear to be any greater than that by normal individuals (52); this might perhaps have been expected if their response to all antigens was abnormally increased and seems to be a feature of patients with SLE, at least with respect to some viral antigens (53, 54).

However, it is likely that a general lack of regulation will be superimposed in some patients on the specific defect contributing to the disease process and possibly responsible for the high antibody titers and raised serum immunoglobulin levels in some individuals (55). Some evidence for a suppressor cell defect has been reported by Aoki et al. (56) for Graves' patients but not for patients with Hashimoto's thyroiditis; these results were based on studies of concanavalin A-induced suppressor cells. Similar conclusions were drawn by Thielemans et al. (57) and Sridama et al. (58) using monoclonal antibodies to delineate T cell subsets; they showed that the number of T cells belonging to the suppressor/cytotoxic subset was reduced in patients with autoimmune thyroid disease compared with normal controls. Preliminary studies of our own suggest that there is considerable overlap between the proportions of the T cell subsets in normal donors and patients with autoimmune thyroid disease. It should also be emphasized that the correlations between subsets

Table 1. Some immunologic features of patients with autoimmune thyroid disease and systemic lupus erythematosus

Parameter	Autoimmune Thyroid Disease	Systemic Lupus Erythematosus
Autoantibodies	Antibodies to thyroglobulin (9), thyroid microsomes (10), TSH receptors (1–8)	Antibodies to nuclear antigens, DNA, RNA (27), lymphocytotoxic antibodies to regulatory T cell subsets (20)
Total serum immunoglobulins	Sometimes increased (55)	Frequently raised (26)
Complement	Within normal range (25)	Reduced in some patients (27)
Immune complexes in serum	Present in 25% of patients (28)	Present in >50% of patients and implicated in the pathogenesis of SLE (29)
T cell function:		
Circulating numbers and subsets	Within normal range (31–37), reduced cytotoxic/suppressor T cells (57, 58), and reduced total T cells (57)	Total T cells decreased compared with controls, especially in the active phase of the disease (17), decrease in suppressor/cytotoxic T subset (21–23), variable numbers of T cell subsets (24)
Proliferative responses in vitro to mitogens or alloantigens	Normal response to PHA (32, 36), to PHA and Candida (30), and to alloantigens (38)	Decreased responses to mitogens PHA, ConA, PWM (18, 19)
ConA-induced suppression of:		
Proliferative response	Reduced in Graves' patients but normal in Hashimoto's disease (56)	Decreased, especially in the active phase of the disease (39–42)
Antibody/immunoglobulin synthesis	Not determined	Decreased (22, 43, 44)
B Cell function:		
Circulating numbers	Within normal range (31, 32, 57), increased (37, 45)	Within normal range (17, 23)
Circulating cells secreting immunoglobulin	Within normal range (113)	Increased numbers (20, 46, 47, 50, 51)
Synthesis in culture without mitogen	Similar to normal donors (113, 132, 136)	Increased compared with normals (47, 48)
Synthesis in culture with PWM	Similar to normal donors (113, 132, 136)	Decreased (47, 49–51)
In vivo antibody synthesis to other antigens	Comparable with normal response to tetanus toxoid (52)	Increased antibody titers to some viruses (53, 54)

defined by monoclonal antisera and the ability of the subsets to induce or suppress is not absolute as originally described (59); for example, the ''inducer'' subset has been shown to be capable of suppressing in an in vitro assay (60).

In this chapter the immune function in patients with autoimmune thyroid disease is considered in terms of a general response— total immunoglobulin synthesis in vitro—and the specific responses to thyroid antigens. The latter include responses thought to be due primarily to T cells (''cell-mediated immune responses'') as well as production of specific thyroid autoantibodies, a process which is likely to involve T cell control of B cell differentiation. Much of the currently available information in man is based on in vitro studies, but immune changes following therapy in patients with autoimmune thyroid disease are also considered.

2. CELL-MEDIATED IMMUNE RESPONSES

The presence of lymphocytes sensitized to specific antigen is commonly assessed in the following ways:

1. Measurement of cell replication (in terms of tritiated thymidine, ^{3}H-TdR, incorporation into DNA) by lymphocytes cultured with the sensitizing antigen.
2. Release of factor(s) termed ''lymphokines'' which have the ability to inhibit the migration of lymphoid cells.
3. Cytotoxicity.

Early studies reported variable results for the incorporation of ^{3}H-TdR in response to thyroglobulin (Table 2), stimulation being shown by some workers for Hashimoto's peripheral blood lymphocytes (61–63) but not by other investigators (30, 64). Recently, De Groot and his colleagues reinvestigated this response in peripheral blood lymphocytes

from Graves' and Hashimoto's patients and showed that significant stimulation occurred in all patients provided that a range of doses from 0.5 to 30 μg/ml was used (65). The situation is somewhat confused by the finding that a higher concentration of thyroglobulin (100 μg/ml) stimulated proliferative responses in both Graves' and normal lymphocytes (66). Lymphocytes from the peripheral blood of Hashimoto's patients and from some Graves' patients have been shown to be stimulated by thyroid membrane preparations (63, 67, 68), and Makinen et al. (69) demonstrated that the response could be inhibited if the thyroid membranes (containing TSH receptors) were incubated with TSH prior to culture. This important point, which provided evidence for the specificity of the response, has been disputed by Wenzel et al. (70); they showed that the same concentration of TSH but not other hormones could inhibit T cell transformation to mitogens (phytohemagglutinin and concanavalin A) and antigens (purified protein derivative and streptokinase/streptodornase) and this suppressive effect appeared to be based on an interaction between monocytes and TSH. It seems likely that although responses to thyroid membranes can be detected in some patients, stimulation by TSH receptors has yet to be conclusively demonstrated. In this context it is of interest to note that TSH receptors have been reported to be present on human peripheral blood mononuclear cells (71).

Investigation of migration inhibition has also produced variable results (Table 3) as summarized by Calder and Irvine (64). Some studies using thyroglobulin reported inhibition for patients with autoimmune thyroid disease (72–75) and some were negative (76). In the presence of a crude thyroid extract or thyroid membranes, migration inhibition was positive in Graves' and Hashimoto's peripheral blood lymphocytes (68, 73, 75, 77–83). As reported in a few studies for proliferative responses to thyroglobulin, lymphocytes from normal donors sometimes gave positive responses in the migration inhibition test; Amino and

Table 2. Proliferative responses to thyroid antigens in patients
with autoimmune thyroid disease

| Antigen | Dose Range | % Positive Responses (n)[a] | | | Ref. |
		Graves' Disease	Hashimoto's Disease	Normal Donors	
Thyroglobulin	Not given	ND	100 (1)	ND	62
	Not given	ND	0 (10)	ND	64
	50–2000 µg/ml	50 (4)	100 (1)	0 (15)	61
Thyroglobulin and	1–2 mg/ml	0 (20)	0 (14)	0 (6)	30
crude extract	150 µg/ml	0 (10)	67 (9)	0 (15)	63
Thyroglobulin	0.5–30µg/ml	69 (13)	71 (7)	9 (11)	65
	100 µg/ml	100 (12)[b]	ND	100 (13)[b]	66
Thyroid extract or	Av. 1.5 mg/ml	20 (15)	ND	0 (12)	67
membranes	50 µg/ml	82 (11)	ND	0 (10)	69
	35–40 µg/ml	100 (19)	100 (15)	0 (10)	68

ND, not determined.
[a] n, number of subjects tested.
[b] No significant difference between Graves' patients and normals.

De Groot (79), for example, observed inhibition by lymphocytes from all patients and normal donors but the extent of inhibition was greater in patients than in the controls. All the results so far considered were based on lymphocytes from the peripheral blood (PBL). Totterman et al. (81) compared the responses of PBL and lymphocytes in thyroid aspirates and showed that whereas PBL from both Hashimoto's and Graves' patients were positive in terms of lymphocyte migration inhibition, only lymphocytes from Graves'

Table 3. Studies of lymphocyte migration inhibition to thyroid antigens
in patients with autoimmune thyroid disease

| Antigen | Dose Range | % Positive Responses (n)[a] | | | Ref. |
		Graves' Disease	Hashimoto's Disease	Normal Donors	
Thyroglobulin	50–2000 µg/ml	75 (4)	80 (5)	41 (17)	74
	100–500 µg/ml	50 (23)	46 (19)	8 (13)	75
	50–200 µg/ml	ND	44 (32)	ND	73
	50–5000 µg/ml	0 (12)	0 (26)	0 (47)	76
	Not given	ND	63 (26)	ND	72
Thyroid microsomes	Not given	ND	80 (15)	0 (25)	77
	500 µg/ml	ND	35 (40)	6 (35)	73
	5–250 µg/ml	100 (12)	100 (34)	0 (47)	76
	0.21 mg/ml[b]	64 (22)	81 (15)	15 (13)	78
	500 µg/ml	100[c] (12)	100[c] (14)	100 (14)	79
	100–500 µg/ml	41 (23)	31 (19)	0 (12)	75
Thyroid homogenate	360 µg/ml	74 (57)	75 (4)	5 (20)	80, 81
Solubilized extract	40 µg/ml	87 (15)	75 (12)	0 (24)	82, 83

ND, not determined.
[a] n, number of subjects tested.
[b] Equivalence of nitrogen.
[c] Extent of inhibition greater in patients with autoimmune thyroid disease than in controls.

thyroid tissue were responsive to thyroid antigens; further cell fractionation studies showed that these cells in Graves' thyroid were T lymphocytes. Similarly Okita et al. (82, 83) demonstrated that the cells in peripheral blood of patients with autoimmune thyroid disease which produced lymphokines and responded in migration tests to thyroid membranes or a soluble preparation of thyroid membranes were T cells. They also showed that T cells from normal donors but not from other patients with autoimmune thyroid disease could suppress the response to thyroid antigens, and they used these data to support the hypothesis that autoimmune thyroid disease is the result of a suppressor cell defect (84, 85).

Sensitization to thyroid antigens has also been demonstrated by cytotoxicity. Podlewski (86) showed that lymphocytes from the peripheral blood of Hashimoto's patients were cytotoxic for target cells coated with thyroglobulin. Calder et al. (87) confirmed the observation and demonstrated that a serum factor was involved since normal PBL incubated with Hashimoto's serum acquired the ability to kill thyroglobulin-coated target cells (88). The cells responsible for this antibody-dependent cytotoxicity are K cells which are non-T, non-B lymphoid cells (64), and in man they are present in peripheral blood, spleen, and bone marrow but not in the thymus, lymph node, or tonsils (89). The components required for antibody-dependent cytotoxicity are present within the thyroid in Hashimoto's disease: plasma cells, some even penetrating thyroid follicles (90); immune complexes present on the basement membrane (25, 90, 91); killer cells (92); and specific antibody (93). As postulated by Allison (89) it is likely that the K cells, complexed with specific antibody secreted by the plasma cells, are responsible for the destruction of thyroid epithelial cells which leads ultimately to the hypothyroidism characteristic of Hashimoto's disease.

The techniques outlined above have shown that at least in some patients with autoimmune thyroid disease there are lymphocytes which recognize and respond to thyroid antigen, and two studies have shown that these are T cells. Using radiolabeled or fluorescent thyroid antigens, lymphocytes capable of binding thyroglobulin (94, 95) and thyroid membranes (96) have been demonstrated in the peripheral blood of Hashimoto patients, and these cells occur more frequently in thyroid aspirates (97, 98). In contrast to the cells involved in cell-mediated immunity, the majority of these thyroid antigen-binding cells were shown to be B lymphocytes (98), presumably the precursors of the lymphocytes which differentiate into thyroid autoantibody-secreting cells.

3. SYNTHESIS OF TOTAL IgG AND THYROID AUTOANTIBODIES IN LYMPHOCYTE CULTURES

In autoimmune disease, tolerance to a variety of self-antigens has been lost. Although a number of hypotheses have been put forward (one of which has already been mentioned), the reason for this breakdown in self-tolerance is not known. An in vitro system in which lymphocytes from patients with autoimmune thyroid disease synthesize thyroid autoantibodies would make it possible to analyze this defect and determine whether the autoimmune response in this group of patients occurs because of changes in the immune system or the thyroid or possibly in both systems.

We have developed a system in which lymphocytes from patients with Graves' disease and Hashimoto's thyroiditis synthesize TSH-receptor antibodies and antibodies to thyroglobulin and thyroid microsomes, respectively (99–101). Synthesis of total IgG is routinely measured in parallel with autoantibody production for several reasons: the production of immunoglobulin indicates that the lymphocytes are functioning in the culture system; the total amount produced is an in vitro measure of the patient's overall immune response; and finally the proportion of total IgG which is thyroid autoantibody, the specific activity, provides an estimate of the number of cells involved in the production of a particular antibody and can be used to assess the contribution made to the in vivo level of autoantibody by lymphocytes from different tissues.

The source of lymphocytes most readily available in man is the peripheral blood and consequently most of the results to be described here are based on these cells. However, lymphocytes may also be extracted in sufficiently large numbers for culture purposes from thyroid tissue removed at operation as well as from spleen tissue available from donors of renal transplants. Observations based on cultures of all three tissue types are considered.

The culture system was designed for peripheral blood lymphocytes, a population of cells characterized by small undifferentiated lymphocytes, predominantly T cells (102). In normal individuals, few of these B lymphocytes are capable of directly secreting immunoglobulin or of developing into cells secreting immunoglobulin in culture. Consequently it is necessary to stimulate the cells in some way, for example, using the plant lectin pokeweed mitogen, which triggers B cells indirectly via T cells to differentiate into lymphoblasts or plasma cells (103, 104). Assay systems for measuring some thyroid autoantibodies, notably TSH-receptor antibodies, often require relatively large amounts of serum IgG (micro- to milligram quantities) for detection of specific antibody. In order to produce sufficient IgG in culture to permit detection of these antibodies, a relatively dense population of cells (7×10^6 to 10×10^6 per milliliter) was incubated with the mitogen in the inner chamber of a Marbrook flask (105), separated by a dialysis membrane from the outer reservoir containing 25 milliliters of culture medium. Under these conditions, the lymphocytes are sufficiently close for cellular interactions to occur; they have access to the nutrients in the reservoir, and most important, toxic waste products (which would otherwise accumulate in the vicinity of the cells) diffuse out into the reservoir (106). Cultures were harvested after 2 weeks, and supernatants were separated from the cell pellet and analyzed for total IgG by a solid phase radioimmunoassay (107, 108). Peripheral blood lymphocytes incubated in Marbrook flasks synthesize relatively large amounts of immunoglobulin, between 35 and 420 milligrams of IgG per 10^7 cells over 21 days (108). Replicate supernatants were usually pooled and the immunoglobulins synthesized in culture concentrated about 8 to 10 times by precipitation with ammonium sulfate (100). TSH-receptor antibodies were analyzed in these "culture concentrates" by radioreceptor assay (5) and cytochemical bioassay (109); thyroglobulin and microsomal antibodies in supernatants and culture concentrates were measured by tanned red cell hemagglutination (110–112). In addition, in some studies, plaque assays were carried out to determine the number of cells secreting total IgG and IgM as well as thyroglobulin antibody (113).

Other studies of thyroid autoantibody synthesis have been described and the results of these investigations are also considered.

3.1. Graves' Disease—Antibody Synthesis by Peripheral Blood Lymphocytes

The ability of peripheral blood lymphocytes from patients with Graves' disease to synthesize total immunoglobulin and TSH-receptor antibody was studied using the plant lectins pokeweed mitogen (PWM) and phytohemagglutinin (PHA). In addition, an attempt was made to specifically stimulate TSH-receptor antibody production by incubation of the lymphocytes for 24 hours with a preparation of thyroid membranes (known to have TSH-receptor activity), washing the cells, and returning the suspensions to fresh medium with or without pokeweed mitogen for 13 days. Considerable amounts of total IgG were produced by lymphocytes from Graves' patients and normal donors cultured with PWM (Table 4). In contrast, lymphocyte cultures that had been incubated with thyroid membranes contained only small amounts of total

Table 4.   Synthesis of total IgG by peripheral blood lymphocytes
from Graves' patients and normal donors cultured for 14 days
with mitogens and thyroid membranes

| Culture Conditions | μg IgG Synthesized per 10^7 Cells (Mean $\pm$ SEM) | |
	Graves' Patients $(n)^a$	Normal Donors $(n)^a$
PWM	50.0 $\pm$ 18.9 (4)	88.7 $\pm$ 20.6 (3)
Thyroid membranes	1.6 $\pm$ 0.2 (3)	1.7 $\pm$ 0.3 (3)
Thyroid membranes plus		
PWM	22.9 $\pm$ 6.5 (4)	30.3 $\pm$ 18.9 (4)
PHA	5.4 $\pm$ 0.9 (3)	15.6 $\pm$ 5.4 (5)

^{a} n, number of donors studied.

immunoglobulin, although this was markedly increased in cultures to which PWM had been added after 24 hours. The presence of PHA was associated with the production of modest amounts of total IgG and clearly the most effective stimulus to immunoglobulin synthesis in both Graves' and normal lymphocyte cultures was PWM present throughout the culture period. Delay in the addition of this mitogen has been shown by others (114) to result in a decreased total IgG response, and similar observations were made in the study described above. No significant differences were observed between the results obtained for PBL from Graves' patients and normal donors in response to the four ''stimulators'' described above.

Culture concentrates prepared from these cultures were examined for the presence of TSH-receptor antibody activity. Using the radioreceptor assay (5), antibody activity was undetectable in cultures of lymphocytes incubated with PHA or thyroid membranes. However, in two Graves' lymphocyte cultures stimulated with PWM (Fig. 1) and two cultures incubated with thyroid membranes and PWM or PHA (Figs. 1 and 2), TSH-receptor antibody activity was detectable as a small but significant inhibition of the binding of labeled TSH to thyroid membranes. Further, the minimum output of serum IgG from each patient that is required to give a positive result in the

receptor assay was known, and this has been compared with the amount of culture IgG assayed (Fig. 1). Clearly, unless the immunoglobulin produced in culture had a greater content of TSH-receptor antibody activity than serum IgG, only cultures from patients FG and DC would be likely to produce significant inhibition in the radioreceptor assay, and these expectations were fulfilled.

The specificity of these TSH-receptor antibodies was demonstrated by the ability of thyroid membranes to absorb out this activity. Lymphocytes from a Graves' patient and a normal donor were incubated with thyroid membranes for the first 24 hours; in some flasks dibutyryl cyclic AMP (db cAMP) was added since there is evidence from experiments in mice that cAMP administered with antigen results in higher numbers of antibody-forming cells (115). After washing to remove antigen, lymphocytes were incubated with PWM or PHA; cells treated with cAMP were resuspended in medium only. Thirteen days later, cultures were harvested and the immunoglobulins synthesized divided into two fractions, one treated with a suspension of thyroid membranes and the other with bovine serum albumin. After centrifugation, aliquots were examined for TSH-receptor antibodies in the radioreceptor assay. The thyroid autoantibody activity present in the albumin-treated fractions of PWM- and PHA-stimulated Graves' lym-

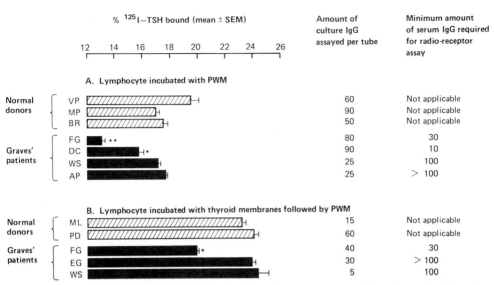

Figure 1. TSH-receptor antibody activity measured by radioreceptor assay in 14-day cultures from Graves' peripheral blood lymphocytes. The presence of TSH-receptor antibody activity is indicated by the inhibition of binding of ^{125}I-labeled TSH to thyroid membranes. Values significantly different from those given by cultures from normal donors: **$p < .01$ and *$p < .05$. The amount of culture IgG assayed per tube is compared with the minimum level of serum IgG required per tube to give significant inhibition in the radioreceptor assay. Adapted from McLachlan et al. (100).

phocyte cultures (Fig. 2a) was specifically absorbed out using the thyroid membranes (Fig. 2b).

Cultures were also examined using the highly sensitive cytochemical bioassay, which is based on the ability of thyroid stimulators to increase the permeability of thyroid lysosomes, and this increase is measured by hydrolysis of a chromogenic lysosomal enzyme substrate (109, 116). As shown in Figure 3, significant stimulation in the cytochemical bioassay occurred in the presence of IgG produced in culture by PWM-stimulated lymphocytes from three Graves' patients; immunoglobulins synthesized by lymphocytes from three normal donors produced only background levels of activity. The amount of total IgG required for this assay is small (Fig. 3 compared with Fig. 1), and it is clearly the most suitable system for studying TSH-receptor antibody synthesis in cultures of lymphocytes from Graves' patients. Pokeweed mitogen is preferable to PHA as a stimulus and, as yet, specific stimulation using antigen

with or without a mitogen has not been achieved.

Other studies have been made to demonstrate TSH-receptor antibody synthesis in vitro using lymphocytes cultured for 6 to 7 days with PHA or thyroid membranes and measuring the activity of these cultures using the McKenzie mouse bioassay (117–119) or cAMP release in thyroid slices (120, 121). No measurements were made of total IgG synthesis in these studies but on the basis of the work reported above, as well as from information on the kinetics of immunoglobulin synthesis in culture (108), it seems likely that only low levels of total IgG (less than 10 micrograms per 10^7 cells) would have been synthesized, amounts which would be unlikely to produce detectable effects in the assay techniques used to measure the presence of TSH-receptor antibodies; for example, 0.1 to 1.0 milligrams of serum IgG is necessary in the assay used by Knox et al. (120, 121). The observations of Rapaport et al. (122) appear to provide a possible explanation for

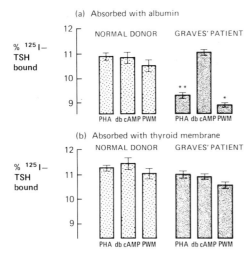

Figure 2. Specificity of TSH-receptor antibody activity measured by radioreceptor assay in 14-day cultures of peripheral blood lymphocytes from a Graves' patient (AB). Immunoglobulins synthesized in culture were assayed after absorption with bovine serum albumin (A) or thyroid membranes (B). Inhibition of binding of ^{125}I-labeled TSH to thyroid membranes significantly greater in Graves' immunoglobulins compared with those from a normal donor: **$p < .001$ *$p < .01$. Adapted from McLachlan et al. (99).

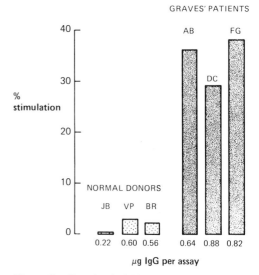

Figure 3. Cytochemical bioassay measurements of TSH-receptor antibody activity in immunoglobulins synthesized in culture by Graves' and normal lymphocytes. Adapted from McLachlan et al. (100).

the reports of TSH-receptor antibody activity in some of these short-term cultures: Rapaport's work showed that cultures of Graves' PBL and thyroid cells synthesized a factor, "human thyroid stimulator" (HTS), which stimulated the release of cAMP from thyroid slices, and was shown to be a prostaglandin (123, 124). HTS was also shown to be produced in PHA-stimulated lymphocyte cultures (122), and this is confirmed by the observations of Goodwin et al. (125) on the synthesis of prostaglandins of the E series by human PBL cultured with this lectin.

Herman et al. (126) showed that corticosteroids suppressed synthesis of HTS in vitro and suggested that, because glucocorticoids induce remission in hyperthyroid Graves' patients more rapidly than can be explained by decreasing immunoglobulins, this provides circumstantial evidence for the suggestion that prostaglandins are involved in the disease. It is possible that both TSH-

receptor antibodies and prostaglandins play a role in Graves' disease (127) and prostaglandins may themselves modulate receptor antibody production by altering lymphocyte activity via intracellular cAMP (128).

3.2. Hashimoto's Disease—Antibody Synthesis by Peripheral Blood Lymphocytes

A variety of preparations has been shown to stimulate immunoglobulin synthesis by peripheral blood lymphocytes including (in addition to PWM) staphylococcal protein A (129) and purified protein derivative (130). However, PWM appears to stimulate more class IgG than IgM than the other polyclonal activators and since most thyroid autoantibodies are of this class, PWM was selected to "trigger" peripheral blood lymphocytes from Hashimoto's patients in studies of microsomal and thyroglobulin antibody synthesis. In addition, some investigations have been carried out using the T-cell independent activator, Epstein Barr virus (131), and the results of these experiments are also considered.

Table 5. Synthesis of total IgG by peripheral blood lymphocytes from patients with Hashimoto's disease and control donors cultured for 14 days with or without PWM

	No. Donors	μg IgG Synthesized per 10^7 Cells (Mean ± SEM)	
		−PWM	+PWM
Hashimoto's patients	22	3.3 ± 0.8	131.8 ± 36.4
Normal donors	14	3.8 ± 1.5	108.0 ± 16.8

Synthesis of total IgG in the presence or absence of PWM has been studied in cultures of peripheral blood lymphocytes from 22 Hashimoto's patients and 14 normal donors (Table 5); the amount of IgG produced with or without the mitogen was not significantly different in cultures from patients and controls. The immunoglobulins synthesized in vitro by Hashimoto's lymphocytes were analyzed for the presence of thyroglobulin and microsomal antibodies by tanned red cell hemagglutination (101). As shown in Figure 4, thyroid auto-antibodies were detectable only in cultures of Hashimoto's lymphocytes and not in immunoglobulins synthesized by lymphocytes from normal individuals despite the production of comparable levels of total IgG. In the ab-

sence of PWM, thyroid autoantibodies were either absent or present in very small amounts (as might have been anticipated from the low levels of total IgG synthesized). In general, there was a correlation between the level of serum thyroid autoantibody and the amount of antibody synthesized in PWM-stimulated cultures, higher titers being found in immunoglobulins secreted by lymphocytes from patients with high serum levels of the autoantibody. However, the ability of lymphocytes to respond to PWM in vitro was also an important factor, as can be seen by comparing the results obtained for patients 1 and 2 who had the same microsomal antibody titer but whose lymphocytes synthesized differing amounts of total IgG and consequently

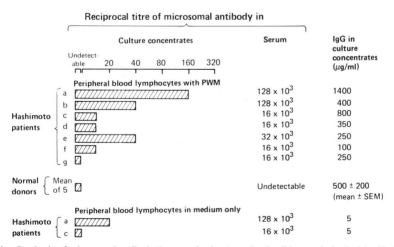

Figure 4. Synthesis of microsomal antibody (measured using tanned red cell hemagglutination) by Hashimoto's peripheral blood lymphocytes cultured in Marbrook flasks for 14 days in the presence or absence of PWM. Adapted from McGregor et al. (101).

differing levels of microsomal antibody in culture. The data considered so far are those for microsomal antibodies and essentially similar results were obtained for the synthesis of thyroglobulin antibodies (data not shown). Immunoglobulins present in serum and synthesized in culture were analyzed by gel chromatography for one patient and microsomal and thyroglobulin autoantibodies were found principally in the 7S (or IgG) fraction; these findings suggest that the immunoglobulins produced in culture are essentially the same as those circulating in vivo (101).

Plaque assays have also been used to study synthesis of total immunoglobulin and thyroglobulin antibody (113). Similar numbers of cells secreting total IgG were detectable by reverse plaque assay in 7 day Marbrook cultures from normal and Hashimoto's peripheral blood lymphocytes. However, cultures of Hashimoto's lymphocytes contained cells actively secreting antibody to thyroglobulin-coated sheep red blood cells, and these antibodies were principally of class IgG (Fig. 5a). The specificity of the response was demonstrated by the lack of plaque-forming cells to sheep red cells coated with an unrelated antigen (bovine serum albumin) and by the inhibition of thyroglobulin antibody plaque-forming cells (but not total IgG plaque-forming cells) using 50 micrograms per milliliter of thyroglobulin (Fig. 5b). There was good agreement between the total numbers of thyroglobulin antibody plaque-forming cells and the amount of thyroglobulin antibody in culture as measured by hemagglutination, but the plaque assay was more sensitive, permitting detection in many patients at an earlier stage in culture (7 days compared with 14 days) and in a greater number of patients than had been possible using hemagglutination tests (113). Weiss and Davies (132) have described a similar system based on lymphocytes cultured for 6 to 7 days in tubes with PWM; thyroglobulin antibody plaque-forming cells were also confined to class IgG and the frequency of specific thyroid antibody plaque-forming cells in the two systems is similar:

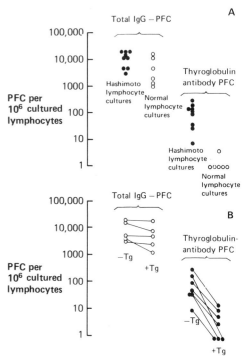

Figure 5. (A) Total IgG plaque-forming cells (PFC) and specific thyroglobulin antibody PFC in 7-day PWM stimulated cultures of peripheral blood lymphocytes from seven Hashimoto's patients and six normal donors. (B) Total IgG PFC and thyroglobulin antibody PFC in cultures of Hashimoto's peripheral blood lymphocytes enumerated in the presence and absence of 50 µg/ml thyroglobulin (Tg). Adapted from McLachlan et al. (113).

0.1 to 1.7% of cells secreting total IgG were found to be thyroglobulin antibody plaque-forming cells by Weiss and Davies (132), compared with 0.3 to 3.8% (mean 1.1%) by McLachlan et al. (113).

Studies of thyroglobulin antibody synthesis in vitro have also been carried out by Beall and Kruger (133) using reconstituted populations of B and T cells cultured for 7 days with PWM and PHA. Thyroglobulin antibodies were measured by a radioimmunoassay and were found to be principally of class IgG. Production of the thyroid autoantibody depended on the presence of T cells although, as shown by others for total IgG synthesis (104, 134), increased numbers of T cells suppressed autoantibody synthesis (135).

Table 6.   Thyroid autoantibody synthesis by PWM-stimulated Hashimoto's peripheral blood lymphocytes cultured alone or cocultured with an equal number of peripheral blood lymphocytes from a normal donor[a]

Hashimoto's Patients	Normal Donors	Type of Auto-antibody	Reciprocal Titer of Thyroid Autoantibody Synthesized		IgG $\left(\% \dfrac{\text{Observed}}{\text{Expected}}\right)$
			Alone or with Autologous T Cells	In Coculture or with Normal T Cells	
Peripheral Blood Lymphocytes Alone or in Coculture					
A	1	Microsomal	80	80[b]	99
B	2	Thyroglobulin	80	80[b]	75
C	3	Thyroglobulin	80	160[b]	68
D	4	Thyroglobulin	10	40[b]	140
E	5	Microsomal	40	80[b]	74
F	2	Thyroglobulin	160	40[b]	150
Hashimoto's B cells + T Cells					
G	6	Microsomal	320	40	12
H	7	Thyroglobulin	10	20	83

Adapted from McLachlan et al. (136).
[a] *Data are also given for Hashimoto's B cells recombined with autologous T cells or T cells from a normal donor. IgG synthesis is given in terms of the observed amount expressed as a percentage of the amount expected on the basis of lymphocytes cultured alone or with autologous T cells.*
[b] *Titer shown is twice the observed value because half as many Hashimoto's peripheral blood lymphocytes were used.*

As discussed earlier, one hypothesis put forward to explain self-tolerance suggests that autoimmune reactions are prevented by populations of suppressor T cells (84, 85), and a defect in a specific clone of T suppressor cells would, therefore, result in autoantibody production. Consequently, if suppressor cells are involved in preventing autoantibody synthesis, normal lymphocytes might be expected to be capable of inhibiting thyroid autoantibody production. This possibility was investigated by culturing peripheral blood lymphocytes or B cells from Hashimoto's patients with lymphocytes or T cells from normal donors (136). A similar approach had previously been used to demonstrate the presence of spontaneously occurring suppressor cells in a number of disease states using cultures of lymphocytes stimulated with PWM, for example, in patients with common variable hypogammaglobulinemia (137, 138) and adult T cell leukemia

(139). As described by these investigators, the amount of total IgG produced by lymphocytes from two normal donors cultured alone or cocultured with equal numbers of lymphocytes from another donor was essentially the same; similarly, when Hashimoto's PBL were cocultured with lymphocytes from normal individuals, the amount of IgG produced compared with the amount expected was about 100% (Table 6). Therefore, total IgG production by Hashimoto's lymphocytes was not inhibited by PBL from normal donors. Further, the presence of lymphocytes from five normal donors did not result in decreased levels of autoantibody synthesis by lymphocytes from five Hashimoto's patients (Table 6). The partial inhibition of thyroglobulin antibody production by lymphocytes from one normal donor (2) whose lymphocytes had no suppressive effect on autoantibody production by lymphocytes from a second Hashimoto's patient could not be explained in terms of HLA similarities or differences (136) and possibly resulted from experimental variation. The combination of normal T cells with B cells of one Hashimoto's patient (G) resulted in less microsomal antibody production than cultures with autologous T cells. However, this did not represent specific suppression of autoantibody synthesis, for total IgG production was reduced by a similar factor (one-eighth). Cultures of normal T cells with Hashimoto's B cells from another Hashimoto's patient (H) synthesized similar amounts of IgG and thyroglobulin antibody compared with cultures of autologous T and B cells (Table 6).

The coculture experiments and cultures involving cross-combinations of B and T lymphocytes indicated that populations of normal PBL or normal T cells do not contain lymphocytes capable of spontaneously suppressing thyroid autoantibody synthesis. Comparable observations were made by Beall and Kruger (140) with combinations of B cells and irradiated T lymphocytes; they demonstrated similar levels of thyroglobulin antibody synthesis using autologous T cells or T cells from normal donors. However, these data are different from those obtained in studies of SLE patients in which normal PBL were able to inhibit immunoglobulin or anti-DNA production in vitro by PBL from patients with SLE (43, 44, 141). As discussed earlier, SLE is an autoimmune disease in which gross immune defects are frequently apparent, which does not generally appear to be the case in Hashimoto's thyroiditis; this may account for the difference in results. It is also possible that the suppressor activity of normal individuals may need to be activated before its presence can be demonstrated. Some support for this comes from studies on rats which develop thyroiditis after thymectomy and sublethal irradiation. This form of thyroiditis could be abrogated by reconstitution with normal syngeneic lymphocytes if the cells were added during the development of the autoimmune response. In contrast, reconsti-

tution with normal lymphocytes had no effect in rats with established thyroiditis (142) and similar observations have been made in NZB/NZW mice with SLE-like autoimmune disease (143).

Attempts have been made to stimulate PBL with autoantigen, that is, thyroglobulin, in the presence and absence of PWM. Lymphocytes were incubated with increasing amounts of thyroglobulin (0 to 240 μg/ml) for 24 hours, washed to remove all thyroglobulin, and incubated for a further 13 days in rinsed flasks. Preliminary experiments suggested that addition of increasing amounts of thyroglobulin (10 to 240 μg/ml) to PWM-treated cultures specifically inhibited synthesis of thyroglobulin antibody, microsomal antibody levels remaining relatively unchanged (Fig. 6a). However, this apparent inhibition was shown to be due to residual thyroglobulin adhering to the culture vessel and complexing with antibody. In a later series of experiments the lymphocytes were transferred to *fresh* Marbrook flasks for the final culture period. Under these conditions, PBL from 4 Hashimoto's patients showed no response to increasing concentrations of thyroglobulin in PWM-stimulated cultures; titers of both thyroglobulin and microsomal antibodies varied irregularly over the range of thyroglobulin concentrations used (Fig. 6b), nor was any significant effect detected on total IgG synthesis (Table 7). These results differ from those obtained by Stevens (144) for the secondary response in vitro to tetanus toxoid by PBL from donors boosted with the antigen; in this study 10 micrograms per milliliter of tetanus toxoid present for as little as 1 hour at the initiation of the culture period resulted in specific inhibition of the tetanus toxoid (but not diphtheria toxoid) antibody response. In some respects in vitro synthesis of IgG class thyroid autoantibody appears to resemble the pattern of antibody production to a non-autoantigen (tetanus toxoid) by human PBL (145, 146); however, the lack of inhibition by autoantigen over a similar concentration range to that of tetanus toxoid in the PWM-

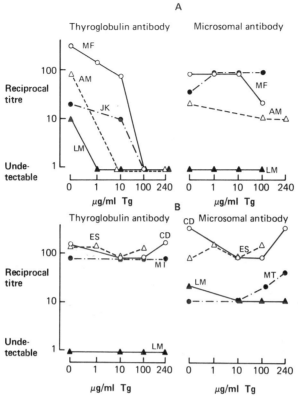

Figure 6. Synthesis of antibodies to thyroglobulin and thyroid microsomes by peripheral blood lymphocytes from Hashimoto's patients incubated for 24 hours with PWM in the presence of increasing concentrations of thyroglobulin (1 to 240 μg/ml), washed and cultured for 13 days. (A) Final culture in rinsed Marbrook flasks (patients MF, AM, JK, and LM). (B) Final culture in a *new* Marbrook flask (patients ES, MT, CD, and LM).

stimulated system appears to be one potentially important difference to be considered in studying regulation of the autoimmune response.

The effect of thyroglobulin was also studied in mitogen-free cultures (Table 7). Again following a 24-hour incubation period, lymphocytes were washed extensively and cultured in medium for 13 days. PBL from one Hashimoto's patient synthesized more total IgG after treatment with 1 and 10 micrograms per milliliter of thyroglobulin than when incubated in medium only; however, lymphocyte cultures from three other patients showed no significant response to thyroglobulin. Thyroid autoantibodies were undetectable in these cultures and it has therefore not proved possible to demonstrate an antigen specific response to

thyroid autoantigen by Hashimoto's PBL. It seems likely that presentation of the antigen in a different way, either on the surface of a red blood cell or for a longer period of time, for example, following the procedure described by Callard (147) in his study of the antibody response to influenza virus, may be required in order to obtain an antigen-dependent response in Hashimoto's PBL. Further, the use of the plaque assay for thyroglobulin antibody-producing cells would overcome the need to remove antigen at some stage during the culture period.

Thyroid autoantibody production has also been studied in Hashimoto's PBL infected with Epstein Barr virus (EBV) (113). Virally infected B lymphocytes differentiate into cells secreting immunoglobulins of all classes. The

Table 7. Synthesis of total IgG by Hashimoto's peripheral blood lymphocytes cultured with or without PWM in the presence of increasing amounts of thyroglobulin (Tg)[a]

Culture Conditions	Patient	μg IgG Synthesized per 10^7 Cells (Mean ± SEM)				
		0 μg/ml Tg	1 μg/ml Tg	10 μg/ml Tg	100 μg/ml Tg	240 μg/ml Tg
		Cultured with PWM				
Final culture in *same* flask	MF	335.4 ± 57.7	320.9 ± 16.6	310.1 ± 21.6	396.7 ± 69.0	—
	AM	95.8 ± 20.8	—	101.5 ± 17.9	129.6 ± 7.6	106.2 ± 23.0
	LM	99.2 ± 23.1	—	145.5 ± 39.3	127.4 ± 28.5	—
	JK	76.2 ± 6.7	—	77.8 ± 8.7	57.9 ± 12.6	93.3 ± 8.0
Final culture in *new* flask	ES	186.3 ± 21.8	151.4 ± 27.2	182.7 ± 11.3	254.0 ± 38.9	—
	CD	134.9 ± 16.6	—	151.7 ± 27.2	151.1 ± 22.3	121.1 ± 9.8
	LM	27.1 ± 6.1	—	20.5 ± 2.1	13.7 ± 2.1	12.0 ± 2.1
	MT	20.0 ± 6.3	—	17.4 ± 5.1	29.4 ± 9.5	23.5 ± 1.6
		Cultured without PWM				
Final culture in *same* flask	MT	2.1 ± 0.1	2.1 ± 0.1	2.2 ± 0.1	1.9 ± 0.1	—
	MF	1.4 ± 0.2	—	2.7 ± 0.9	2.2 ± 0.6	—
Final culture in *new* flask	JC	2.0 ± 0.2	2.9 ± 0.2[b]	3.3 ± 0.2[b]	—	—
	IW	1.4 ± 0.8	—	2.8 ± 0.4	2.1 ± 0.3	—
	MT	0.5 ± 0.1	—	0.3 ± 0.1	0.6 ± 0.1	0.8 ± 0.1

[a] *After 24 hours, lymphocytes were washed and cultured for a further 13 days in the same Marbrook flask (rinsed) or in new flasks.*
[b] *Significantly greater than the amount of IgG synthesized in the absence of thyroglobulin,* $p < .05$.

Table 8.   Synthesis of thyroglobulin antibody (measured by plaque assay) in cultures of Hashimoto's peripheral blood lymphocytes infected with EBV and cultured with or without cyclosporin A (CSA)[a]

Donor	Culture Conditions	Plaque-Forming Cells (PFC) per 10^6 Cultured Lymphocytes		
		Total IgG-PFC	PFC to Thryoglobulin-coated Red Blood Cells	PFC to Red Blood Cells
Hashimoto's Peripheral Blood Lymphocytes				
1	Medium only	487	0	0
	EBV	1,903	530	0
2	Medium only	2,431	2	ND
	EBV	4,152	40	0
	EBV + CSA	15,568	252	43
3	Medium only	0	0	0
	EBV	3,808	1	22
	EBV + CSA	64,737	84	9
4	Medium only	435	0	ND
	EBV + CSA	30,369	116	0
5	Medium only	655	0	ND
	EBV + CSA	6,267	275	5
Normal Peripheral Blood Lymphocytes				
a	Medium only	640	0	ND
	EBV	9,069	0	14
b	Medium only	307	0	0
	EBV	8,410	4	4

ND, not determined.
[a] *Adapted from McLachlan et al.*[113]

response does not require T cells and in this sense EBV is a T-independent mitogen (131). However, in cultures from donors previously exposed to EBV, the presence of virally infected B cells after 10 to 14 days stimulates the development of cytotoxic T cells which then destroy the transformed B lymphocytes (148). This problem can be overcome by the use of purified B cell populations or by the addition of the drug cyclosporin A which functionally deletes T cells (149). Hashimoto's PBL "triggered" by infection with EBV resulted in a dramatic increase in the number of total immunoglobulin-secreting plaque-forming cells, particularly IgM class (Table 8). This increase was associated with a rise in the number of specific thyroglobulin antibody plaque-forming cells, which were principally of class IgG. The addition of cyclosporin A to EBV-infected Hashimoto's

cultures was accompanied by a further increase in total immunoglobulin synthesis and also in the number of plaques to thyroglobulin-coated red cells. Despite comparable levels of stimulation of total immunoglobulin plaque-forming cells by lymphocyte cultures of EBV-transformed normal PBL, specific thyroglobulin antibody plaque-forming cells were not detectable in cultures from the two donors studied (Table 8).

It has been suggested that polyclonal activation induced by a virus such as EBV could be responsible for the initiation of autoimmune responses (89). This possibility was investigated by Sutton et al. (150) by studying serial samples from patients with infectious mononucleosis, a disease which appears to result from EBV infection (151). Although antibodies (usually IgM class) to a number of autoantigens were detected in the initial stages of the disease, these were directed at antigens on the lymphocyte membrane, to smooth muscle, or to contractable fibers, and the small number of sera positive for thyroid autoantibodies was no higher than in a control group of donors. Therefore, on the basis of these results it seems unlikely that the autoimmune response to thyroid antigens in Hashimoto's or Graves' patients is initiated by a polyclonal B cell activator such as EBV. If this is correct, then it would be unlikely for it to be possible to initiate synthesis of thyroid autoantibody in vitro using lymphocytes from normal donors (as shown above and to be considered further in the next section). However, there is evidence for such polyclonal stimulation of rheumatoid factors in mice using lipopolysaccharide (152) and in man with EBV (153). A report has also appeared on the production of IgM class thyroglobulin antibody production by EBV-infected PBL from normal donors, particularly in individuals over 70 years of age (154). Evidence that the antibodies being measured were directed against the antigenic determinants of thyroglobulin were lacking, however, and until such information is available it seems preferable to leave open the question of viral involvement in autoimmune thyroid disease.

3.3. Synthesis of Antibody by Lymphocytes from Thyroid and Spleen

Infiltration of the thyroid by lymphoid tissue is a feature common to both Graves' and Hashimoto's thyroiditis (85). In untreated thyrotoxic patients, the thyroid parenchyma is hypertrophied; the cuboidal cells found in normal thyroid tissue are greatly increased in height, forming a columnar epithelium, and other signs of increased activity are present, such as a well-developed Golgi apparatus (155). In Hashimoto's disease, however, the original parenchyma appears to be destroyed following invasion by lymphoid tissue and the "gland" ultimately develops the histological features of a lymph node including

lymphocytes, lymphoblasts, and plasma cells (156) as well as the structural pattern of cortex, paracortex, and medulla typical of lymph nodes (157). Associated with these basic elements of the immune system are features specific to autoimmune thyroid disease. Plasma cells containing antithyroglobulin activity of 7S type have been recorded in thyroid tissue from a patient with Hashimoto's disease (93) and γ-globulins extracted from Hashimoto's tissue have been shown to contain thyroglobulin antibodies of IgG class (158).

These studies suggest that thyroid autoantibodies are synthesized by lymphocytes localized in the thyroid. Consequently we have extracted lymphocytes from thyroid tissue obtained at operation and cultured these cell suspensions to assess their capacity to produce IgG and thyroid autoantibodies (159).

Subtotal thyroidectomy may be the treatment of choice in many patients with Graves' disease (160), and in some cases this is preceded by the use of the antithyroid drug carbimazole. Comparison of thyroid glands from Graves' patients treated with carbimazole or the β-receptor blocker propranolol showed that the extent of lymphocytic infiltration was considerably reduced by carbimazole therapy (161). This appears to be reflected in the small yield of mononuclear cells obtained from thyroid tissue of Graves' patients treated with carbimazole alone or carbimazole followed by propranolol shortly before operation: $0.5 \pm 0.1 \times 10^6$ (mean $\pm$ SEM, $n = 4$) cells were obtained per gram of tissue. In contrast, more than 30 times as many lymphocytes were extracted from thyroid tissue of a Graves' patient on propranolol only (29.6×10^6 per gram), and this yield of cells was similar to that obtained from four Hashimoto's glands ($22.4 \pm 4.1 \times 10^6$ cells per gram). The contribution made by tissues other than lymphoid to autoimmune thyroid glands can be assessed by comparing the yield of lymphocytes from thyroid tissue and the spleen; a mean of $170.2 \pm 25.5 \times 10^6$ cells were isolated per gram of spleen tissue from five renal transplant donors. Despite this difference, it is clear that the lymphocyte content of thyroid glands from patients with autoimmune thyroid disease may be considerable.

Synthesis of total IgG and thyroid auto-antibodies were studied in thyroid and spleen cell suspensions cultured with and without PWM and in some cases after EBV infection (Fig. 7). Lymphocytes from the thyroid of two Hashimoto's patients produced relatively large amounts of total IgG in the absence of PWM and in both cases this was slightly reduced in the presence of the lectin. Although immunoglobulin synthesis by thyroid lymphocytes from Hashimoto's patient 3 was considerably lower, this was also decreased when PWM was added. However, infection of these thyroid lymphocytes with EBV followed by culture resulted in the production of considerable amounts of total IgG, suggesting that the two polyclonal B cell activators, PWM and EBV, affect different subsets of B lymphocytes. In contrast to the relatively large amounts of IgG synthesized by Hashimoto's thyroid lymphocytes, the production of IgG by thyroid lymphocytes from carbi-

mazole-treated Graves' patients was usually small, a mean value of 7.4 ± 3.0 micrograms per 10^7 cells being obtained from PWM-stimulated cultures from six patients; thyroid lymphocytes from one patient were incubated with and without the mitogen but under both conditions only 3.5 micrograms of IgG were produced by 10^7 cells. As discussed later (Section 4) it seems likely that this was associated with the effects of carbimazole treatment. Variable amounts of total IgG were synthesized by lymphocytes from three spleens incubated in culture medium only (Fig. 7); however, in all cases increased amounts of total IgG were observed when PWM was present in the cultures as well as in cultures of lymphocytes infected with EBV.

It is not known why the response of Hashimoto's thyroid lymphocytes to PWM is so different from that of PBL in patients and normal donors. However, the cell types present in suspensions extracted from thyroid tissue differ considerably from those in peripheral blood, containing not only plasma cells but higher numbers of B cells (44% compared

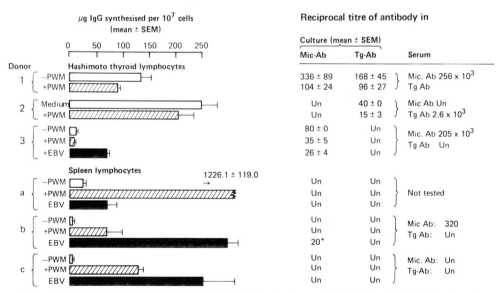

Figure 7. Synthesis of total IgG and thyroglobulin (Tg) and microsomal (Mic) autoantibodies by lymphocytes from Graves' and Hashimoto's thyroid tissue and spleen lymphocytes from renal transplant donors. Lymphocytes were cultured in the presence or absence of PWM or after infection with EBV. Un, thyroid autoantibodies undetectable by hemagglutination tests; *, titer measured in culture concentrate.

with 17% in blood) and fewer T cells (98) (39% compared with 71%); it is likely that the T cell subsets also vary. Pokeweed mitogen stimulates both helper and suppressor T cells in peripheral blood (162), and it is possible that the existing ratio of helper:suppressor T cells, favorable to the production of total IgG, is upset by the activation of T cells caused by the mitogen. A similar inhibitory effect of PWM has been observed by Stevens et al. (163) in studies of IgG class antitetanus toxoid antibody secreted spontaneously by lymphoblastoid cells present in the peripheral blood of donors between 4 and 14 days after boosting with tetanus toxoid.

The supernatants from thyroid lymphocyte cultures were examined directly for the presence of thyroid autoantibodies (Fig. 7). Hashimoto's lymphocytes spontaneously synthesized thyroglobulin and/or microsomal antibodies (depending on the autoantibody present in serum) and in all cases the level of thyroid autoantibody was significantly decreased in cultures containing PWM. Despite the synthesis of considerable amounts of total IgG by Hashimoto's lymphocytes infected with EBV, only small amounts of microsomal antibody were produced. There is evidence that PWM and EBV trigger different B lymphocyte subsets in the peripheral blood, EBV infection tending to result in the production mainly of subclasses IgG3 and little if any IgG4, whereas synthesis of IgG1 predominated in PWM-treated cultures (164). On the basis of these results and the data in Figure 3, it seems likely that Hashimoto's thyroid tissue contains a variety of B cell subsets and it also indicates that the thyroid autoantibody may be largely of subclass IgG1. It is important to note that although it is possible, using tanned red cell hemagglutination, to detect thyroid autoantibody production by peripheral blood lymphocytes directly in the culture supernatants in some patients, in many cases it was necessary to concentrate the immunoglobulins about 8 to 10 times (Section 3.2). However, thyroid autoantibodies were detectable directly in the supernatants from all three Hashimoto patients; further, patient 2

had a relatively low serum thyroglobulin antibody titer (1:2560), less than that found generally necessary (>1:10,000) to study thyroid autoantibody production by peripheral blood lymphocytes in vitro using hemagglutination tests.

Despite the large amounts of total IgG synthesized by spleen lymphocytes in culture after infection with EBV or addition of PWM, no thyroid autoantibodies were detectable in cultures from donors a or c. However, donor b had low levels of serum microsomal antibody and synthesis of this thyroid autoantibody was just detectable in the culture concentrates prepared from immunoglobulins synthesized after infection with EBV (Fig. 7). Therefore, even with lymphocytes obtained from a tissue other than peripheral blood it has so far not proved possible to initiate a detectable autoimmune response using a viral polyclonal B cell activator.

The ability of thyroid lymphocytes to synthesize antibody without PWM provided the opportunity for examining thyroglobulin antibody synthesis in the presence of increasing amounts of thyroglobulin. As described for peripheral blood lymphocytes, cell suspensions were incubated for 24 hours in the presence of thyroglobulin (from 1 to 100 μg/ml) and washed, and incubation was continued in medium only for a further 13 days. No change was observed in the amount of total IgG produced at increasing concentrations of thyroglobulin, but significantly higher levels of thyroglobulin autoantibody were detectable in cultures incubated with 100 micrograms per milliliter than in cultures treated with 1 microgram per milliliter (Fig. 8). This increase was seen even more clearly when the values obtained for culture concentrates were considered. These studies showed that thyroid lymphocytes not only have the ability to produce immunoglobulins, including thyroid autoantibodies, spontaneously, but in addition thyroid autoantibody synthesis can be stimulated by autoantigen.

The relative contributions made to the in vivo concentration of thyroid autoantibodies may be assessed by comparison of the specific

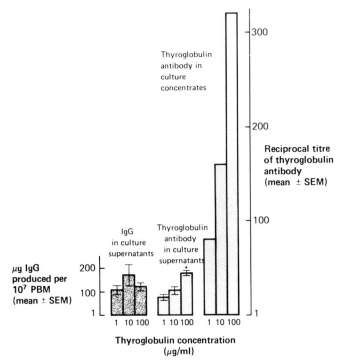

Figure 8.   Stimulation of thyroglobulin antibody synthesis by thyroid lymphocytes. IgG production and reciprocal autoantibody titers are shown as mean ± SEM for culture supernatants and as a single determination for culture concentrates. *, Thyroglobulin antibody level significantly greater in cultures treated with 100 μg/ml thyroglobulin than with 1 μg/ml thyroglobulin: $p < .01$. Adapted from McLachlan et al. (159).

activity of the autoantibody synthesized by lymphocytes from different tissues with the values obtained for serum autoantibody. The specific activity, that is, the reciprocal titer per 10 milligrams per milliliter of IgG, is shown for immunoglobulin present in serum and immunoglobulin synthesized in culture for some Hashimoto's patients in Table 9. Thyroid lymphocytes from three Hashimoto's patients produced IgG in culture with a specific activity as high as that of serum and these values were reduced in immunoglobulins synthesized in the presence of pokeweed mitogen. In contrast PBL (which usually required the stimulus of PWM to produce detectable levels of autoantibody) generally synthesized IgG with a very much lower specific activity than that present in the patient's serum. The exception was patient MS, whose PBL produced immunoglobulin with a specific activity similar to that in serum. In general, however,

it appears that the thyroid in Hashimoto's patients contains considerably more lymphocytes capable of synthesizing thyroid autoantigens than the peripheral blood.

The results of the in vitro studies, together with evidence from animal models and clinical observations (to be described in Section 4), support the suggestion that the thyroid is a major site of autoantibody synthesis in Hashimoto's thyroiditis. It might be expected that the thyroid should also be a major site of synthesis of TSH-receptor antibodies in Graves' disease as well.

4.   EFFECT OF TREATMENT ON THE AUTOIMMUNE RESPONSE

Basically two approaches are used in the treatment of patients with Graves' disease: (1) by using drugs which have a direct effect

Table 9. Specific activity of IgG in serum and synthesized in culture by lymphocytes from thyroid tissue and peripheral blood of Hashimoto's patients

Donor	Thyroid Autoantibody	Specific Activity (Reciprocal Titer per 10 mg/ml IgG)		
		Serum IgG	IgG in Culture −PWM	IgG in Culture +PWM
Thyroid Lymphocytes				
JH	Thyroglobulin	2,560	3,200	1,450
DJ	Microsomal	25,600	49,800	23,200
MS	Microsomal	204,800	198,000	106,000
Peripheral Blood Lymphocytes				
CD	Thyroglobulin	32,000	Undetectable	9,200
GB	Thyroglobulin	64,000	Undetectable	700
MF	Thyroglobulin	128,000	Not determined	11,050
MS	Microsomal	204,800	129,000	61,500
MT	Thyroglobulin	256,000	Undetectable	3,190

on the thyroid, generally by interfering with the synthesis and/or release of thyroid hormones and including carbimazole, propylthiouracil, iodides, lithium, perchlorate, and thiocyanate; and (2) thyroid ablation by subtotal thyroidectomy or using radioactive iodine (summarized in Ref. 160). Hashimoto's thyroiditis is normally treated with a replacement dose of thyroxine but in a few cases thyroidectomy is required (165). Many of these forms of therapy are accompanied by changes in thyroid autoantibodies.

Ablation of the thyroid by ^{131}I is commonly used to treat older Graves' patients (160). During the 3 months following therapy a transient rise in thyroid autoantibodies has been observed for TSH-receptor antibodies (166) and for TSH-receptor antibodies and microsomal antibodies (167). It has been suggested that the release of thyroid antigens following damage to the thyroid might be responsible for this rise in autoantibodies (166). The possibility that irradiation could affect the autoimmune response was explored using the culture system described for thyroid autoantibody synthesis (168). Previous work on irradiation of normal PBL had shown that this treatment destroys B lymphocytes; however, coculture of equal proportions of irra-

diated and untreated autologous cells resulted in a considerable increase in total immunoglobulin synthesis, since helper T cells (unlike suppressor T lymphocytes) are radiation resistant (169, 170). McGregor et al. (168) confirmed that irradiation of Hashimoto's B cells prevented their development into thyroid autoantibody secreting cells and further showed that untreated Hashimoto's PBL, cocultured with autologous PBL exposed to 2000 to 3000 rads, synthesized increased amounts of total IgG and microsomal or thyroglobulin autoantibodies in PWM stimulated cultures.

It seems possible, therefore, that following localization of ^{131}I in the thyroid, B cells and suppressor cells in that area are destroyed by the radiation. When the thyroid tissue is repopulated by circulating lymphocytes, antigen-specific B cells, provided with an excess of helper T cells, are stimulated to synthesize large amounts of thyroid autoantibodies. The role of antigen in this process is uncertain; however, the in vitro studies indicated that stimulation of autoantibody synthesis can occur in the absence of antigen. It might be argued that the levels of irradiation in the thyroid in a patient exposed to 15 millicuries of ^{131}I are in excess of the amounts required to destroy helper T cell activity as well as the suppressor subsets. Although the thyroid appears to be a major site of autoantibody synthesis (as seems likely from the evidence put forward in Section 3.3), thyroid autoantibodies may well be produced in other lymphoid organs such as the spleen and bone marrow (171). The destruction by radiation of all T cells is likely to be confined to the thyroid but cells in the peripheral circulation are exposed to lower doses, including the range over which suppressor cell activity is lost and the helper element remains intact. The increased availability of helper cells, possibly in association with autoantigen, could result in a transient increase in synthesis of thyroid autoantibodies in the bone marrow or spleen which then appear transiently in the serum.

The reduction of lymphocytic infiltration in the thyroid of Graves' patients treated with antithyroid drugs has already been referred to (161); it seems likely that this reduction was responsible for the low yield of lymphoid cells from Graves' thyroid tissue obtained at operation from patients treated with carbimazole (Section 3.3). It was also observed that these lymphocyte suspensions generally synthesized very small amounts of total IgG. In some Graves' patients treated with methimazole, a decrease in TSH-receptor antibodies was observed (166). Similarly, carbimazole therapy was associated with a fall both in TSH-receptor antibody and microsomal antibody in Graves' and Hashimoto's patients (172, 173), but not in patients treated with the β-receptor blocker propranolol (173). Using our in vitro system the effect of methimazole (the active metabolite of carbimazole) on synthesis of total IgG and thyroid autoantibodies by PBL from Hashimoto's patients was investigated. Carbimazole at a concentration of 10^{-4} M inhibited IgG and thyroglobulin/microsomal antibody synthesis without affecting the viability of cells cultured for 14 days; at higher concentrations the drug was clearly cytotoxic for PBL. In contrast, propranolol over the same concentration range had little effect or slightly stimulated immunoglobulin synthesis (173). Plaque assays

have also been used to study the effects of methimazole and propylthiouracil, and similar decreases in total IgG and thyroglobulin antibody synthesis were observed in Hashimoto's lymphocytes cultured for 6 days in the presence of the drugs (174). These data suggest that carbimazole has a general immunosuppressive effect on immunoglobulin production by human PBL. However, since carbimazole is concentrated in the thyroid (175) it seems likely that this form of therapy may have a specific immunosuppressive effect on thyroid autoantibody synthesis.

Partial thyroidectomy in Graves' patients is frequently associated with clinical improvement and surgery is the treatment of choice in some patients (160). Removal of the thyroid is also associated with a gradual decrease in the level of TSH-receptor antibodies as might have been anticipated if the thyroid is not only a source of antigen but also a major site of thyroid autoantibody synthesis. In some patients, a sharp short-lived increase in the level of thyroid autoantibody is observed a few days after surgery; thereafter values return to preoperative levels and fall slowly over a period of months.

Plasmapheresis has been used to treat a patient with acute exophthalmic Graves' disease; a decrease in the level of TSH-receptor antibodies coincided with clinical improvement, but after a period of 9 weeks the symptoms reappeared and plasmapheresis in association with immunosuppressive drugs was used to control the disease (177). It would appear that, as in myasthenia gravis (178), plasmapheresis may be of benefit in the treatment of acute cases but long-term plasmapheresis without the use of immunosuppressive drugs has no advantage over drugs alone.

5. CONCLUSIONS

Studies of thyroid autoantibody synthesis *in vitro* have been used to elucidate some of the immunological changes observed in Graves' patients undergoing treatment. It is likely that the *in vitro* system can be used to develop immunospecific forms of therapy for Graves' and Hashimoto's diseases perhaps based on toxins conjugated to thyroid autoantigens or linked to anti-idiotype antibodies. Further it should be possible to use the system to dissect the processes involved in the development of the autoimmune response to thyroid antigens in man.

REFERENCES

1. D. D. Adams and H. D. Purves, *Proc. Univ. Otago Med. Sch.* **34**, 11–12 (1965).

2. G. Fayet, B. Verrier, A. Giraud, S. Lissitsky, A. Pinchera, J. H. Romaldini, and G. Fenzi, *FEBS Lett.* **32**, 299–302 (1973).

3. S. W. Manley, J. R. Bourke, and R. W. Hawker, *J. Endocrinol.* **61**, 437–445 (1974).

4. S. Q. Mehdi and S. S. Nussey, *Biochem. J.* **145**, 105–111 (1975).

5. B. R. Smith and R. Hall, *Lancet* **2**, 427–431 (1974).

6. E. D. Mukhtar, B. Rees Smith, G. A. Pyle, R. Hall, and P. Vice, *Lancet* **1**, 713–715 (1975).

7. R. Clague, E. D. Mukhtar, G. A. Pyle, J. Nutt, F. Clark, M. Scott, D. Evered, B. Rees Smith, and R. Hall, *J. Clin. Endocrinol. Metab.* **43**, 550–556. (1976).

8. B. Rees Smith, in R. J. Lefkowitz, Ed., *Receptors and Recognition, Series B: Receptor Regulation*, Vol. 13, Chapman & Hall, London, 1981, pp. 217–244.

9. I. M. Roitt, D. Doniach, P. N. Campbell, and R. V. Hudson, *Lancet* **2**, 820–821 (1956).

10. G. Belyavin and W. R. Trotter, *Lancet* **2**, 648–652 (1959).

11. J. M. McKenzie, *J. Biol. Chem.* **237**, PC 3571–3572 (1962).

12. G. Torrigiani, I. M. Roitt, and D. Doniach, *Clin. Exp. Immunol.* **3**, 621–630 (1968).

13. H. A. Drexhage, G. F. Bottazzo, D. Doniach, L. Bitensky, and J. Chayen, *Lancet* **2**, 287–292 (1980).

14. K. F. R. Schiller, G. H. Spray, A. G. Wangel, and R. Wright, in C. Cassano and M. Andreoli, Eds., *Current Topics in Thyroid Research*, Proceedings of the 5th International Thyroid Conference, Academic Press, New York, 1965.

15. M. M. B. Kay, *Mech. Age. Dev.* **9**, 39–59 (1979).

16. J. K. Portaro, G. I. Glick, and J. Zighelboim,

Clin. Immunol. Immunopathol. **11**, 339–345 (1978).

17. R. Michalevicz, A. Many, and B. Ramot, *Acta Heamatol.* **57**, 199–205 (1977).

18. D. A. Horwitz and M. A. Garret, *Clin. Exp. Immunol.* **27**, 92–99 (1977).

19. P. D. Utsinger and W. J. Yount, *J. Clin. Invest.* **60**, 626–638 (1977).

20. A. J. Strelkauskas, T. Callery, J. McDowell, Y. Borel, and S. F. Schlossman, *Proc. Natl. Acad. Sci. USA* **75**, 5150–5154 (1978).

21. D. Alarcón-Segovia and A. Ruiz-Argüelles, *J. Clin. Invest.* **62**, 1390–1394 (1978).

22. S. Fauci, A. D. Steinberg, B. F. Haynes, and G. Whalen, *J. Immunol.* **121**, 1473–1479 (1978).

23. M. E. Hamilton and J. B. Winfield, *Arthritis Rheum.* **22**, 1–6 (1979).

24. K. Matsumoto, K. Osakabe, H. Ohi, N. Yoshizawa, M. Harada, and M. Hatano, *Scand. J. Immunol.* **11**, 187–193 (1980).

25. H. Fujiwara, M. Torisu, Y. Koitabashi, T. Baba, and H. Esak, *Clin. Immunol. Immunopathol.* **19**, 98–108 (1981).

26. R. M. Cass, E. S. Mongan, R. F. Jacox, and J. H. Vaughan, *Ann. Int. Med.* **69**, 649–656 (1968).

27. D. Glass and P. H. Schur, in N. Talal, Ed., *Autoimmunity. Genetic, Immunologic, Virologic and Clinical Aspects*, Academic Press, New York, (1977), pp. 532–568.

28. D. Brohee, G, Delespesse, M. J. Debisschop, and M. Bonnyns, *Clin. Exp. Immunol.* **36**, 379–383 (1979).

29. K. S. K. Tung, R. J. DeHoratius, and R. C. Williams, *Clin. Exp. Immunol.* **43**, 615–625 (1981).

30. L. J. De Groot and S. Jaksina, *J. Clin. Endocrinol.* **29**, 207–212 (1969).

31. S. J. Urbaniak, W. J. Penhale, and W. J. Irvine, *Clin. Exp. Immunol.* **18**, 449–459 (1974).

32. C. Mulaisho, N. I. Abdou, and R. D. Utiger, *J. Clin. Endocrinol. Metab.* **41**, 266–270 (1975).

33. R. Volpé and V. V. Row, *N. Engl. J. Med.* **293**, 44 (1975).

34. E. A. Calder, W. J. Irvine, N. McD. Davidson, and F. Wu, *Clin. Exp. Immunol.* **25**, 17–22 (1976).

35. K. Hackenberg, E. Cohnen, and D. Reinwein, *Klin. Wochenschr.* **54**, 987–993 (1976).

36. G. Lundell, J. Wasserman, P. O. Granberg, and H. Blomgren, *Clin. Exp. Immunol.* **23**, 33–39 (1976).

37. C. C. S. Hsu, Y. Chen, and R. Paterson, *Clin. Exp. Immunol.* **26**, 431–440 (1976).

38. E. P. Noel, J. M. Barnard, and N. R. Farid, *IRCS Med. Sci.* **5**, 180 (1977).

39. T. Sakane, A. Steinberg, and I. Green, *Arthritis Rheum.* **21**, 657–664 (1978).

40. S. Horowitz, W. Borcherding, A. V. Moorthy, R. Chesney, H. Schulte-Wisserman, R. Hong, and A. Goldstein, *Science* **197**, 999–1001 (1977).

41. B. Newman, S. Blank, R. Lomnitzer, P. Disler, and A. R. Rabson, *Clin. Immunol. Immunopathol.* **13**, 187–193 (1979).

42. D. B. Kaufman and E. Bostwick, *Clin. Immunol. Immunopathol.* **13**, 9–18 (1979).

43. C. Morimoto, *Clin. Exp. Immunol.* **32**, 125–133 (1978).

44. N. I. Abdou, A. Sagawa, E. Pascual, J. Hebert, and S. Sadeghee, *Clin. Immunol. Immunopathol.* **6**, 192–199 (1976).

45. H. Mori, N. Amino, Y. Iwatani, O. Kabutomori, S. Asari, S. Motoi, K. Miyai, and Y. Kumahara, *Clin. Exp. Immunol.* **42**, 33–40 (1980).

46. D. R. Budman, E. B. Marchant, A. D. Steinberg, B. Doft, M. E. Gershwin, E. Lizzio, and J. Patton Reeves, *Arthritis Rheum.* **20**, 829–833 (1977).

47. K. M. Nies and J. S. Louie, *Arthritis Rheum.* **21**, 51–57 (1978).

48. K. Okudaira, K. Tanimoto, T. Nakamura, and Y. Horiuchi, *Clin. Immunol. Immunopathol.* **16**, 267–278 (1980).

49. A. M. Bobrove, *Arthritis Rheum.* **19**, 790 (1976).

50. W. W. Ginsburg, F. D. Finkelman, and P. E. Lipsky, *Clin. Exp. Immunol.* **35**, 76–88 (1979).

51. A. I. Levinson, A. Dziarski, R. Pincus, R. J. De Horatius, and B. Zweiman, *J. Clin. Lab. Immunol.* **5**, 17–22 (1981).

52. M. Barr, W. W. Buchanan, D. Doniach, and I. M. Roitt, *Scott. Med. J.* **9**, 295–298 (1964).

53. E. R. Hurd, W. Dowdle, H. Casey, and M. Ziff, *Arthritis Rheum.* **15**, 267–274 (1972).

54. D. Stancek and J. Rovensky, *Acta Virol.* **23**, 168–169 (1979).

55. R. W. Luxton and R. T. Cooke, *Lancet* **2**, 105–109 (1956).

56. N. Aoki, K. M. Pinnamaneni, and L. J. DeGroot, *J. Clin. Endocrinol. Metab.* **48**, 803–810 (1979).

57. C. Thielemans, L. Vanhaelst, M. De Waele, M. Jonckheer, and B. Van Camp, *Clin. Endocrinol.* **15**, 259–263 (1981).

58. V. Sridama, F. Pacini, and L. De Groot, *Ann. d'Endocrinol.* t. **42**, 29A (1981).

59. E. L. Reinherz, C. Morimoto, A. C. Penda, and S. F. Schlossman, *Eur. J. Immunol.* **10**, 570–572 (1980).

60. Y. Thomas, L. Rogozinski, O. H. Irigoyen, S. M. Friedman, P. C. Kung, G. Goldstein, and L. Chess, *J. Exp. Med.* **154**, 459–467 (1981).

61. G. Delespesse, J. Duchateau, H. Collet, A. Go-vaerts, and P. A. Bastenie, *Clin. Exp. Immunol.* **12**, 439–445 (1972).

62. R. R. Lycette and G. E. Pearmain, *N. Z. Med. J.* **64**, 81–82 (1965).

63. E. N. Ehrenfeld, E. Klein, and D. Benezra, *J. Clin. Endocrinol.* **32**, 115–116 (1971).

64. E. A. Calder and W. J. Irvine, *Clin. Endocrinol. Metab.* **4**, 287–318 (1975).

65. N. Aoki and J. De Groot, *Clin. Exp. Immunol.* **38**, 523–530 (1979).

66. H. Blomgren and G. Lundell, *Acta Endocrinol.* **90**, 227–232 (1979).

67. J. R. Wall, S. L. Fang, S. H. Ingbar, and L. E. Braverman, *J. Clin. Endocrinol. Metab.* **43**, 587–590 (1976).

68. A. Galluzo, C. Filardo, C. Giordano, G. Sparacino, and G. D. Bompiani, *J. Endocrinol. Invest.* **4**, 173–176 (1981).

69. T. Makinen, G. Wagar, L. Apter, E. von Willebrand, and F. Pekonen, *Nature* **275**, 314–315 (1978).

70. B. Wenzel, K. W. Wenzel, P. Kotulla, and H. Schleusener, in J. R. Stockigt and S. Nagataki, Eds., *Thyroid Research VIII*, 8th International Thyroid Congress, Pergamon, Elmsford, N.Y., 1980, pp. 785–788.

71. O. Chabaud and S. Lissitzky, *Mol. Cell Endocrinol.* **7**, 79–87 (1977).

72. J. Brostoff, *Proc. Roy. Soc. Med.* **63**, 905–906 (1970).

73. E. A. Calder, D. McLemen, E. W. Barnes, and W. J. Irvine, *Clin. Exp. Immunol.* **12**, 429–438 (1972).

74. G. Delespesse, J. Duchateau, B. Kennes, A. Govaerts, and P. A. Bastenie, *Hormone Metab. Res.* **5**, 176–179 (1973).

75. K. Ikekubo, *Folia Endocrinol. Jap.* **51**, 840–855 (1975).

76. J. Wartzenberg, D. Doniach, J. Brostoff, and I. M. Roitt, *Int. Arch. Allergy Appl. Immunol.* **44**, 396–408 (1973).

77. M. Søberg and P. Hallberg, *Proc. Roy. Soc. Med.* **63**, 903–905 (1968).

78. L. Lamki, V. V. Row, and R. Volpé, *J. Clin. Endocrinol. Metab.* **36**, 358–364 (1973).

79. N. Amino and L. De Groot, *Metabolism* **24**, 45–56 (1975).

80. T. H. Totterman, T. Makinen, and A. Gordin, *Acta Endocrinol.* **86**, 89–98 (1977).

81. T. H. Totterman, L. C. Anderson, and P. Hayry, *Clin. Endocrinol.* **11**, 59–68 (1979).

82. N. Okita, A. Kidd, V. V. Row, and R. Volpé, *J. Clin. Endocrinol. Metab.* **51**, 316–320 (1980).

83. N. Okita, V. V. Row, and R. Volpé, *J. Clin. Endocrinol. Metab.* **52**, 528–533 (1981).

84. A. C. Allison and A. M. Denman, *Br. Med. Bull.* **32**, 124–129 (1976).

85. R. Volpé, *Clin. Endocrinol. Metab.* **7**, 3–29 (1978).

86. W. K. Podlewski, *Clin. Exp. Immunol.* **11**, 543–548 (1972).

87. E. A. Calder, W. J. Penhale, E. W. Barnes, and W. J. Irvine, *Clin. Exp. Immunol.* **14**, 19–23 (1973).

88. E. A. Calder, D. McLeman, and W. J. Irvine, *Clin. Exp. Immunol.* **15**, 467–470 (1973).

89. A. C. Allison, in N. Talal, Ed., *Autoimmunity. Genetic, Immunologic and Clinical Aspects*, Academic Press, New York, 1977, pp. 91–139.

90. A. E. Kalderon and H. A. Bogaars, *Am. J. Med.* **63**, 729–734 (1977).

91. H. Fujiwara, M. Torisu, T. Sugisaki, and H. Okano, *Clin. Immunol. Immunopathol.* **19**, 109–117 (1981).

92. A. C. Allison, in D. H. Katz and B. Benacerraf, Eds., *Immunological Tolerance*, Academic Press, New York, 1974, pp. 25–55.

93. R. C. Mellors, W. J. Brzosko, and L. S. Sonkin, *Am. J. Pathol.* **41**, 425–437 (1962).

94. A. D. Bankhurst, G. Torrigiani, and A. C. Allison, *Lancet* **1**, 226–230 (1973).

95. G. B. Salabé, H. Salabé, L. Acinni, and R. Dominisi, *Clin. Exp. Immunol.* **32**, 159–168 (1978).

96. B. A. K. Khalid, N. T. Hamilton, and M. N. Cauchi, *Clin. Exp. Immunol.* **23**, 28–32 (1976).

97. S. J. Urbaniak, W. J. Penhale, and W. J. Irvine, *Clin. Exp. Immunol.* **15**, 345–354 (1973).

98. T. H. Totterman, *Clin. Immunol. Immunopathol.* **10**, 270–277 (1978).

99. S. M. McLachlan, B. Rees Smith, V. B. Petersen, T. F. Davies, and R. Hall, *Nature* **270**, 447–449 (1977).

100. S. M. McLachlan, B. Rees Smith, V. B. Petersen, T. F. Davies, and R. Hall, *J. Clin. Lab. Immunol.* **1**, 45–50 (1978).

101. A. McGregor, S. M. McLachlan, F. Clark, B. Rees Smith, and R. Hall, *Immunology* **36**, 81–85 (1979).

102. G. Brown and M. F. Greaves, *Scand. J. Immunol.* **3**, 161–172 (1974).

103. L. Y. F. Wu, A.R. Lawton, and M. D. Cooper, *J. Clin. Invest.* **52**, 3180–3189 (1973).

104. G. Janossy, E. Gomez de la Concha, M. J. Waxdal, and T. Platts-Mills, *Clin. Exp. Immunol.* **26**, 108–117 (1976).

105. J. Marbrook, *Lancet* **2**, 1279–1281 (1967).

106. R. M. Maizels and D. W. Dresser, *Immunology* **32**, 793–801 (1977).

107. L. Wide, S. J. Nillius, O. Gemzell, and P. Roos, *Acta Endocrinol. Suppl.* **174**, 1–58 (1974).

108. S. M. McLachlan, B. Rees Smith, and R. Hall, *J. Immunol. Meth.* **21**, 211–216 (1977).

109. L. Bitensky, J. Alaghband-Zadeh, and J. Chayen, *Clin. Endocrinol.* **3**, 363–374 (1974).

110. T. Bird and J. Stephenson, *J. Clin. Pathol.* **26**, 623–627 (1973).

111. N. Amino, S. R. Hagen, N. Yamada, and S. Refetoff, *Clin. Endocrinol.* **5**, 115–125 (1976).

112. I. Cayzer, S. R. Chalmers, D. Doniach, and G. Swana, *J. Clin. Pathol.* **31**, 1147–1151 (1978).

113. S. M. McLachlan, A. G. Bird, A. P. Weetman, B. Rees Smith, and R. Hall, *Scand. J. Immunol.* **14**, 233–242 (1981).

114. P. E. Lipsky, W. W. Ginsburg, F. D. Finkelman, and M. Ziff, *J. Immunol.* **120**, 902–910 (1978).

115. Y. Weinstein and K. L. Melmon, *Immunol. Commun.* **5**, 401–416 (1976).

116. V. Petersen, B. Rees Smith, and R. Hall, *J. Clin. Endocrinol. Metab.* **41**, 199–202 (1975).

117. J. M. McKenzie and J. Gordon, in C. Cassano and M. Andreoli, Eds., *Current Topics in Thyroid Research*, Proceedings of the 5th International Thyroid Conference, Academic Press, New York, 1965, pp. 445–454.

118. K. Miyai, M. Fukuchi, U. Kumahara, and H. Abe, *J. Clin. Endocrinol. Metab.* **27**, 855–860 (1967).

119. J. R. Wall, B. F. Good, I. J. Forbes, and B. S. Hetzel, *Clin. Exp. Immunol.* **4**, 555–561 (1973).

120. A. J. S. Knox, C. von Westarp, V. V. Row, and R. Volpé, *Metabolism* **25**, 1217–1223 (1976).

121. A. J. S. Knox, C. von Westarp, V. V. Row, and R. Volpé, *J. Clin. Endocrinol. Metab.* **43**, 330–337 (1976).

122. B. Rapoport, R. J. Pillarisetty, E. A. Herman, O. H. Clark, and E. G. Congco, *J. Biol. Chem.* **253**, 631–640 (1978).

123. B. Rapoport, R. J. Pillarisetty, E. A. Herman, and E. G. Congco, *Biochem. Biophys, Res. Commun.* **77**, 1245–1250 (1977).

124. M. Yamamoto, E. A. Herman, and B. Rapoport, *J. Biol. Chem.* **254**, 4046–4051 (1979).

125. J. S. Goodwin, A. D. Bankhurst, and R. P. Messner, *J. Exp. Med.* **146**, 1719–1733 (1977).

126. E. A. Herman, R. J. Pillarisetty, and B. Rapoport, *J. Biol. Chem.* **25**, 641–644 (1978).

127. D. Doniach, G. F. Bottazzo, and R. C. G. Russell, *Clin. Endocrinol. Metab.* **8**, 63–79 (1979).

128. C. W. Parker, *N. Engl. J. Med.* **295**, 1183–1186 (1976).

129. O. Ringden and B. Rynnel-Dagoo, *Eur. J. Immunol.* **8**, 47 (1978).

130. S. Nishikawa, T. Hirata, T. Nagai, M. Mayumi, and T. Izumi, *J. Immunol.* **122**, 2143–2149 (1979).

131. A. G. Bird and S. Britton, *Immunol. Rev.* **45**, 41–67 (1979).

132. I. Weiss and T. F. Davies, *J. Clin. Endocrinol. Metab.* **53**, 1223–1228 (1981).

133. G. N. Beall and S. R. Kruger, *Clin. Immunol. Immunopathol.* **16**, 485–497 (1980).

134. A. Saxon, R. H. Stevens, and R. F. Ashman, *J. Immunol.* **118**, 1872–1879 (1977).

135. G. N. Beall and S. R. Kruger, *Clin. Immunol. Immunopathol.* **16**, 498–503 (1980).

136. S. M. McLachlan, S. L. Wee, A. M. McGregor, B. Rees Smith, and R. Hall, *J. Clin. Lab. Immunol.* **3**, 15–21 (1980).

137. T. A. Waldmann, S. Broder, R. M. Blaese, M. Blackman, and W. Strober, *Lancet* **2**, 609–613 (1974).

138. F. P. Siegal, M. Siegal, and R. A. Good, *J. Clin. Invest.* **58**, 109–122 (1976).

139. T. Uchiyama, K. Sagawa, K. Takatsuki, and H. Uchino, *Clin. Immunol. Immunopathol.* **10**, 24–34 (1978).

140. G. N. Beall and S. R. Kruger, *J. Clin. Endocrinol. Metab.* **48**, 712–714 (1979).

141. C. Morimoto, T. Abe, M. Hara, and M. Homma, *Scand. J. Immunol.* **6**, 575–579 (1977).

142. W. J. Penhale, W. J. Irvine, J. R. Inglis, and A. Farmer, *Clin. Exp. Immunol.* **25**, 6–16 (1976).

143. J. G. Knight and D. D. Adams, *J. Clin. Lab. Immunol.* **1**, 151–158 (1978).

144. R. H. Stevens, *J. Immunol.* **127**, 968–972 (1981).

145. R. H. Stevens and A. Saxon, *J. Clin. Invest.* **62**, 1154–1160 (1978).

146. R. H. Stevens and A. Saxon, *Cell. Immunol.* **45**, 142–150 (1979).

147. R. E. Callard, *Nature* **282**, 734–736 (1979).

148. D. J. Moss, A. B. Rickinson, and J. H. Pope, *Int. J. Cancer* **22**, 662–668 (1978).

149. A. G. Bird, S. M. McLachlan, and S. Britton, *Nature* **289**, 300–301 (1981).

150. R. N. P. Sutton, R. T. D. Edmond, D. B. Thomas, and D. Doniach, *Clin. Exp. Immunol.* **17**, 427–436 (1974).

151. G. Henle, W. Henle, and V. Diehl, *Proc. Natl. Acad. Sci.* **59**, 94–101 (1968).

152. S. Izui, R. A. Eisenberg, and F. J. Dixon, *J. Immunol.* **122**, 2096–2102 (1979).

153. L. Slaughter, D. A. Carson, F. C. Jensen, T. L. Holbrook, and J. H. Vaughan, *J. Exp. Med.* **148**, 1429–1434 (1978).

154. S. Fong, C. D. Tsoukas, L. A. Frincke, S. K. Lawrence, T. L. Holbrook, J. H. Vaughan, and D. A. Carson, *J. Immunol.* **126**, 910–914 (1981).

155. P. Heimann, *Acta Endocrinol.* **53** (Suppl. 110), 1–102 (1966).

156. A. Biorklund and N. Söderstrom, *Acta Otolaryngol.* **82**, 204–207 (1976).

157. N. Söderstrom and A. Biorklund, *Scand. J. Immunol.* **3**, 295–302 (1974).

158. S. B. Salabé, C. Davoli, and M. Andreoli, *Int. Arch. Allergy Appl. Immunol.* **47**, 63–79 (1974).

159. S. M. McLachlan, A. McGregor, B. Rees Smith, and R. Hall, *Lancet* **1**, 162–163 (1979).

160. L. E. Braverman, *Clin. Endocrinol. Metab.* **7**, 221–240 (1978).

161. J. Swanson Beck, J. R. Young, J. G. Simpson, E. S. Gray, A. G. Nicol, C. A. S. Pegg, and W. Michie, *Br. J. Surg.* **60**, 679–771 (1973).

162. L. Moretta, M. C. Mingari, A. Moretta, and M. D. Cooper, *J. Immunol.* **122**, 984–990 (1979).

163. R. H. Stevens, E. Macy, C. Morrow, and A. Saxon, *J. Immunol.* **122**, 2498–3404 (1979).

164. U. Andersson, G. Bird, and S. Britton, *Immunol. Rev.* **57**, 5–38 (1981).

165. D. Doniach, *Clin. Endocrinol. Metab.* **4**, 267–285 (1975).

166. A. Pinchera, P. Liberti, E. Martino, G. F. Fenzi, L. Grasso, L. Rovis, and L. Baschieri, *J. Clin. Endocrinol. Metab.* **29**, 231–238 (1969).

167. A. M. McGregor, M. M. Petersen, R. Capiferri, D. C. Evered, B. Rees Smith, and R. Hall, *Clin. Endocrinol.* **11**, 437–444 (1979).

168. A. M. McGregor, S. M. McLachlan, B. Rees Smith, and R. Hall, *Lancet* **2**, 432–444 (1979).

169. F. P. Siegal and M. Siegal, *J. Immunol.* **118**, 642–647 (1977).

170. A. S. Fauci, K. R. Pratt, and G. Whalen, *Immunology* **35**, 715–720 (1978).

171. R. Benner, W. Hijmans, and J. J. Haaijman, *Clin. Exp. Immunol.* **46**, 1–8 (1981).

172. A. M. McGregor, M. M. Petersen, S. M. McLachlan, P. Rooke, B. Rees Smith, and R. Hall, *N. Engl. J. Med.* **303**, 302–307 (1980).

173. A. M. McGregor, H. K. Ibbertson, B. Rees Smith, and R. Hall, *Br. Med. J.* **281**, 968–969 (1980).

174. I. Weiss and T. F. Davies, *J. Clin. Endocrinol. Metab.*, **54**, 282–285 (1982).

175. B. Marchant, W. D. Alexander, J. H. Lazarus, J. Lees, and D. H. Clark, *J. Clin. Endocrinol.* **34**, 847–851 (1972).

176. A. M. McGregor, M. M. Petersen, S. M. McLachlan, B. Rees Smith, and R. Hall, *J. Mol. Med.* **4**, 119–127 (1980).

177. P. Dandona, N. J. Marshall, S. P. Bidey, A. Nathan, and C. W. H. Havard, *Br. Med. J.* **1**, 374–376 (1979).

178. J. Newsom-Davis, S. G. Wilson, A. Vincent, and C. D. Ward, *Lancet* **1**, 464–468 (1979).

8

The Spectrum of Islet Cell Antibodies

George K. Papadopoulos
Åke Lernmark

Hagedorn Research Laboratory
Gentofte, Denmark

Contents

1. INTRODUCTION

Antibodies reactive with a variety of cellular antigens are often found in disorders of au-toimmune character. A high incidence of antibodies against the pancreatic islet cells seems to be associated with insulin-dependent (or type 1) diabetes (1, 2). Insulin-dependent diabetes (IDD), which is not restricted to onset in childhood or adolescence, is designated (3, 4) based on its association with certain HLA antigens, autoimmune features, presence of islet cell antibodies, and insulin dependence. We have abandoned the term juvenile diabetes and instead refer to insulin-dependent diabetes (IDD) throughout this chapter.

Noninsulin-dependent (type 2) diabetes (NIDD), formerly called maturity onset diabetes, appears to represent a different set of disorders. NIDD presents a heterogeneous set of disorders and is strongly associated with obesity, onset at maturity, and absence of ketone bodies despite hyperglycemia.

The presence of islet cell antibodies in IDD offers new means by which to understand its etiology and pathogenesis. Evidence has accumulated in recent years suggesting that immune mechanisms may contribute to the development of IDD (Table 1). A variety of

Table 1.   Immune mechanisms in IDD

Humoral
Islet cell antibodies
    Cytoplasmic antibodies
    Cell surface antibodies
    Cytotoxic antibodies
    Immunoprecipitating antibodies
Other organ-specific autoantibodies

Cell-Mediated
Leukocyte migration inhibition by pancreatic
    antigens
Inflammatory infiltrates, insulitis, in the pan-
    creas of newly diagnosed diabetic children

phenomena, both humoral and cell mediated, have been observed. The different phenomena are most obvious in patients of recent diagnosis, at the time when the ability of the pancreatic β cells to release insulin to potent stimuli is markedly diminished (5, 6). This functional derangement is associated with a loss of β cells, representing a diminished volume to about 10 to 30% of normal (7, 8). The loss of β cells at the time of diagnosis can be associated with the presence of inflammatory cells within the islets of Langerhans (9, 10). The process of β cell destruction is not known. IDD has long been known to be associated with autoimmune disorders such as Hashimoto's disease, Graves' disease, Addison's disease, or pernicious anemia. In analogy to the organ-specific antibodies present in these diseases it is of particular interest to determine the extent to which the appearance of islet cell antibodies signifies islet cell destructive processes. Autoantibodies against β cells may in addition interfere with cellular functions by binding to specific sites such as receptors or other effector structures on the surface of the cell. Destruction of β cells may also be caused by islet cell antibodies with a capacity to mediate immunocytolytic reactions such as complement-mediated cytotoxicity or antibody-dependent cellular cytotoxicity.

Pancreatic β cell destruction may result not only in stimulation of antibody production but also in formation of circulating immune complexes. The facets of autoimmunity in IDD have recently been reviewed (11–13). It is not known how immunologic mechanisms against self are induced and result in a specific disease or disorder. We review the spectrum of islet cell antibodies and speculate about their possible relevance to the pathogenesis of IDD.

2. ISLET CELL ANTIBODIES IN DIABETES MELLITUS

The spectrum of islet cell antibodies in IDD encompasses several types of molecules with differing antigen specificities and other immunoreactive properties. Thus the antibodies from the sera of newly diagnosed IDD patients react with antigen(s) in the islet cell cytoplasm or on the cell membrane. Furthermore, both types of antibody can fix complement and hence participate in a cytotoxic reaction. Finally, sera of newly diagnosed IDD patients have been shown to immunoprecipitate antigens from human islet cells. We treat each category of antibodies separately, according to the immune phenomena they exhibit, even though some of the antibodies may participate in more than one type of immune reaction. The putative antibodies in the circulating immune complexes found in many newly diagnosed IDD patients (14) have not been sufficiently characterized; therefore we do not deal with them here.

2.1.   Cytoplasmic Antibodies

Cytoplasmic antibodies to pancreatic islet cells were first discovered in the sera of IDD patients suffering from polyendocrine autoimmune disorders (15, 16). Frozen sections of human pancreatic tissue (from blood type O kidney donors to prevent interference from isoagglutinins) were incubated with sera from IDD patients and antihuman fluorescently labeled IgG. The fluorescence from such sections appeared only within the endocrine portion of the gland, but was not originating exclusively from the β cells. On the contrary, it appears that the cytoplasmic antigen(s) is shared by all four known types of pancreatic endocrine cells (i.e., producers of insulin, glucagon, somatostatin, and pancreatic polypeptide) (1). In addition, the cytoplasmic islet cell antibodies cannot be absorbed by insulin, glucagon, or somatostatin (1).

At the time of onset of IDD, cytoplasmic islet cell antibodies are found in the sera of approximately 90% of the patients (17) (Fig. 1). However, in most cases these antibodies are evanescent and tend to disappear within a year after onset, so that only 20% of the patients show such antibodies 3 years hence (17). By contrast, patients that suffer from endocrine autoimmune disorders demonstrate stable titers of cytoplasmic islet cell antibodies several years after the onset of IDD (18, 19).

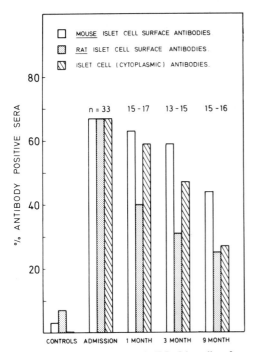

Figure 1. Islet cell antibodies in IDD. Islet cell surface antibodies were determined by an indirect immunofluorescence test on suspensions of either mouse or rat islet cells. Islet cell cytoplasmic antibodies were determined by indirect immunofluorescence on frozen sections of a human pancreas. The number of patient sera analyzed are indicated along with the results in analyzing sera from 74 healthy controls.

It appears that most of these patients belong to families in which several members suffer from autoimmune endocrinopathies. Bottazzo et al. (1) cite one case in which the sibling of a diabetic child from a "polyendocrine family" was regularly monitored for cytoplasmic islet cell antibodies. The antibodies were present at least 7 months before onset and could still be detected 1 year after the onset, showing apparently the same immunofluorescent intensity against pancreatic sections.

Approximately 55% of the positive islet cell antibody sera are capable of fixing complement (1, 20). It is also apparent that not all the IgG subclasses are represented in the cytoplasmic islet cell antibodies (21). Specifically, in some sera there may be islet cell antibodies in the IgG_2 subclass while the IgG_3 and IgG_4 may not be present at all (21). Thus the complement-fixing ability of a portion of the islet cell antibodies from a given serum may only reflect the fact that particular subclasses of IgG are synthesized that can bind to C3b. In order to study this one would have to examine the origins of these subclasses from individual clones of B lymphocyte subsets (see Section 4).

The islet cell antibodies, whether complement fixing or otherwise, do not appear to contribute to the pathogenesis of IDD since they are not specific to β cells and cannot conceivably damage such cells if they were solely directed against a cytoplasmic antigen. Cytoplasmic islet cell antibodies have been detected also in some patients where the onset of IDD was preceded by a viral infection (Coxsackie B, mumps, influenza) (1, 22). Since only a minute fraction of newly diagnosed diabetics shows direct association with viral infection, the significance of the cytoplasmic islet cell antibodies in such cases must remain in doubt. In summary, the absence of β cell specificity from the cytoplasmic islet cell antibodies leads us to conclude at present that such antibodies are probably an epiphenomenon, associated with the onset of IDD but not causative of the disease.

2.2. Islet Cell Surface Antibodies

Surface antibodies to pancreatic islet cells in IDD were demonstrated with dispersed islet cells from rats or mice by the indirect immunofluorescence test (23). Earlier attempts to demonstrate islet cell surface antibodies in IDD with human insulinoma cells (24) remain uncertain because the insulinoma cells did not produce insulin (25). When tested on living rodent islet cells positive sera resulted in a patchy cell-surface reaction which sometimes fused to form a continuous zone of fluorescence at the cell margin (23) (Fig. 2). Nonviable cells showed a bright cytoplasmic immunofluorescence which could be caused by exposing the cells to fresh plasma or serum.

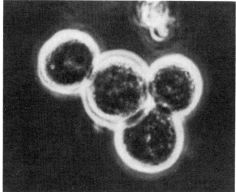
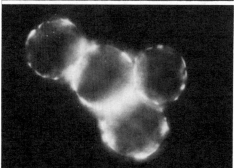

Figure 2. Islet cell surface antibodies demonstrated by indirect immunofluorescence on dispersed islet cells incubated in an antibody-positive serum sample. The upper part of the figure shows the appearance of the cells in the phase contrast microscope. The lower part of the figure shows the patchy immunofluorescent reaction on the cells. × 1800.

The indirect immunofluorescence technique for detecting islet cell surface antibodies is only semiquantitative. Using ^{125}I-protein A which detects surface-bound IgG, a quantitative and reproducible method for detecting surface antibodies in IDD was developed (26). However, it is not clear to what extent such antibodies react with the different endocrine islet cell types. The antibodies are likely to react with the β cells since rat or mouse islet cell suspensions are composed of 60 to 90% β cells and since positive sera induced fluorescence on up to 75% of the cells (23). Evidence has also been presented that IDD sera can induce surface immunofluorescence on a monolayer culture of human fetal β cells (1, 27). Absorption experiments with a variety of cells and tissue powders suggested that the islet cell surface antibodies are organ specific but not species specific (23, 26).

Islet cell surface antibodies were present in 2 to 4% of control subjects (23, 28, 29) and in about 30% of patients with IDD (23). Prior to the initiation of insulin therapy more than 60% of IDD children had surface antibodies and the prevalence diminished with increasing duration of diabetes (28) (Fig. 1). The assays for cytoplasmic and surface antibodies did not yield concordant results (29), indicating that the antibodies may occur independently of one another. The use of both methods increased the prevalence of islet cell antibodies in IDD (28, 29). The existing knowledge of islet cell surface antibodies is incomplete, for example, with regard to antibody subclasses and antigenic specificity. It will be necessary to determine the variability and precision of the antibody assays before the rate of islet cell surface antibodies in the pathogenesis of IDD can be clearly understood.

2.3. Cytotoxic Antibodies

Antibodies bound to the surface of living cells are often recognized by components of the complement system. Binding of complement induces the complement cascade reaction leading to a proteolytic attack on the plasma membrane. The resulting lesion is expressed as an increased permeability to cations, influx of macromolecules, or loss of intracellular components. Complete lysis of the target cell may follow cell death. Whole sera from different species, including man, induce a prompt release of insulin, block K^+ accumulation, or increase the release of chromium-51 from pre-labeled β cells (30). These effects were prevented by heating (50 or 56°C for 30 minutes) and an extended series of experiments demonstrated that islet cells can activate complement via the alternative pathway (31). Care must, therefore, be taken in interpreting effects of complement-mediated cytotoxic phenomena. Recent studies with guinea pig serum as a source of complement indicate that islet cell (surface) antibodies in human serum can mediate cytotoxicity measured as an increase in chromium-51 release from labeled rat islet cells (32, 33), rat insulinoma cells (34, 35), or dispersed human islet cells (Soderstrum, personal communication). The complement-dependent cytotoxic effect of serum from a newly diagnosed diabetic patient relative to the serum concentration is shown in Figure 3. Cytotoxic islet cell antibodies correlated with islet cell surface but not with cytoplasmic antibodies (33). The viability of collagenase-isolated hamster islets decreased when kept in culture with complement and diabetic serum (36). Furthermore, in a similar system with rat islets, insulin release induced by glucose and theophylline was inhibited (37). Cytotoxic sera were mainly found among patients with a concomitant autoimmune disease. Islet cell cytotoxic antibodies need to be characterized in terms of immunoglobulin class, species, and cell specificity as well as prevalence in newly diagnosed diabetic patients and their relatives. It is difficult to ignore the possible pathogenic significance of cytotoxic islet cell antibodies in view of their in vitro biologic effects.

Antibodies reacting with antigens exposed on the surface of a cell may also be the target of natural killer cells (K cells). The K cell can be found among circulating monocytes

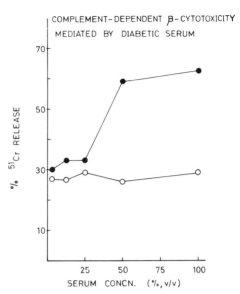

Figure 3.   Release of radioactive chromium in percent of total releasable radioactivity from prelabeled dispersed rat islet cells. The rat islet cells were first incubated with serum at various concentrations. After washing by centrifugation the cells were incubated with guinea pig serum as the source of complement and the amount of radioactivity released into the medium from damaged cells determined. The cells were exposed to serum from a healthy individual (○ ———— ○) or from a patient with newly diagnosed IDD (● ———— ●).

and possesses surface molecules capable of binding the constant portion of an antibody molecule. The attack of a killer cell, either as an armed cell with antibodies on its surface or against a target cell with a surface-bound antibody, is referred to as antibody-dependent cellular cytotoxicity. Serum from 1 out of 14 newly diagnosed insulin-dependent diabetic children was found to induce antibody-dependent cellular cytotoxicity against dispersed rat islet cells (Soderstrum, personal communication). Increased levels of K cells are found in early diabetes (38), but it is not clear to what extent this observation is relevant to the presumed destruction of β cells.

2.4.   Immunoprecipitating Antibodies

The limited availability of pancreatic islets hampers studies on cell specificity and subcellular distribution of the self-antigen targets of islet cell antibodies. Unlike other tissues, it is not known whether the pancreatic islet endocrine cells express cell-specific proteins. Such proteins may be target antigens in an autoaggressive reaction and perhaps explain the specific loss of the β cells in IDD. In recent experiments human pancreatic islets, isolated from kidney cadaver donors, were biosynthetically labeled with ^{35}S-methionine and solubilized in a detergent (39). The detergent lysate was subjected to immunoprecipitation with human serum and the labeled antigen in resulting immune complexes analyzed by slab-gel electrophoresis and autoradiography. Serum from 8 out of 10 newly diagnosed diabetic children immunoprecipitated a protein of molecular mass about 64,000. An additional protein (M_r 38,000) is also precipitated by some sera from labeled lysates of islets from an HLA-DR3 positive donor. None of these components was found in experiments with labeled human lymphocytes. Some sera of diabetic children also immunoprecipitated the 64,000 and 38,000 components from detergent lysates of labeled mouse or rat islets. Experiments are in progress to determine the cell specificity and subcellular location of these self-antigens.

3. EFFECTS OF ANTIBODIES ON THE β CELL FUNCTION

The blood glucose concentration in man is controlled by many hormonal responses. Insulin is the sole hormone to clearly effectuate a decrease in blood glucose, whereas an increase can be caused by the action of a variety of hormones. Since the control of blood glucose is influenced by alterations of the amount of insulin released rather than by the metabolism of insulin in the peripheral tissues (40), the β cells must possess a secretory system which responds effectively to changes in blood glucose. Several excellent reviews are available (41–43) to which the reader is referred to get a fuller discussion of the β cell phys-

iology. The following serves as a short introduction.

It is generally accepted that glucose is the major stimulus controlling β cell function and insulin release. A large number of carbohydrates, amino acids, hormones, and drugs are also known to affect the release of insulin. Two propositions are made to explain the recognition of D-glucose as a stimulus. The *regulator-site model* suggests that the β cell plasma membrane harbors a glucoreceptor; the binding of ligand to this receptor would elicit a secretory response. There is no direct evidence for the existence of a plasma membrane glucoreceptor. In the *substrate-site* model, initiation of insulin release is explained by the formation of an appropriate signal by metabolism of D-glucose. The glycolytic flux between glyceraldehyde 3-phosphate and pyruvate seems particularly important for formation of a trigger molecule (42). In addition, although not directly implicated in the initiation event, the adenylate cyclase-cyclic AMP system has the capacity to mediate potentiation of insulin release (44). The adenylate cyclase along with surface receptors for various ligands are known to reside in the plasma membrane.

Binding of a ligand to its surface receptor results in a specific response conveyed to the interior of the cell by unknown mechanisms of transmembrane signaling. Antibodies have been shown to be capable of mimicking the effect of certain ligands. Antibodies reactive with the acetylcholine receptor at the neuromuscular junction are present in serum from patients with myasthenia gravis (45, 46). Monoclonal antibodies against the acetylcholine receptor induce a myasthenic syndrome when injected into rats (47). Autoantibodies in Graves' disease seem to compete with thyroid-stimulating hormone for its receptors (48). Autoantibodies (49) or anti-idiotypic antibodies (50) against the insulin receptor not only compete with insulin binding but also have insulin-like effects. Transmembrane signals may also be triggered by antibodies simply binding to cell surface antigens. An isoimmune sheep antierythrocyte serum was found to contain two populations of antibodies; whereas one of them stimulated the active potassium transport, the other inhibited passive transport of the same cation (51). Antibodies specific for cell surface antigens stimulate blast formation in lymphocytes (52). Antibodies against transplantation antigens can activate membrane-associated enzymes such as Na^+/K^+ ATPase and $5'$-nucleotidase (53), presumably due to the possibility that the antigen is intimately linked to these enzyme systems. The effector molecules in the sequence of events resulting in secretion of insulin from the pancreatic cells are not known. As discussed in Section 2.3 certain islet cell antibodies have the capacity to mediate complement-dependent as well as antibody-dependent cellular cytotoxicity.

The assay for islet cell surface antibodies is normally carried out with dispersed living islet cells. These cell preparations are capable of releasing insulin in a biphasic manner after glucose stimulation (54, 55), synthesizing proinsulin/insulin (56), accumulating Rb^+, and retaining the stereospecific transport system for D-glucose (57, 58).

Little information is yet available on the possible effects of antibodies binding to the β cell surface. Rat islet cells were found to synthesize less (pro) insulin when incubated with immunoglobulin from IDD serum containing islet cell surface antibodies (59). A decrease in insulin synthesis was also observed in response to a rabbit anti-rat islet cell serum with a high titer of surface antibodies. Preliminary studies suggested that this antiserum did not influence initial glucose uptake in rat islet cells (Freedman and Lernmark, unpublished observation) nor the glucose transport in the rat adipose cell (Cushman and Lernmark, unpublished observations).

The technique of cell column perifusion (60) was utilized to examine the dynamics of insulin release from dispersed rat pancreatic islet cells (55). The rate of insulin release was not affected by a rabbit anti-rat islet cell serum alone, but after addition of complement the glucose-stimulated insulin release was blocked (55). We have recent evidence that immunoglobulin from newly diagnosed diabetic children ($n = 6$) can inhibit glucose-stimulated insulin release from rat islet cells (Kanatsuna and Lernmark, unpublished observations). In addition, lymphocytes from diabetic subjects with an associated autoimmune disease were found to inhibit insulin release from dispersed mouse islet cells (61). The mechanism and possible pathogenic importance of this observation needs further investigation.

4. MONOCLONAL AND EXPERIMENTAL ISLET CELL ANTIBODIES

The techniques described by Köhler and Milstein (62) allow the construction of hybrid cell lines secreting antibody of preselected specificity. A number of such monoclonal antibody-secreting hybridomas have been produced after immunizing mice with rat insulinoma cells (63, 64). The antibodies reacted with insulinoma cells but not always with normal rat islet cells. Some antibodies also cross-reacted with other rat cells. The antigens were not identified but indirect evidence suggested that gangliosides or glycolipids were possible antigenic determinants (63, 64). An important development toward the understanding of autoantibody formation in IDD was also reported by Eisenbarth and co-workers (65), who fused human myeloma cells with lymphocytes from a diabetic child. One hybridoma culture, B6, produced an IgM antibody which bound to the cytoplasm of islet cells in sections of frozen human pancreas. The experiments demonstrate that B lymphocytes which have differentiated into islet cell antibody-producing cells can circulate in the blood of a patient. The B6 antibody induced a finely granular cytoplasmic fluorescence in some islet endocrine cells. This fluorescence pattern differed from that induced by IDD sera. Production of human monoclonal antibodies against islet cells in IDD patients should now make it possible to study the composition and antigenic characteristics of the islet cells, genetic regulation of autoantibody formation, as well as the role of autoantibodies in IDD.

Xenogenic islet cell surface antisera have also been produced (66). Leiter et al. (67) have reported cytotoxic β cell antibodies after allogenic immunization. An immunochemical investigation showed that in addition to islet cells, the islet alloantiserum also stained a macrophage-like cell in spleen and lymph nodes (67). The multiple specificity of the islet antibody might be explained by the presence of passenger leukocytes in the islet homogenates used to immunize the mice. In contrast, immunoprecipitation of ^{35}S-methionine labeled mouse islet cells with a preabsorbed xenogenic antiserum (66) revealed the presence of antibodies precipitating a protein of M_r 38,000 (68). This antigen was also precipitated after elution from a Lens Culinaris lectin affinity column. In addition, the antigen was labeled after surface iodination of living islet cells. Electron microscopic immunocytochemistry indicated that the xenogenic islet cell surface antibodies predominantly bound to the pancreatic β cells.

5.   OTHER AUTOANTIBODIES IN DIABETES

There are many studies demonstrating a clinical association of diabetes with diseases of autoimmune character such as Addison's disease, thyrotoxicosis, or Hashimoto's thyroiditis. These demonstrations led to studies on the prevalence of a variety of organ-specific autoantibodies in diabetes. Since often neither the stimulus for antibody formation nor the antigens are known, the presence of such autoantibodies in diabetes may be of clinical and etiologic as well as pathogenetic relevance. The presence of organ-specific antibodies have been much discussed in attempts to reach an agreement on an appropriate classification of diabetes mellitus (3, 4). In this section we

consider autoantibodies observed in IDD and NIDD along with some of the problems of insulin antibody formation. Finally, we discuss islet cell and other antibodies in experimental diabetes.

5.1.   Noninsulin-Dependent (Type 2) Diabetes

Noninsulin-dependent diabetes (NIDD) occurs at all ages but is associated in 60 to 90% with obesity. The glucose intolerance is usually improved by weight loss. Studies of the serum from NIDD patients reveal a slightly higher prevalence (3 to 5%) of islet cell antibodies compared to controls. Irvine and coworkers (69) have described islet cell antibody positive NIDD patients who were treated with oral hypoglycemic agents and later developed IDD. This observation indicates that the islet cell antibody test may become useful in predicting future insulin dependency. It has been suggested that members of families with organ-specific autoimmunity develop a late-onset, mild form of IDD which can be controlled with oral hypoglycemic agents for some time (70).

Autoantibodies in NIDD are regarded as a rare event. Mirakian et al. (71) found that 7 out of 50 NIDD sera stained duodenal endocrine cells by immunofluorescence. Four of the positive sera stained cells positive for an antiserum against gastric inhibitory polypeptide. A small group of NIDD patients may thus have gut-associated endocrine cell antibodies. It is of interest to note that antibodies against glucagon or somatostatin cells have been found in diabetic patients, often with an associated endocrine disease (72). Further studies are necessary to delineate a hypothetical autoimmune disorder owing to the loss of other islet cell types.

5.2.   Insulin-Dependent (Type 1) Diabetes

There is evidence to suggest that different endocrinopathies are 4 to 5 times more prevalent among IDD patients than in the general population. The prevalence of subclinical primary thyroid failure in IDD was found to be close to 12%, with the overall prevalence of clinically unrecognized and recognized thyroid disease being about 20% (73). The serum from IDD patients contains several organ-specific autoantibodies in an increased frequency (Table 2). Thyroid, gastric, and adrenal antibodies were more frequent among young, female patients (12). In newly diagnosed insulin-dependent diabetic children ($n = 17$) the prevalence of thyroid cell (thyroglobulin and microsomal), gastric-parietal cell, smooth muscle cell, reticulin, or mitochondrial antibodies did not differ from that observed among 74 age- and sex-matched controls (66). Prospective studies will be necessary to determine to what extent a polyendocrine disease may develop during the course of IDD.

Lymphocytotoxic antibodies, demonstrated in several diseases of autoimmune character (74), were found to be present in patients with IDD of short duration (75). The HLA antigens B8 and B18 were associated with

an increased risk for these antibodies although they did not correlate with islet cell cytoplasmic antibodies. The pathogenic importance of autoantibodies against peripheral lymphocytes is not known but such antibodies may be responsible for a specific removal of lymphocyte subpopulations.

In patients with systemic lupus erythematosus, for example, antibodies to T lymphocytes mediate complement-dependent as well as antibody-dependent cellular cytotoxicity against human T lymphocytes (76). It is important to determine to what extent pancreatic islet cells and immune system cells may share antigenic determinants.

Nearly all IDD patients develop insulin antibodies in response to the insulin therapy. Commercial insulin preparations contain not only insulin but also glucagon, pancreatic polypeptide, and somatostatin. Recent studies demonstrate that commercial insulin stimulates the production of antibodies to all four hormones (77, 78). Purification of insulin has resulted in considerable reduction of insulin antibody production. The clinical importance of insulin antibodies has been much discussed

Table 2. Autoantibodies in IDD

Antibody	Overall Prevalence (%)	
	IDD	Controls
Organ Specific		
Thyroid globulin antibody	9	7
Thyroid microsomal antibody	16	7
Parietal cell antibody	19	9
Intrinsic factor antibody	2	0
Adrenal antibody	2	0
Lymphocytotoxic antibodies	19	4
Non-Organ Specific		
Antinuclear antibody	No difference	
Smooth muscle cell antibody	No difference	
Reticulin antibody	No difference	
Mitochondrial antibody	No difference	
Antibodies Due to Insulin Treatment		
Insulin antibodies	>90	0
Glucagon antibodies	10–15	0
Somatostatin antibodies	5–10	0
Pancreatic polypeptide antibodies	50–80	0

(79). Insulin antibodies may alter the time course of insulin action. It was suggested that diabetic children with glucagon antibodies have a greater tendency to develop hypoglycemia than do glucagon antibody negative children (80). The ability of IDD patients to develop antibodies against insulin preparations may be influenced by the immune response genes since HLA-DR3 positive IDD patients carry an increased risk of developing insulin antibodies (81, 82). The antibody production may also be controlled by the immunoglobulin gene complex since a significant correlation between the G_m (1, 2, 13, 15, 16, 21) phenotype and the presence of insulin antibodies was demonstrated in IDD patients (83).

A better understanding of possible pathophysiological effects of hormone antibodies may come from studies of patients with humoral hormone autoantibodies. Insulin autoantibodies have been detected in several patients (84, 85) with clinical symptoms of hypoglycemic attacks (81, 82). In contrast, glucagon autoantibodies were found only in one mildly diabetic patient (86). The underlying mechanisms responsible for the appearence of hormonal autoantibodies remain to be identified. In vitro techniques are available to study the influence of immune response genes on the formation of insulin antibodies (87, 88). It should be possible to apply these techniques to human immune system cells as well.

5.3.   Experimental Diabetes

A large number of experimental animals are known to develope diabetes either spontaneously or after treatment with different viruses of drugs; several reviews are available (89–91). An insulin-dependent ketosis-prone type of diabetes develops in the Chinese hamster (92), the BB rat (93), and in the NOD mouse (94).

Although diabetes in the Chinese hamster seems not to be associated with autoimmune mechanisms, massive round cell infiltration of the pancreatic islets is observed in both the BB rat and the NOD mouse at the time of onset of diabetes. Antilymphocyte serum was found to cause a marked decrease in the incidence of diabetes among BB rats (95). We have recently observed that the serum of newly diagnosed diabetic BB rats can contain islet surface antibodies (96).

The serum of BB rats can also contain thyroid antibodies (97), and spleen cells from diabetic BB rats induces insulitis after transfer to nude mice (98). The precipitating cause of diabetes in this strain of rats remains to be determined but may not necessarily be caused by environmental factors since the incidence of diabetes was not affected in BB rats raised in a gnotobiotic environment (99).

Diabetes can also be induced in mice by a variety of viruses (100, 101). Although the diabetes often is associated with insulitis, islet cell surface antibodies may not always be present (102). Onodera and co-workers (103) have reported the appearance of growth hormone and insulin autoantibodies in mice infected with reovirus type 1. Insulitis can also be induced in certain strains of mice after injection of multiple small doses of streptozotocin (104). Passive transfer of disease by splenic lymphocytes has been reported (105, 106) but it is not known whether the appearance of insulitis and hyperglycemia is associated with formation of islet cell antibodies. Deposition of IgG in the pancreatic islets as well as antibody to nucleic acid, polyadenylic-polyuridylic acid, single-stranded DNA were found in non-inbred CD-1 mice treated with a single low dose of streptozotocin (107). The pathogenic importance of insulitis in mice treated with varying doses of streptozotocin is not clear since a major loss in islet volume and cell function was found to precede the appearance of insulitis (108).

6.   SUMMARY

The onset of IDD in man is associated with the presence of antibodies against the pancreatic islet cells. Lymphocytic infiltrations of the pancreatic islets, evidence of cellular hypersensitivity against pancreatic islet cell antigens, and the association of IDD with certain alleles of the major histocompatibility complex provide further suggestions that the disease may develop after an environmental insult, perhaps a virus, which could cause an autoimmune response leading to the destruction of the patients' own β cells. The spectrum of islet cell antibodies in IDD includes antibodies reactive with cytoplasmic components, antibodies binding to the surface of living cells, cytotoxic islet cell antibodies, and antibodies immunoprecipitating detergent-solubilized islet cell proteins. The latter may represent β cell specific antigens.

Islet cell cytoplasmic antibodies are unlikely to be of pathogenetic importance if they solely react with intracellular components which are inaccessible to these antibodies in the living cell. In contrast, serum containing islet cell surface antibodies mediates complement-dependent cytotoxicity. However, it remains to be determined whether this phenomenon is operative in vivo since it is not known to what extent antibodies and complement components can reach the β cells from the bloodstream. In the future, however, direct biological effects of islet cell antibodies must be documented since preliminary evidence suggests that islet cell antibodies in IDD may inhibit glucose-induced insulin release. Additional experiments, preferably with human cells, are necessary to test the hypothesis that certain islet cell antibodies may be directed against component(s) of the glucoreceptor mechanism in the β cells.

The different procedures for detecting islet cell antibodies that utilize a variety of tissue preparations argue that the autoantibodies are directed against several antigens. Monoclonal antibodies against human islet cell antigens should provide means by which to analyze islet cell specific antigens and their ability to elicit an autoimmune reaction. In this respect, it has been possible to produce human monoclonal antibodies after fusing human myeloma cells with B-lymphocytes from diabetic patients. It would be worth investigating whether an anti-idiotypic antiserum administered to susceptible persons would prevent an ongoing β cell destruction from resulting in IDD.

It is clear that future attempts to identify susceptible persons require sensitive and specific assays for β cell damage. The isolation and use of β cell specific target antigens in a sensitive immunoassay may allow prospective analysis in individuals at risk. Although the mechanisms by which the antiself reaction(s) is initiated remain to be identified, we expect that the identification of the putative antigens will shed some light on these mechanisms. Future studies will certainly involve an examination of immunocompetent cells responsible for antigen presentation, induction, and help to cytotoxic T cells and antibody-producing B-lymphocytes as well as those T cell subsets responsible for suppressing the immune response.

ACKNOWLEDGMENTS

The studies at the authors' laboratory were supported in part by grant AM 26190 from the National Institutes of Health and from Vera and Carl Johan Michaelsen's Legat.

REFERENCES

1. G. F. Bottazzo, R. Pujol-Borrell, and D. Doniach, *Clin. Immunol. Allergy* **1**, 139 (1956).

2. Å. Lernmark, V. Bonnevie-Nielsen, S. Baekkeskov, T. Dyrberg, T. Kanatsuna, and J. Scott, in J. M. Martin, R. M. Ehrlich, and F. J. Holland, Eds., *Etiology and Pathogenesis of Insulin-Dependent Diabetes Mellitus*, Raven Press, New York, 1981, p. 61.

3. National Diabetes Data Group, *Diabetes* **28**, 1039 (1979).

4. WHO Expert Committee on Diabetes Mellitus: Second Report, *WHO Tech. Rep. Ser. 646* (1980).

5. A. H. Rubenstein, D. F. Steiner, D. L. Horwitz, M. E. Mako, M. B. Block, J. I. Starr, H. Kuzuya, and F. Melani, *Recent Prog. Horm. Res.* **33**, 435 (1977).

6. C. Binder and O. Faber, *Diabetes* **27** (Suppl. 1), 226 (1978).

7. B. W. Volk and K. F. Wellman, Eds., *The Diabetic Pancreas*, Plenum Press, New York, 1977.

8. W. Gepts and P. LeCompte, *Am. J. Med.* **70**, 105 (1981).

9. W. Gepts, *Diabetes* **14**, 619 (1965).

10. W. Gepts and J. De Mey, *Diabetes* **27** (Suppl. 1), 251 (1978).

11. A. C. MacCuish and W. J. Irvine, *Clin. Endocrinol. Metab.* **4**, 435 (1975).

12. J. Nerup, M. Christy, T. Deckert, and J. Egeberg, in M. Samter, Ed., *Immunological Diseases*, Little, Brown, Boston, 1978, p. 1330.

13. J. Nerup and Å. Lernmark, *Am. J. Med.* **70**, 135 (1981).

14. U. DiMario, M. Iavicoli, and D. Andreani, *Diabetologia* **19**, 89 (1980).

15. G. F. Bottazzo, A. Florin-Christensen, and D. Doniach, *Lancet* **2**, 1279 (1974).

16. A. C. MacCuish, J. Jordan, C. J. Campbell, L. J. P. Duncan, and W. J. Irvine, *Lancet* **2**, 1529 (1974).

17. R. Lendrum, G. Walker, A. G. Cudworth, C. Theophanides, D. A. Pyke, A. Bloom, and D. R. Gamble, *Lancet* **2**, 1273 (1976).

18. W. J. Irvine, C. J. McCallum, R. S. Gray, G. J. Campbell, L. J. P. Duncan, J. W. Farquhar, H. Vaughan, and P. J. Morris, *Diabetes* **26**, 138 (1977).

19. G. F. Bottazzo, J. I. Mann, M. Thorogood, J. D. Baum, and D. Doniach, *Br. Med. J.* **2**, 165 (1978).

20. G. F. Bottazzo, B. M. Dean, A. N. Gorsuch, A. G. Cudworth, and D. Doniach, *Lancet* **1**, 668 (1980).

21. B. M. Dean, J. M. McNally, and D. Doniach, *Diabetologia* **19**, 268 (1980).

22. K. Helmke, A. Otten, and W. Willems, *Lancet* **2**, 211 (1980).

23. Å. Lernmark, Z. R. Freedman, C. Hofmann, A. H. Rubenstein, D. F. Steiner, R. L. Jackson, R. J. Winter, and H. S. Traisman, *N. Engl. J. Med.* **299**, 375 (1978).

24. N. K. MacLaren, S. W. Huang, and J. Fogh, *Lancet* **1**, 997 (1975).

25. N. K. MacLaren and S. W. Huang, in J. Irvine, Ed., *Immunology of Diabetes*, Teviot Scientific Publications, Edinburgh, 1980, p. 193.

26. A. H-J. Huen, M. Haneda, Z. Freedman, and Å. Lernmark, *Diabetes* **30** (Suppl. 1), 65A (1981).

27. R. Pujol-Borrell, G. F. Bottazzo, E. L. Khoury, and D. Doniach, *Diabetologia* **19**, 308 (1980).

28. Å. Lernmark, B. Hägglöf, Z. R. Freedman, W. J. Irvine, J. Ludvigsson, and G. Holmgren, *Diabetologia* **20**, 471 (1981).

29. Z. R. Freedman, C. M. Feed, W. J. Irvine, Å. Lernmark, A. H. Rubenstein, D. F. Steiner, and A. Huen, *Trans. Assoc. Am. Physicians* **96**, 64 (1979).

30. Å. Lernmark, J. Sehlin, I.-B. Täljedal, H. Kromann, and J. Nerup, *Diabetologia* **14**, 25 (1978).

31. L.-Å. Idahl, J. Sehlin, I.-B. Täljedal, and L.-E. Thornell, *Diabetes* **29**, 636 (1980).

32. W. K. Soderstrum, Z. R. Freedman, and Å. Lernmark, *Diabetes* **28**, 397 (1979).

33. M. J. Dobersen, J. E. Scharff, F. Ginsberg-Fellner, and A. L. Notkins, *N. Engl. J. Med.* **303**, 1493 (1980).

34. G. S. Eisenbarth, M. A. Morris, and R. M. Scearce, *J. Clin. Invest.* **67**, 403 (1981).

35. M. Kende, M. J. Dobersen, F. Ginsberg-Fellner, and A. L. Notkins, *Diabetes* **30** (Suppl. 1), 65A (1981).

36. H. G. Rittenhouse, D. L. Oxender, S. Pek, and D. Ar, *Diabetes* **29**, 317 (1980).

37. P. Sai, M. Debray-Sachs, C. Boitard, and R. Assan, *C. R. Acad. Sci [D]* **292**, 21 (1981).

38. M. Sensi, P. Pozzilli, A. N. Gorsuch, G. F. Bottazzo, and A. G. Cudworth, *Diabetologia* **20**, 106 (1981).

39. S. Baekkeskov, J. H. Nielsen, B. Marner, T. Bilde, J. Ludvigsson and Å. Lernmark, *Nature* **298**, 167 (1982).

40. E. Cerasi, *Q. Rev. Biophys.* **8**, 1 (1975).

41. A. E. Lambert, *Rev. Physiol. Biochem. Pharmacol.* **75**, 97 (1976).

42. C. J. Hedeskov, *Physiol. Rev.* **60**, 442 (1980).

43. W. J. Malaisse and I.-B. Täljedal, Eds., *Biochemistry and Biophysics of the Pancreatic B-Cell*, Horm. Metab. Res., Suppl. No. 10, 1980, pp. 1–171.

44. J. E. Gerich, M. A. Charles, and G. M. Grodsky, *Annu. Rev. Physiol.* **38**, 353 (1976).

45. A. Aharonov, O. Abramsky, R. Tarrab-Hazdai, and S. Fuchs, *Lancet* **2**, 340 (1975).

46. K. V. Toyka, D. B. Drachman, D. E. Griffin, A. Pestronk, J. A. Winkelstein, K. H. Fischbeck, and I. Kao, *N. Engl. J. Med.* **296**, 125 (1977).

47. D. P. Richman, C. M. Gomez, P. W. Berman, S. A. Burres, F. W. Fitch, and B. G. W. Arnason, *Nature* **286**, 738 (1980).

48. T. F. Davies and E. DeBernardo, Chapter 6, this book.

49. L. C. Harrison and P. Heyma, Chapter 5, this book.

50. K. Sege and P. A. Peterson, *Proc. Natl. Acad. Sci. USA* **75**, 2443 (1978).

51. P. B. Dunham, *Biochim. Biophys. Acta* **443**, 219 (1976).

52. S. Sell, D. S. Rowe, and P. G. H. Gell, *J. Exp. Med.* **122**, 823 (1965).

53. J. Aubry, A. Zachowski, A. Paraf, and J. Colombani, *Ann. Immunol. (Inst. Pasteur)* **130c**, 17 (1979).

54. L.-Å. Idahl, Å. Lernmark, J. Sehlin, and I.-B. Täljedal, *Pflügers Arch.* **366**, 185 (1976).

55. T. Kanatsuna, Å. Lernmark, A. H. Rubenstein, and D. F. Steiner, *Diabetes* **30**, 231 (1981).

56. Å. Lernmark, S. J. Chan, R. Choy, A. Nathans, R. Carrol, H. S. Tager, A. H. Rubenstein, H. H. Swift, and D. F. Steiner, *The Peptide Hormones: Molecular and Cellular Aspects*, Ciba Symposium 41, London, 1976, pp. 7–30.

57. Å. Lernmark, J. Sehlin, and I.-B. Täljedal, *Anal. Biochem.* **63**, 73 (1975).

58. B. Hellman, J. Sehlin, and I.-B. Täljedal, *Biochim. Biophys. Acta* **241**, 147 (1971).

59. Å. Lernmark, T. Kanatsuna, A. H. Rubenstein, and D. F. Steiner, *Adv. Exp. Med. Biol.* **119**, 157 (1979).

60. P. J. Lowry and C. McMartin, *Biochem. J.* **142**, 287 (1974).

61. C. Boitard, M. Debray-Sachs, A. Pouplard, R. Assan, and J. Hamburger, *Diabetologia* **21**, 41 (1981).

62. G. Köhler and C. Milstein, *Nature* **256**, 495 (1975).

63. G. S. Eisenbarth, H. Oie, A. Gazdar, W. Chick, J. A. Schultz, and R. M. Scearce, *Diabetes* **30**, 226 (1981).

64. M. Crumps, M. J. Dobersen, R. Scearce, and G. S. Eisenbarth, *Endocrinology*, in press (1982).

65. G. S. Eisenbarth, A. Linnenbach, R. Jackson, and C. Croce, *Clin. Res.* **29**, 404A (1981).

66. Å. Lernmark, T. Kanatsuna, C. Patzelt, K. Diakoumis, R. Carroll, A. H. Rubenstein, and D. F. Steiner, *Diabetologia* **19**, 445 (1980).

67. E. H. Leiter, D. Simon, M. Cherry, and C. A. Phillips, *Diabetes* **30**, 30 (1981).

68. T. Dyrberg, S. Baekkeskev, and Å. Lernmark, *J. Cell Biol.* **94**, 472 (1982).

69. W. J. Irvine, R. S. Gray, C. J. McCallum, and L. J. P. Duncan, *Lancet* **2**, 1025 (1977).

70. A. N. Gorsuch, B. M. Dean, G. F. Bottazzo, J. Lister, and A. G. Cudworth, *Br. Med. J.* **1**, 145 (1980).

71. R. Mirakian, G. F. Bottazzo, and D. Doniach, *Clin. Exp. Immunol.* **41**, 38 (1980).

72. G. F. Bottazzo and R. Lendrum, *Lancet* **2**, 873 (1976).

73. R. S. Gray, D. Q. Borsey, J. Seth, R. Herd, N. S. Brown, and B. F. Clarke, *J. Clin. Endocrinol. Metab.* **50**, 1034 (1980).

74. G. Ozturk and P. I. Terazaki, *Tissue Antigens* **14**, 52 (1979).

75. S. Serjeantson, J. Theophilus, P. Zimmet, J. Court, J. R. Crossley, and R. B. Elliott, *Diabetes* **30**, 26 (1981).

76. S. Kumagai, A. D. Steinberg, and I. Green, *J. Clin. Invest.* **67**, 604 (1981).

77. S. R. Bloom, T. E. Adrian, A. J. Barnes, and J. M. Polak, in W. J. Irvine, Ed., *Immunology of Diabetes*, Teviot Scientific Publications, Edinburgh, 1980, p. 291.

78. D. Fitz-Patrick and Y. C. Patel, *J. Clin. Endocrinol. Metab.* **52**, 948 (1981).

79. K. G. M. M. Alberti and M. Nattrass, *Diabetologia* **15** 77 (1980).

80. S. Villalpando and A. Drash, *Diabetes* **28**, 294 (1979).

81. G. Schernthaner, H. Ludwig, and W. R. Mayr, *J. Clin. Endocrinol. Metab.* **48**, 403 (1979).

82. J. Ludvigsson, J. Säfwenberg, and L. G. Heding, *Diabetologia* **13**, 13 (1977).

83. Y. Nakao, H. Matsumoto, T. Miyazaki, N. Mizuno, N. Arima, A. Wakisaka, K. Okimoto, Y. Akazawa, K. Tsuji, and T. Fujita, *N. Engl. J. Med.* **304**, 407 (1981).

84. I. Følling and N. Norman, *Diabetes* **21**, 814 (1972).

85. J. H. Anderson, W. G. Blackard, J. Goldman, and A. H. Rubenstein, *Am. J. Med.* **65**, 868 (1978).

86. S. Baba, S. Morita, N. Mizumo, and K. Okada, *Lancet* **2**, 586 (1976).

87. A. S. Rosenthal, *Immunol. Rev.* **40**, 136 (1978).

88. R. P. Bucy and J. A. Kapp, *J. Immunol.* **126**, 603 (1981).

89. L. Herberg and D. L. Coleman, *Metabolism* **26**, 59 (1977).

90. G. M. Grodsky, *Diabetes*, **31** (Suppl. 1), 45 (1982).

91. J. P. Mordes and A. A. Rossini, *Am. J. Med.* **70**, 353 (1981).

92. G. C. Gerritsen and W. E. Dulin, *Diabetologia* **3**, 74 (1967).

93. A. F. Nakhooda, A. A. Like, C. I. Chappel, F. T. Murray, and E. B. Marliss, *Diabetes* **26**, 100 (1977).

94. S. Makino, K. Kunimoto, Y. Muraoka, Y. Mi-

zushima, K. Katagiri, and Y. Tochino, *Exp. Anim.* **29**, 1 (1980).

95. A. A. Like, A. A. Rossini, D. L. Guberslei, M. C. Appel, and R. M. Williams, *Science* **206**, 1421 (1979).

96. T. Dyrberg, A. F. Nakhooda, S. Baekkeskov, Å. Lemmark, P. Poussier, and E. B. Marliss, *Diabetes* **31**, 278 (1982).

97. M. Elder, N. MacLaren, W. Riley, and T. McConnell, *Diabetes* **31**, 313 (1982).

98. A. F. Nakhooda, A. A. F. Sima, and E. B. Marliss, *Diabetes* **30**, 66A (1981).

99. A. A. Rossini, R. M. Williams, J. P. Mordes, M. C. Appel, and A. A. Like, *Diabetes* **28**, 1031 (1979).

100. J. E. Craighead, in P. J. Fitzgerald and A. B. Morrison, Eds., *The Pancreas*, Waverly Press, Baltimore, 1980, pp. 166–176.

101. A. L. Notkins, in S. Podolsky and M. Viswan-athan, Eds., *Secondary Diabetes, The Spectrum of the Diabetic Syndromes*, Raven Press, New York, 1980, pp. 471–486.

102. H. Kromann, Å. Lemmark, B. F. Vestergaard, J. Egeberg, and J. Nerup, *Diabetologia* **16**, 107 (1979).

103. T. Onodera, A. Toniolo, U. R. Ray, A. B. Jenson, R. A. Knazek, and A. L. Notkins, *J. Exp. Med.* **153**, 1457 (1981).

104. A. A. Like and A. A. Rossini, *Science* **193**, 415 (1976).

105. S. G. Paik, N. Fleischer, and S-I Shin, *Proc. Natl. Acad. Sci. USA* **77**, 6129 (1980).

106. U. Kiesel, G. Freytag, J. Biener, and H. Kolb, *Diabetologia* **19**, 516 (1980).

107. S.-W. Huang and G. E. Taylor, *Clin. Exp. Immunol.* **43**, 425 (1981).

108. V. Bonnevie-Nielsen, M. W. Steffes, and Å. Lemmark, *Diabetes* **30**, 424 (1981).

9

Steroid Hormone Cell Autoimmunity

Melissa Elder
Noel K. Maclaren

Division of Clinical Chemistry
Department of Pathology
University of Florida College of Medicine
J. Hillis Miller Health Center
Gainesville, Florida

Contents

1. INTRODUCTION

By 1855, Addison recognized many of the characteristics of adrenocortical failure and realized that many cases were not due to identifiable causes such as tuberculosis, histoplasmosis, or metastatic disease (13). Although the term "idiopathic" Addison's disease was originally applied to these cases of unknown etiology, many of these instances of adrenocortical failure are now considered to result from the autoimmune destruction of the steroid hormone-producing cells of the adrenal cortex. Additional autoimmunity to the steroid hormone-producing cells of the gonads may occasionally occur in this disease. "Autoimmune" Addison's disease is uncommon with an incidence of only 40 per million adults in one series (18); however, there has been great interest in this disease as a model for other organ-specific autoimmune conditions (13).

Principal reasons why "idiopathic" adrenal insufficiency is considered to be autoimmune in origin include evidence of mononuclear infiltration of the affected organ (adrenalitis), presence of autoantibodies specific for the adrenal cortex in the patients' sera, association of the disease with other endocrinopathies that are thought to be autoimmune, and disturbances in the frequencies of certain HLA antigens in affected patients in comparison with that of the general population.

2.   ADDISON'S DISEASE IN TWO POLYGLANDULAR SYNDROMES

Endocrine disorders most frequently associated with autoimmune Addison's disease include autoimmune thyroid diseases (chronic lymphocytic thyroiditis and Graves' disease) (1–3), hypoparathyroidism (4), and insulin-dependent diabetes mellitus (IDDM) (2, 5). Based on the age of onset of Addison's disease, the associated diseases, and HLA data, two autoimmune polyglandular syndromes (APS) involving Addison's disease have been proposed (6, 7).

In type I APS, Addison's disease is seen in association with chronic mucocutaneous candidiasis and hypoparathyroidism. Other frequently associated diseases include alopecia, malabsorption, juvenile onset pernicious anemia, chronic active hepatitis, and gonadal failure. In many cases, the sequence of appearance of the major diseases in type I APS is chronic mucocutaneous candidiasis followed by hypoparathyroidism and then Addison's disease. Autoimmune thyroid diseases and IDDM are infrequent in this syndrome. Type I APS occurs exclusively in children and young adults with the peak age of onset of overt Addison's disease being approximately 10 years.

In type II APS, Addison's disease is strongly associated with autoimmune thyroid diseases (Schmidt's syndrome) (1) and IDDM (Carpenter's syndrome) (2), and an increase in late-onset pernicious anemia may be found. Chronic active hepatitis, malabsorption, chronic mucocutaneous candidiasis, and hypoparathyroidism are not found in type II APS. This syndrome may occur in all stages of life, but is most common during midlife, especially among women.

Type I APS may result from a thymic or T lymphocyte dysfunction (8). The disease is occasionally familial and may be inherited as an autosomal recessive trait (11), but is probably not associated with disturbed frequencies of any particular HLA antigen (8). The numbers of patients with this rare condition studied by HLA typing to date, however, remain small. In contrast, significant increases in the frequencies of HLA A1 and HLA B8 have been found in patients with Addison's disease and type II APS (9, 10). This syndrome complex is usually familial, with thyrogastric and/or pancreatic islet cell autoimmunity being commonly found among first-degree relatives of such patients (12).

3.   ADRENOCORTICAL AUTOANTIBODIES

Approximately 65% (13) of patients with "idiopathic" Addison's disease, regardless of syndrome classification, have autoantibodies that react specifically with a cytosolic antigen found in the cells of the adrenal cortex. Anderson and co-workers (14) first reported the presence of such *adrenocortical autoantibodies* in the sera of two patients with Addison's disease. Since then many articles describing adrenal autoantibodies have been published (13, 15, 16). The current method for the detection of adrenal autoantibodies is the indirect immunofluorescence technique (IFL) using frozen, unfixed sections of human or monkey adrenal tissue. The presence of adrenal antibodies in the patient's serum does not correlate with disease duration or age of onset of Addison's disease (13, 16). The autoantibodies are absent in cases of tuberculous Addison's disease and are found at a rate of 0.5% in the general population (13). Adrenal antibodies are found in the sera of approximately 2% of insulin-dependent diabetics and in the sera of about 6% of those patients with both IDDM and autoimmune thyroid disease (Table 1). [Patients with IDDM and adrenal antibodies had a greatly increased frequency of B8-bearing HLA haplotypes (17).] Most striking, however, are the findings

Table 1. Frequencies and significances of adrenal and steroid cell autoantibodies

Condition	Adrenal Autoantibodies	Addison's Disease	SCA	Hypogonadism
Idiopathic Addison's disease	27/37 (73%)	37/37 (100%)	11/37 (29.7%)[a]	7/37 (18.9%)
Type I APS	7/7 (100%)	7/7 (100%)	6/7 (85.7%)[a]	6/7 (85.7%)
Type II APS	22/23 (95.6%)	19/23 (82.6%)	3/23 (13.0%)[a]	1/23 (4.4%)
IDDM	8/505 (1.6%)	2/505 (0.4%)	0/505	0/505
IDDM and autoimmune thyroid disease	5/77 (6.5%)	2/77 (2.6%)	0/77	0/77
Hypogonadism associated with Addison's disease	0/15	0/15	0/15	0/15
Turner's syndrome	0/21	0/21	0/21	0/21
Controls	2/235 (0.6%)	0/325	1/325 (0.3%)[a]	0/325

From Refs. 17 and 25.

[a] SCA only found in sera also positive for adrenocortical autoantibodies. Thus, for example, of the 27 patients with both idiopathic Addison's disease and adrenal autoantibodies, 11 (40.7%) patients also had SCA in their sera.

183

that adrenal autoantibodies occurred in the sera of 25–30% of patients with idiopathic hypoparathyroidism (18).

Adrenal autoantibodies are exclusively IgG immunoglobulins (18) and are usually present in low titers in the serum. These antibodies react with cells of the zona glomerulosa and/ or with cells in all three layers of the adrenal cortex (19) (Figure 1a). Antibodies readily visualized as reacting with the entire adrenal cortex tend to be of higher titer than antibodies detected principally by immunofluorescence of only the zona glomerulosa and are more often associated with overt Addison's disease (17).

The cytosolic antigen to which the adrenal autoantibodies are directed has been widely demonstrated in the adrenal cortex of many

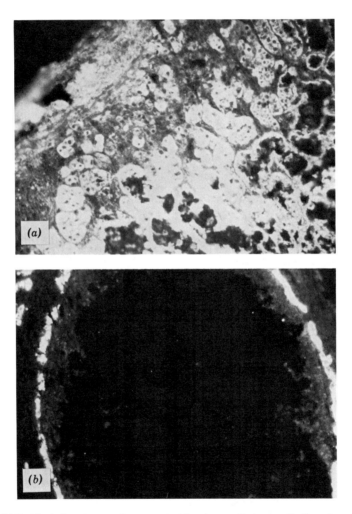

Figure 1. (a) Positive indirect immunofluorescent test for adrenocortical autoantibodies using a human adrenal cortex section. (b) Positive indirect immunofluorescent test for steroid hormone cell autoantibodies using a rabbit ovarian section. The fluorescent cells are in the theca interna/granulosa layer of the Graafian follicle. (c) Positive indirect immunofluorescent test for steroid hormone cell autoantibodies using a human placental section. The fluorescent cells are those of the syncytiotrophoblast. (d) Positive indirect immunofluorescent test for steroid hormone cell autoantibodies using a human testis section from a prepubertal boy with testicular feminization syndrome. The fluorescent cells are the Leydig cells.

species, except rat and mouse (16), and is not found in other organs such as thyroid, pancreas, stomach, and liver (16, 21). The antigen is thought to be a membrane lipoprotein, probably of microsomes, but it may be of mitochondrial origin also (13, 20).

3.1.   Steroid Cell Autoantibodies

Steroid cell autoantibodies (SCA) that react with all steroid hormone-producing cells of the adrenal cortex, ovary (Figure 1b), placenta (Figure 1c), and testis (Figure 1d) have also been demonstrated in the sera of some patients with Addison's disease. Anderson and co-workers (22) first demonstrated autoantibodies that reacted with cells of the theca interna and corpus luteum of the ovary, Leydig cells of the testis, and syncytiotrophoblasts of the placenta in two patients with Addison's disease who did not have obvious symptoms of gonadal insufficiency. Irvine and Barnes (13) later described SCA in the sera of all patients with Addison's disease and primary amenorrhea, and in about 60% of the sera from patients with both Addison's disease and secondary amenorrhea. However, SCA were not detected in sera from any patients with gonadal dysgenesis occurring in association with chromosomal abnormalities, ovarian failure not

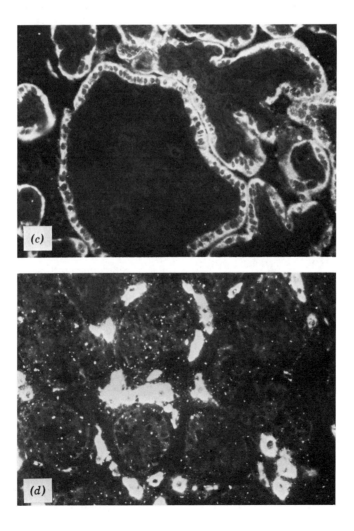

associated with Addison's disease, or normal controls. Similar reports of the presence of SCA in some patient sera have been made by others (23, 24) but there has been some controversy. Questions have been raised as to whether specific gonadal autoantibodies exist separately from the previously described SCA, whether SCA necessarily react with adrenocortical cells, and whether SCA can be demonstrated in patients with gonadal failure who do not have autoimmune Addison's disease. In our own studies (25), no patients were found to have gonadal-reactive autoantibodies that were not identifiable as SCA. SCA were found in 40% of patients with both adrenocortical autoantibodies and Addison's disease, but were not found in subjects without adrenal antibodies (including patients with Addison's disease), in patients with ovarian insufficiency unrelated to Addison's disease, or among normal controls. SCA were found in the majority (86%) of patients with type I Addison's disease (most of which had clinical features of gonadal insufficiency). In comparison, SCA were detected in only 13% of patients with type II Addison's disease. Since SCA are rare in patients who do not have autoimmune Addison's disease, only patients with adrenal autoimmunity are at risk to develop autoimmune hypogonadism (Table 1). At the time of this writing, however, we have additionally examined sera from two siblings with primary hypogonadism and optic atrophy. Both siblings had SCA which were of low titer but which were not identifiable as reacting with adrenal sections. However, specific absorptions of the sera with adrenal tissue have yet to be performed.

From our studies involving various tissue absorptions of sera containing SCA, two distinct adrenocortical autoantibodies detectable by IFL can be demonstrated in some patients with Addison's disease: one type of antibody that is specific for the adrenal cortex and a second antibody type (SCA) that cross-reacts with all steroid hormone-producing tissues including the adrenal cortex. Most patients with Addison's disease have only adreno-

cortical-specific reactive immunoglobulins in their serum, however, that do not react with other steroid hormone-producing cells.

3.2.   Precipitating Antibodies

Precipitating antibodies directed against adrenal homogenates, as detected by the Ouchterlony gel diffusion technique, have also been found in patients with Addison's disease (26). These adrenal antibodies are IgG and specifically react with the adrenal cortex, for no cross-reaction with other steroid hormone-producing tissues has been found. These precipitating adrenal antibodies react with two adrenal antigens: one in mitochondria and another found in all subcellular fractions (27). The presence of these precipitating antibodies did not correlate well with the presence of adrenal antibodies detected by tissue IFL in patients' sera. There are more patients in addition to those with precipitating antibodies that have adrenal autoantibodies detectable by IFL (26). The precipitating adrenal antibodies may be detected only in sera from patients with type I Addison's disease (26, 28).

3.3.   Adrenal Antibodies

Adrenal antibodies have also been produced *in experimental animals* following injections of either heterologous or homologous adrenal tissue homogenates in complete Freund's adjuvant. Both antibodies reacting specifically with adrenal tissue (29, 31) and antibodies cross-reacting with ovary and testis (30) have been demonstrated, primarily by complement fixation, but also by tanned red cell agglutination and precipitation reactions.

4.   ADRENOCORTICAL AUTOANTIBODIES AND PATHOGENESIS OF ADDISON'S DISEASE

It is difficult to imagine how autoantibodies reacting with antigens found in the cytoplasm of steroid hormone-producing cells can play a direct role in the pathogenesis of autoimmune steroid cell failure. These antibodies are not thought to be able to penetrate living, undamaged cells and thus are considered by some to be produced only as a result of the exposure of the relevant intracellular antigens to the immune system after tissue destruction by immunologic or other means. Supporting evidence for a noncausal role for adrenal autoantibodies includes findings that infants of mothers with Addison's disease and circulating adrenocortical autoantibodies have, in general, not developed even transient impaired adrenocortical function, even though the autoantibodies can be detected in the umbilical cord blood after transplacental passage (13, 32). Notwithstanding, Irvine and colleagues reported that one such infant died from an illness suggestive of adrenocortical insufficiency (13). We recently examined an infant who developed Addison's disease at 15 months of age. The child's mother had adrenal autoantibodies in her sera, but the infant did not. Other evidence indicating a passive role for adrenal autoantibodies in the etiology of autoimmune Addison's disease includes the finding that transfers of adrenal antibodies from animals with experimental adrenalitis have not resulted in autoimmune adrenal disease in the recipient animals.

Adrenal autoantibodies directed against cell surface antigens, which could participate in complement-dependent lysis and/or antibody-dependent cell-mediated cytotoxicity, have not yet been conclusively demonstrated. However, McNatty et al. (33) described the cytotoxic effects on cultured human granulosa cells of 9 SCA-positive sera from 23 patients with Addison's disease and autoimmune ovarian failure. The cytotoxicity was complement dependent (and thus most likely due to the presence of antibodies directed against cell surface antigens in the sera) and was related to the immunofluorescent staining properties of the serum and the titer of antibody present.

5. CELL-MEDIATED AUTOIMMUNITY AND ADDISON'S DISEASE

Certain common *histopathological findings* are found upon examination of the adrenals from patients with autoimmune adrenal failure. In contrast to the entire gland destruction seen in tuberculous or other nonautoimmune types of Addison's disease, ony the adrenal cortex is destroyed in adrenal autoimmunity (18). Characteristically, the adrenal cortex is extremely atrophied, with the medulla being separated from the thickened fibrous capsule by only a collapsed stroma which is almost devoid of cortical cells. The remaining adrenocortical cells are enlarged or pleomorphic and are lacking lipid. Some evidence of mononuclear infiltration is always found, with mostly small lymphocytes and some plasma cells and macrophages being present. Germinal center formations are seen in some cases. The presence of this typical chronic mononuclear infiltration in the adrenal cortex along with the selective cortical destruction is considered to be specific to autoimmune Addison's disease. Some autopsy cases of patients with Addison's disease have also revealed mononuclear infiltrations in the thyroid and pancreatic islets as well as in the adrenal cortex (2).

The *leukocyte migration inhibition test* (LMIT) is the technique that has been used most often to detect positive cell-mediated immunity to adrenocortical antigens in patients with Addison's disease. Using this technique, Nerup and Bendixen first demonstrated organ-specific antiadrenal cellular hypersensitivity in many patients with idiopathic Addison's disease (34). Moulias et al. (35) also reported abnormal LMIT tests to adrenal extracts in more than 80% of patients with the disease, whereas negative results were obtained in patients with tuberculous Addison's disease. Positive delayed-type hypersensitivity skin tests to adrenal extracts have been demonstrated in a few patients with Addison's disease. The findings correlated with the results obtained using the in vitro LMIT tests (36). However, blast transformation of lymphocytes from patients with Addison's disease as measured by ³H-thymidine incorporation was not induced after stimulation with adrenal antigen (36, 37). The adrenal antigen responsible for the positive LMIT test was not species specific (35, 38) and was thought to be located in the mitochondrial subcellular fraction.

Absolute lymphocyte numbers and proportions of T and B lymphocytes in peripheral blood are usually normal in patients with autoimmune Addison's disease; however, in at least one instance, the percentage of B cells in the peripheral blood was reported as increased in two siblings with Addison's disease (39). *Suppressor cells* from these two brothers were also unable to inhibit the activity of either mitogen-induced B cell polyclonal immunoglobulin biosynthesis or T cell proliferation. Yet in our preliminary studies of two children with type I APS, no deficiency was seen in the relative proportion of T lymphocytes that react with the OKT8 monoclonal antibody. The T lymphocytes that react with this antisera are thought to represent the cytotoxic/suppressor subpopulation (45). In patients with type I Addison's disease, elevated levels of IgG (9) and IgE (8), decreased levels of IgA (8), abnormal skin tests to several ubiquitous antigens (9), and decreased suppressor cell functions (8) have been noted. Although current methods for assessing immunoregulatory T cell functions are crude and unable to detect subtle changes, results to date suggest that the hypothesis of disordered immunoregulation in some patients with autoimmune adrenal failure remains attractive.

Adrenalitis has also been produced in *experimental animals* following injections of adrenal extracts in complete Freund's adjuvant. Colover and Glynn (40) reported necrosis and round cell invasion of the adrenal cortex in guinea pigs following such immunizations with homologous adrenal tissue. Similar results have been reported by others (41, 29), usually only after injections of heterologous adrenal tissue in adjuvant. The mononuclear infiltrates

observed in these experiments consisted of lymphocytes and histiocytes, with some plasma cells and eosinophils also present. The inflammatory lesions were most numerous and extensive in the deeper layers of the cortex, and degenerative changes of the adrenocortical cells were noted. No histopathological changes were noted in the gonads. Using autoradiographic tracings of ³H-thymidine and ³H-adenosine labeled cells, Wederlin (42) suggested that the adrenalitis was initiated by a few specifically sensitized lymphocytes which had emigrated from antigen-stimulated lymph nodes. Monocytes were then recruited by released chemotactic factors, with most lymphocytes appearing later after local vascular changes had occurred.

Other markers of cell-mediated immunity such as the production of macrophage migration inhibition factor also occur in experimental adrenalitis (31). Analogous to human autoimmune adrenal disease, lymphocyte transformation in experimental adrenalitis has not been demonstrated (31). However, most importantly, successful passive transfer of experimental adrenalitis in the rat using lymphoid cells has been reported (43). Thus, at least as far as the animal model of adrenal autoimmunity is concerned, cell-mediated immune mechanisms may in fact be more important than humoral immunity in the histopathological changes noted in the adrenal cortex and thus in the development of adrenalitis.

If autoimmune Addison's disease is due to cell-mediated immune mechanisms, the experimental work of Zinkernagel and Doherty (44) as a conceptual model of antigenic recognition in association with histocompatibility antigens may be implicated. In their experiments, immunocompetent mice infected intracerebrally with lymphocytic choriomeningitis virus (LCMV) develop fatal disease, while immunoincompetent or athymic mice were protected and instead became chronic virus carriers. Thus the lymphocytic choriomeningitis was due to the immunologic responses of the mice to the LCMV infection. Sensitized T lymphocytes (CTL) from virally infected mice were cytotoxic to LCMV-infected fibroblasts or macrophages in vitro, but only if these target cells shared major histocompatibility antigens with the LCMV-bearing cells that originally stimulated the production of the sensitized CTL. In the natural situation of an immune response to an environmental stimulus such as a virus infection, the target cells and the CTL are both self, with the CTL thus recognizing the foreign antigens in context of self major histocompatibility complex products. This model has appeal for translation to autoimmune steroid cell failure as seen in man. It reconciles the need for some environmental trigger (to alter self-antigens on steroid cell membranes), the HLA requirement (for T lymphocyte cytolysis of the target steroid hormone-producing cells), and the necessity for an immune response to produce the resulting autoimmune disease. At present, evidence for such a sequence of events in human steroid cell autoimmunity remains to be demonstrated. Parenthetically, it may be noted that both adrenocortical auto-antibodies and the sensitized lymphocytes from experimental animals referred to above react with normal unaltered adrenal cell antigens.

The HLA requirement, an assumption made by the increased association of type II Addison's disease with HLA B8 and probably because of linkage disequilibrium with HLA Dw3/DRw3 and HLA A1, may be due instead to other reasons. A disease-specific gene for adrenocortical autoimmunity may be closely linked to HLA B8 or HLA Dw3/DRw3 which has not yet reached equilibrium throughout the general population by natural recombinant events. Since HLA D/DR antigens are known to be intimately involved in antigen recognition and immune responsiveness, it is also possible that patients with HLA Dw3/DRw3 antigens may mount an overproductive immune response to some innocuous foreign antigens expressed on the membranes of their steroid hormone-producing cells. In such individuals, this intensive immune response could lead to extensive tissue destruction, resulting in steroid cell autoimmunity. However, it would thus be necessary to suggest that most people who

are HLA Dw3/DRw3 would either never encounter the environmental trigger that would lead to the expression of immunizing foreign or altered self-antigens on their cell membranes or, alternatively, they are not otherwise genetically susceptible to adrenal autoimmunity. Those people not possessing HLA Dw3/DRw3 antigens that contact the environmental factor would either not recognize the foreign antigens or, although recognizing the antigens, would not respond immunologically. The findings of disordered immunologic regulation, as indicated by decreased suppressor cell functions, in some patients with Addison's disease tend to indicate that these hypotheses are plausible. However, there is no strong conclusive evidence to date for these possibilities.

6. CONCLUSIONS

Idiopathic Addison's disease and some cases of gonadal failure are clearly of autoimmune origin. However, definitive findings of how and why autoimmune destruction of these steroid hormone-producing cells occurs remains indirect and circumstantial. Proof of underlying autoimmunity could come from immunologic transferability of adrenalitis from affected patients to experimental animals. However, since there may be requirement for some HLA homology between effector lymphocytes and target adrenocortical cells for adrenocortical cell cytolysis to occur, such experiments may not be feasible for demonstration of cell-mediated autoimmunity in Addison's disease.

We see need for several areas of investigation. More patients with Addison's disease and type I APS must be studied by HLA typing to learn the extent of the differences from those seen in patients with type II APS. More of the latter must be HLA typed for A, B, C, and DR locus antigens to learn whether the primary association of adrenal autoimmunity is with HLA B8 or HLA DRw3. We recently had a patient who was Black, with both acute Addison's and Hashimoto's diseases, who was typed as being HLA B8 and

HLA DRw2 but not HLA DRw3. (Interestingly, HLA DRw2 has been thought to be protective for another autoimmune endocrine disease, IDDM.)

It also seems probable that there are surface-reactive autoantibodies to adrenocortical cells as have been described for thyroid and pancreatic islet cell autoimmunities. Since cell surface reacting autoantibodies have the potential to mediate adrenocortical tissue destruction, and such a mechanism is currently enjoying experimental favor in the pathogenesis of IDDM, such autoantibodies should be looked for in patients with Addison's disease. The nature of the cytosolic antigen to which adrenocortical autoantibodies react also needs definition and chemical identification. Could such an antigen be present on the cell surface as well?

More clinical effort is needed to classify the syndrome complexes that occur with autoimmune Addison's disease as many genetic and environmental factors may be involved. An animal model for spontaneous Addison's disease of immunologic origin is also required. In several respects, knowledge of autoimmune Addison's disease had preceded that of other organ-specific autoimmune diseases. The dramatic picture of a patient in Addisonian crisis may be one reason for this. In any event, it is reassuring to reflect that the disease may be readily diagnosed by current methodologies and the patient satisfactorily maintained by appropriate hormone replacement therapy. One wonders whether we will soon reach the point of elucidation of the various mechanisms involved in the etiology of autoimmune Addison's disease so that preventive therapies to arrest the disease short of complete adrenocortical failure could be devised.

ACKNOWLEDGMENTS

We thank Patricia Johnson for her assistance in preparing this manuscript and to William Riley, M.D. for his critical review. Support from NIH Grants AM2178203 and JDF 229H16 is gratefully acknowledged.

REFERENCES

1. M. B. Schmidt, *Verh. Dtsch. Ges. Pathol.* **21**, 212 (1926).
2. C. C. J. Carpenter, N. Solomon, S. G. Silverberg, T. Bledsoe, R. C. Northcutt, J. R. Klinenberg, I. L. Bennett, and A. M. Harvey, *Medicine* **43**, 153 (1964).
3. J. Nerup, *Acta Endocrinol.* **76**, 127 (1974).
4. W. J. Irvine and E. W. Barnes, "Addison's disease and associated conditions: with particular reference to premature ovarian failure, diabetes mellitus and hypoparathyroidism," in P. Gell, R. Coombs, and P. Lachman, Eds., *Clinical Aspects of Immunology*, Blackwell, Oxford, England, 1975, p. 1301.
5. J. Nerup, in P. Basterie and W. Gepts, Eds., *Immunity and Autoimmunity in Diabetes Mellitus*, Excerpta Medica, 1974.
6. M. Neufeld, N. K. Maclaren and R. Blizzard, *Pediatr. Ann.* **9**, 43, (1980).
7. M. Neufeld, N. K. Maclaren, and R. Blizzard, *Clin. Res.* **27**, 812A, (1979).
8. K. Arulanantham, J. J. Dwyer, and M. Genel, *N. Engl. J. Med.* **300**, 164 (1979).
9. G. S. Eisenbarth, P. W. Wilson, F. Ward, C. Buckley, and H. E. Lebowitz, *Ann. Int. Med.* **91**, 528 (1979).
10. G. S. Eisenbarth, P. W. Wilson, F. Ward, and H. E. Lebovitz, *N. Engl. J. Med.* **298**, 92 (1978).
11. M. W. Spinner, R. M. Blizzard, J. Gibbs, H. Abbey, and B. Childs, *Clin. Exp. Immunol.* **5**, 461 (1969).
12. M. Neufeld and R. M. Blizzard, in *Symposium on Autoimmune Aspects of Endocrine Disorders*, Academic Press, New York, 1979.
13. W. J. Irvine and E. W. Barnes, *Clin. Endocrin. Metabol.* **4**, 379 (1975).
14. J. R. Anderson, R. B. Goudie, K. G. Gray, and G. C. Tinbury, *Lancet* **1**, 1123 (1957).
15. R. M. Blizzard, D. Chee, and W. Davis, *Clin. Exp. Immunol.* **2**, 19 (1967).
16. J. Nerup, *Acta Endocrinol.* **76**, 142 (1974).
17. W. J. Riley, N. K. Maclaren, and M. Neufeld, *J. Pediatr.* **97**, 191 (1980).
18. J. Nerup, *Dan. Med. Bull.* **21**(6), 201 (1974).
19. N. K. Maclaren and M. Neufeld, in R. Collu, Ed., *Pediatric Endocrinology*, Raven Press, New York, 1981, Chapter 16.
20. R. B. Goudie, E. MacDonald, J. R. Anderson, and K. Gray, *Clin. Exp. Immunol.* **3**, 119 (1968).
21. W. J. Irvine, A. G. Steward, and L. Scarth, *Clin. Exp. Immunol.* **2**, 31 (1967).
22. J. R. Anderson, R. B. Goudie, K. Gray, and D. A. Stuart-Smith, *Clin. Exp. Immunol.* **3**, 107 (1968).

23. M. de M. Ruehesen, R. M. Blizzard, R. Garcia-Bunnuel, and G. S. Jones, *Am. J. Obstet Gynecol.* **112**, 693 (1972).

24. P. Kamp, P. Platz, and J. Nerup, *Acta Endocrinol.* **76**, 729 (1974).

25. M. Elder, N. Maclaren, and W. Riley, *J. Clin. Endocrinol. Metab.* **52**, 1137 (1981).

26. K. Krohn, J. Perheentupa, and E. Heinonen, *Clin. Immunol. Immunopathol.* **3**, 59 (1974).

27. E. Heinonen and K. Krohn, *Med. Biol.* **55**, 48 (1977).

28. E. Heinonen, K. Krohn, J. Perheentupa, A. Aro, and R. Pelkonen, *Ann. Clin. Res.* **8**, 262 (1976).

29. E. V. Barnett, D. C. Dumonde, and L. E. Glynn, *Immunol.* **6**, 382 (1963).

30. E. Witebsky and F. Milgrom, *Immunol.* **5**, 67 (1962).

31. S. Ishizawa and J. C. Daniels, *Immunol. Commun.* **9**, 437 (1980).

32. T. R. Gamlen, A. Aynsley-Green, W. J. Irvine, and C. J. McCallum, *Clin. Exp. Immunol.* **28**, 192 (1977).

33. K. McNatty, R. V. Short, E. W. Barnes, and W. J. Irvine, *Clin. Exp. Immunol.* **22**, 378 (1975).

34. J. Nerup and G. Bendixen, *Clin. Exp. Immunol.* **5**, 341 (1969).

35. R. Moulias, J. M. Goust, A. Deville Chabrolle, C. Buffets, and C. N. Muller-Berat, *Chez l' homme Presse Med.* **73**, 2315 (1970).

36. J. Nerup, V. Anderson, and G. Bendixen, *Clin. Exp. Immunol.* **6**, 733 (1970).

37. J. Nerup, V. Anderson, and G. Bendixen, *Clin. Exp. Immunol.* **4**, 355 (1969).

38. J. Nerup and G. Bendixen, *Clin. Exp. Immunol.* **5**, 355 (1969).

39. R. S. Fairchild, R. N. Schimke, and N. I. Abdou, *J. Clin. Endocrinol. Metab.* **51**, 1074 (1980).

40. J. Colover and L. E. Glynn, *Immunology* **1**, 172 (1958).

41. J. W. Steiner, B. Langer, D. L. Schatz, and R. Volpe, *J. Exp. Med.* **112**, 187 (1960).

42. O. Werdelin, *Acta Pathol. Microbiol. Scand. A*, Suppl. 232 (1972).

43. S. Levine and E. J. Wenk, *Am. J. Pathol.* **52**, 41 (1967).

44. R. M. Zinkernagel and P. C. Doherty, *J. Exp. Med.* **141**, 1427 (1975).

45. E. L. Reinherz and S. F. Schlossman, *J. Immunol.* **122**, 1335 (1979).

10

Polyglandular Failure Syndromes

George S. Eisenbarth
Nelson Rassi

Research Division
Joslin Diabetes Center
Department of Medicine
Brigham Hospital
Harvard Medical School
Boston, Massachusetts

Contents

1. THE CLINICAL SYNDROME

The polyglandular failure diseases are linked by autoimmune phenomena, by similar immunogenetics, and by the occurrence of multiple illnesses in the same individual. These associated diseases include primary hypothyroidism, Addison's disease, type I diabetes mellitus, primary hypogonadism, Graves' disease, pernicious anemia, vitiligo, alopecia totalis, myasthenia gravis, mucocutaneous candidiasis, chronic active hepatitis, and celiac disease. This group of illnesses has been termed Schmidt's syndrome (1), the polyglandular failure syndrome, organ-specific autoimmune disease, the syndrome of multiple endocrine gland insufficiency, autoimmune polyglandular syndrome, polyendocrinopathy diabetes, and candidiasis endocrinopathy. Despite its lack of reference to Graves' disease and nonendocrine components of the syndrome, we use the term polyglandular failure to describe the syndrome with two major subgroups, polyglandular failure type I (PGF I) and polyglandular failure type II (PGF II) to designate two genetically and clinically distinct syndromes (Table 1).

In a recent review we referenced articles tabulating disease and autoantibody prevalence in the PGF syndrome (2). Several recent reports add to our knowledge of the diseases

Table 1.   PGF subtypes

	Type I	Type II
Common disease associations	Addison's disease	Addison's disease
	Hypoparathyroidism	Graves' disease
	Mucocutaneous candidiasis	Type I diabetes mellitus
	Chronic active hepatitis	Atrophic thyroiditis
Immunogenetics	Not HLA associated	HLA-B8 population association
	Occurs in siblings unrelated to inheritance of HLA haplotypes	Multiple generations with disease. Often inherited with common HLA haplotypes
Peak age of onset of Addison's disease	Less than 10	20–40

associated with Addison's disease and illustrate the clinical information which initially led to the definition of the PGF syndrome. Table 2, which is adapted from a review by Irvine (3), lists illnesses associated with idiopathic Addison's disease. The high prevalence of type I diabetes mellitus (insulin-dependent diabetes mellitus, IDDM) and "autoimmune" thyroid disease in patients with idiopathic Addison's disease is apparent. In contrast, patients with adrenal insufficiency secondary to tuberculosis have a much lower prevalence of "autoimmune" endocrinopathy. In patients with Addison's disease without overt thyroid failure a report by Jens and co-workers (4) indicates that subclinical hypothyroidism is very common.

In addition to overt autoimmune endocrine disease, patients with Addison's disease frequently have autoantibodies to other tissues.

Table 2.   The principal clinical disorders associated with Addison's disease in a series of 383 patients

Disorder	Idiopathic	Tuberculosis	Other
Number of patients	321	58	4
Amenorrhea/oligomenorrhea	59 (18%)	1	
Thyrotoxicosis	16 (5%)	1 (1.7%)	
Hypothyroidism	28 (8.7%)		
Hashimoto's thyroiditis	7 (2.2%)		
Goiter	9 (2.8%)		
Pernicious anemia	12 (3.7%)		
Diabetes mellitus			
Type I	32 (10%)		
Type II	6 (1.9%)	2 (3.4%)	
Hypoparathyroidism	18 (5.6%)		
Vitiligo	22 (6.8%)	1 (1.7%)	
Asthma	9 (2.8%)		
Celiac disease	2 (0.6%)		
Renal tubular acidosis	2 (0.6%)		
Primary biliary cirrhosis	1 (0.3%)		
Myasthenia gravis	1 (0.3%)		

From Irvine (3).

Furthermore, patients with PGF illnesses without Addison's disease have antiadrenal antibodies. In an extensive study by Riley and co-workers (5), antiadrenal antibodies were found in 7 (1.5%) of 466 patients with type I diabetes mellitus. Two of the seven had Addison's disease, three were clinically hypothyroid, and one was thyrotoxic. All of the seven, in addition to their antiadrenal antibodies, had other organ-specific autoantibodies. Furthermore, lymphocytes from all seven patients expressed the HLA-B8 histocompatibility antigen (5).

Another important clinical feature of the PGF syndrome is that the age of onset of multiple diseases in the same individual can vary by more than 20 years. Shown in Figure 1a is the correlation of the age of diagnosis of type I diabetes compared with idiopathic Addison's disease. Figure 1b (from our own studies) plots the onset of several PGF illnesses versus the age of onset of Addison's disease (6). In Figure 1b each vertical group of dots represents the onset of one patient's multiple PGF illnesses. In both studies, age of onset of disease is statistically correlated, but there

is extensive variation about the line. This variation plus genetic studies to be discussed suggest that individuals with PGF inherit susceptibility to a number of autoimmune diseases, with environmental factors influencing the development of overt disease.

2. IMMUNOGENETICS

Similar to the manner in which diabetes mellitus has recently been divided into two distinct disease categories (type I, insulin-dependent diabetes mellitus which is HLA-B8, Dr3 associated, and type II, noninsulin-dependent diabetes mellitus which is not HLA associated) on the basis of clinical, immunologic, and genetic considerations, PGF has also been recently subdivided (7, 8).

As discussed in detail in Chapter 3, the majority of the component illnesses of PGF II in Caucasians are HLA-B8 and Dr3 associated. These illnesses include Addison's disease, Graves' disease, myasthenia gravis (9, 10), and atrophic hypothyroidism. It is noteworthy that goitrous hypothyroidism is

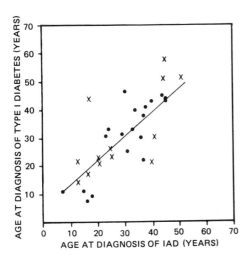
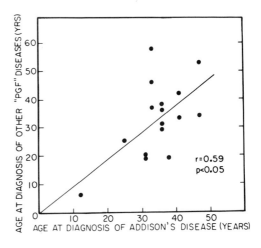

Figure 1. (left) Age at diagnosis of diabetes correlated with age at diagnosis of idiopathic (autoimmune) Addison's disease (IAD). From Irvine (3). (right) Each point represents a patient with Addison's disease and some other PGF disease. The age at which the diagnosis of Addison's was made is plotted on the abscissa. The age at which diagnosis of other diseases of PGF was made is plotted on the ordinate. This shows a positive correlation between age of diagnosis of Addison's disease and age of diagnosis of other PGF illnesses.

not HLA-B8 associated, and pernicious anemia is HLA-B8 associated only in the presence of other endocrine diseases (11–14). Vitiligo is a clinically recognized PGF illness which is not HLA-B8 associated. The association of individual illnesses with HLA-B8 has led to the HLA typing of patients with PGF. Figure 2 is a composite of HLA-A and B locus typing of 136 PGF patients (7, 15–21). Several disease associations, particularly IDDM (type I) with Addison's disease, Graves' disease,

or atrophic thyroiditis, are highly associated with HLA-B8.

In contrast, patients with chronic mucocutaneous candidiasis or hypoparathyroidism and idiopathic Addison's disease (termed type I autoimmune polyglandular syndrome) do not have an increased prevalence of the HLA-B8 histocompatibility antigen.

PGF I and II can be distinguished by the HLA associations discussed, inheritance patterns, and disease associations. More than 70

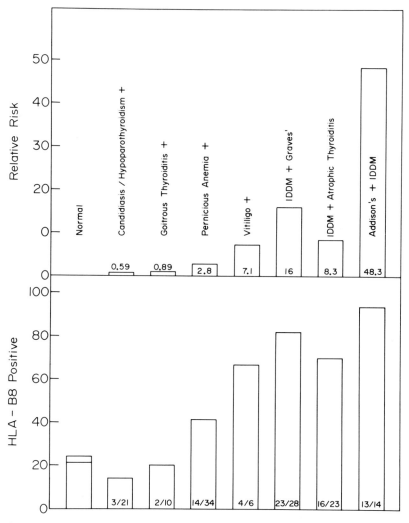

Figure 2. Results of HLA typing for antigen B8 in 136 patients with PGF from our studies and from the literature, subdivided by specific illnesses. A plus sign indicates one or more additional PGF illnesses in addition to the illnesses specified. The lower panel depicts the percentage of HLA-B8 positive, and the upper panel depicts the calculated HLA-B8 relative risk.

patients with Addison's disease and idiopathic hypoparathyroidism (usually with mucocutaneous candidiasis) have been reported (2). This syndrome aggregates within sibships, suggesting an autosomal recessive mode of inheritance (23). We are unaware of any report describing this form of PGF in several generations of a family, as is common with PGF II. In a few families whose HLA typing has been reported, inheritance of PGF I did not correlate with HLA inheritance (6, 24, 25), as occurs frequently with PGF II. Thus clinically and immunogenetically, PGF I is distinct from other PGF syndromes.

In several PGF II families (5, 6, 18, 20; Fig. 3) inheritance of PGF parallels inheritance of a common sixth chromosome, the chromosome coding for HLA antigens. In such families, with disease appearing in three or four generations, an autosomal dominant mode of inheritance is suggested. Even in such families (Fig. 3), susceptibility to a PGF illness and organ-specific autoantibodies rather than the specific PGF illness appears to be inherited. In the family shown in Figure 3, the proband has five diseases, whereas her mother does not have the proband's Addison's disease,

myasthenia gravis, or pernicious anemia. Furthermore, only the mother and aunt have alopecia totalis. In addition to the striking pattern of inheritance in selected PGF families, sharing of HLA haplotypes is common in family members with PGF illness (Table 3). The marked prevalence of PGF illness in relatives of PGF patients is noteworthy. It is common for such relatives to have unrecognized disease, in particular, unrecognized hypothyroidism (6). We found, by screening families, six of eight PGF probands had a relative with a PGF illness, 26% of all relatives had disease, and seven relatives (one in six) were unaware of their illness prior to screening (6).

At present, the pathogenic link between the HLA region of chromosome 6 and PGF II, or for that matter, the component illnesses, is not known. Because alleles in this area of chromosome 6 are not randomly associated (linkage disequilibrium), most hypotheses postulate an allele in linkage disequilibrium with HLA-B8 and HLA-Dr3 which confers disease susceptibility. The number of genes involved in the pathogenesis of these disorders is not known. Furthermore, it is not known

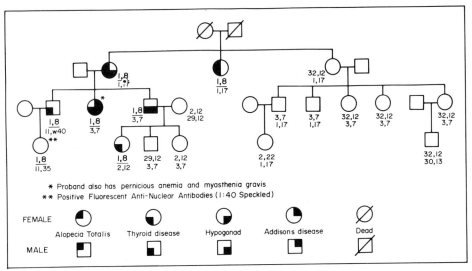

Figure 3. Results of HLA typing and clinical evaluation of one of the families we studied. Asterisks indicate proband. Haplotypes, depicted one above the other, were deduced from HLA typing and the pattern of inheritance. The HLA-A1 B8 haplotype is underlined. Occurrence of disease is as noted.

Table 3.   Relatives with a PGF illness

		Siblings, Shared HLA Haplotypes			
Father	Mother	None	One	Two	Children
3/9[a]	6/11[a]	1/11	6/10	7/13	2/13
33%	55%	9%	60%	54%	17%

From Eisenbarth et al. (2).

[a] In none of the families did both the mother and father have a PGF illness. Information was available on 13 families, but data on the health of six parents were not reported.

whether one gene (or a group of genes) is etiologic for the multiple diseases or whether a single gene confers susceptibility for several individual PGF diseases (6). The HLA region of chromosome 6 certainly controls many immune functions, and the hypothesis we favor is that a single gene or group of genes by their influence on generalized immune function confer susceptibility to many, if not all, of the PGF II illnesses (2). Environmental and probably other genetic influences then determine the particular overt illness that develops. It is noteworthy that an individual with a rare PGF illness, such as Addison's disease or myasthenia gravis, most often develops a PGF illness which is common in the general population (e.g., autoimmune thyroid disease > IDDM > Addison's disease > myasthenia gravis). The prevalence of each of these illnesses is greatly increased relative to the general population. A similar hierarchy of disease prevalence is seen in relatives of PGF patients.

It is unlikely that the histocompatibility alleles, HLA-B8 or Dr3, are directly pathogenic. In non-Caucasian populations PGF illnesses are associated with other HLA alleles (22).

3.   DISEASES WITH SIMILAR IMMUNOGENETICS

A number of diseases are associated with HLA-B8 or Dr3 but are not part of the classic PGF syndrome. These diseases include juvenile dermatomyositis (26, 27), dermatitis herpetiformis (28–32), systemic lupus erythematosus (33–36), celiac disease (28–31, 37–38), IgA deficiency (39), chronic active hepatitis (40), Sjorgren's syndrome (41–46), and possibly asthma (47) and hayfever (48). Does the occurrence of one HLA-B8 or Dr3 associated disease increase an individual's risk for developing another HLA-B8 or Dr3 associated disease?

There are a few reports in the literature linking a number of the above illnesses with endocrine disease. The coexistence of celiac disease and diabetes was reported by Pynton and Cole (49) and subsequently this association was reported in both children and adults (50–56). Walsh et al. (57) described 14 adults with IDDM with coexistent celiac disease (biopsy proven). Cooper et al. (58) studied 314 patients with celiac disease and found that 64 had associated disease of known or suspected immunologic cause such as diabetes mellitus, thyroid disease (Graves' disease and Hashimoto's thyroiditis), and ulcerative colitis. In view of the clinical association of IDDM and celiac disease we consider celiac disease a PGF illness. The association of celiac disease with type I diabetes is clinically important. Severe diarrhea in a patient with type I diabetes may result from celiac disease, which is treatable with a gluten-free diet, and not "diabetic enteropathy," which often defies therapy.

Severe progressive systemic sclerosis (PSS) has been reported to be HLA-B8 associated (59). Gordon et al. (60) have reported the association of primary hypothyroidism and Hashimoto's thyroiditis with progressive systemic sclerosis.

Systemic lupus erythematosus (SLE) has been associated in some instances with thyroiditis (61). There are two case reports of the association of SLE with diabetes mellitus, one by Freeman (62), who described a HLA-B8-positive girl with systemic lupus erythematosus, anti-islet antibodies, and diabetes mellitus. The second report by O'Regan (63) describes an HLA-B8-positive patient with PGF (diabetes mellitus and hypothyroidism) who developed SLE. We have found a high prevalence of anti-islet antibodies in patients with polyclonal B cell activation, including SLE (64).

Holt and Blockwell (65), from a series of 102 patients with dermatitis herpetiformis, found four with IDDM (one also had primary hypothyroidism). Three of those four patients developed severe diabetic nephropathy. The authors postulated that the association of IDDM and dermatitis herpetiformis may occur more often than one would expect by chance and such patients may be at higher risk for diabetic nephropathy.

The association of Sjorgren's syndrome with PGF (autoimmune thyroid disease and premature ovarian failure) has been reported. Other authors have reported an association of PGF with other autoimmune disease such as rheumatoid arthritis (66), juvenile rheumatoid arthritis (67, 68), and autoimmune thrombocytopenia purpura (69–71).

4. IMMUNE FUNCTION

Patients with PGF syndrome have reported abnormalities of both B and T cell function.

4.1. Humoral Immunity

"Organ-specific" autoantibodies (e.g., anti-islet, antiadrenal, antimelanocyte) are present in patients with PGF and often react with glands that are not overtly diseased. In addition, asymptomatic relatives of PGF patients frequently have detectable organ-specific autoantibodies. These autoantibodies have

been described in detail in other chapters, and we highlight these studies only briefly.

Seventy percent of patients with "idiopathic" Addison's disease are reported to have antibodies to the adrenal cortex (73, 74). Such antibodies are absent in patients with adrenal failure secondary to tuberculosis. Sometimes these antibodies cross-react with steroid-producing cells in gonads. These antibodies can be transported across the placenta into the fetal circulation, but they apparently do not damage the fetal adrenal gland (74).

In Graves' disease the autoantibodies appear to play a major role in pathogenesis. Graves' disease antibodies react with the TSH receptor and can be detected by their inhibition of the binding of TSH. Such antibodies stimulate thyroidal adenylate cyclase or may inhibit the activation of adenylate cyclase by TSH.

Islet cell antibodies were first described in patients with IDDM and PGF (75, 76). Patients with type I diabetes in the absence of PGF lose their anti-islet antibodies, whereas patients with PGF retain such antibodies for years. In addition, Irvine et al. have reported that 5.6% of patients with at least one of the PGF illnesses in the absence of diabetes had anti-islet antibodies (77). Thirty percent of these patients developed a diabetic glucose tolerance test during 1 to 11 years of follow-up. The presence of islet cell antibodies in gestational diabetes may predict which patients with gestational diabetes will become insulinopenic on follow-up (78).

Myasthenia gravis is another component of the PGF syndrome in which autoantibodies appear to be pathogenic. Infants of mothers with myasthenia gravis frequently have transient myasthenia secondary to the transplacental passage of antibodies. The anti-acetylcholine receptor antibodies of myasthenia gravis have been studied extensively, including the production of monoclonal antiacetylcholine antibodies which can create acute myasthenia in rodents. It is noteworthy that an intact thymus appears to be of importance for the production of myasthenia gravis by these monoclonal antibodies. In patients with myasthenia gravis, their disease frequently remits post-thymectomy despite high titers of circulating anti-acetylcholine receptor antibodies.

Other diseases of the PGF syndrome such as pernicious anemia are associated with autoantibodies, but such antibodies do not correlate with clinical status (79).

In addition to specific autoantibodies we found generalized abnormalities of immunoglobulin levels in 15 patients with PGF (80) with elevation of IgG and IgA despite normal lGM levels (Fig. 4). Complement-fixing antibodies to a series of common viruses were also studied in these patients and controls. There was no significant difference in the titer between the two groups except for antibodies against Coxsackie B4 and B5 viruses, which were depressed in the PGF patients (80).

4.2.   Cellular Immunity

Several abnormalities in T cell function have been detected in patients with the PGF syndrome. Cutaneous hypersensitivity studied with skin tests utilizing common antigens was assessed in a group of patients with PGF (80), and it was found that they had a decreased delayed cutaneous responsiveness (Fig. 5). Lymphocytes from 22 out of 24 patients with type I diabetes, including 18 with PGF, when incubated with mouse islet cells were able to inhibit insulin release (81). It has also been

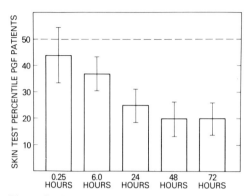

Figure 5.   Skin test responses in PGF patients compared to response for our control populations. Each bar represents the mean percent response from all skin tests of the patient relative to those of age- and sex-matched controls.

found that patients with type I diabetes and PGF have an increased number of B lymphocytes (82). Cell-mediated immune responses have been shown to be impaired in many of the PGF illnesses such as Addison's disease (83), type I diabetes (84), and myasthenia gravis (85). Supressor cell activity has been reported to be depressed in type I diabetes (86, 87).

Utilizing an in vitro bioassay of the suppressor function of concanavalin A-stimulated lymphocytes in patients with PGF, we have found that their suppressor function is, on the average, less than that of normal individuals (88). There was, however, marked overlap of suppressor function utilizing different combinations of human stimulator and responder cells, and the majority of the patients exhibited some suppression in the assays utilized. Two of the PGF patients we have studied were unique. Lymphocytes from one patient (PGF II) could not suppress his own lymphocytes or those of other individuals, whereas lymphocytes from another patient with PGF I could suppress lymphocytes from other people but not her own (Fig. 6).

Pozilli and co-workers (89) studied K cell levels (mononuclear cells forming low affinity rosettes with sheep erythrocytes and which kill IgG-sensitized target organs) in 44 patients with PGF. Forty percent of these patients had

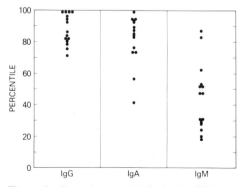

Figure 4.   Serum immunoglobulin levels of PGF patients compared to values for our control population. Each dot represents the percentile of one patient.

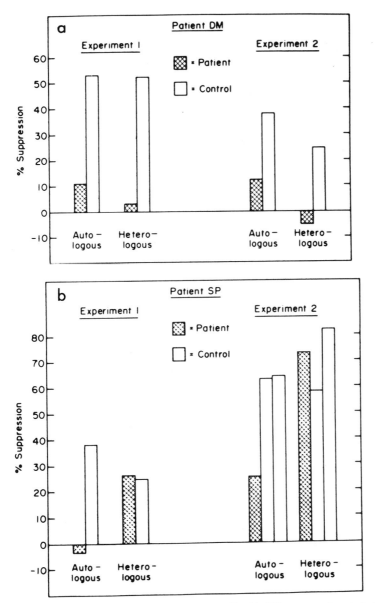

Figure 6. Sets of two experiments for PGF patients DM and SP with different normal controls determining concanavalin A-induced suppressor activity. Both suppression of the patients' own lymphocytes and suppression of other individuals' lymphocytes were studied (autologous and heterologous suppression).

high K cell levels and the percentage of K cells correlated with the level of in vitro antibody-dependent cytotoxicity.

Monoclonal antibody reagents are now available which define a series of human lymphocyte antigens (90). Antibodies we have utilized react with the majority of T cells

(OKT3), subsets of T cells (3A1, OKT4, OKT8), or activated T cells (L243, 4F2, 5E9). Utilizing this panel of monoclonal antibodies in the study of patients with type I diabetes and untreated Graves' disease, we have only found an abnormality of the percentage and absolute number of T cells reacting with antibody L243 or other anti-Ia antibodies (91). Antibody L243 reacts with the Ia antigen which is normally expressed on B lymphocytes, but appears on T lymphocytes after activation. The presence of an increased percentage of Ia-positive T cells early in the course of type I diabetes and Graves' disease probably reflects activation of these cells. The ease of measuring T cell subsets with monoclonal antibodies should aid in defining cellular immune processes in PGF patients.

5. ANIMAL MODELS

A number of inbred strains of animals are now available which develop diabetes mellitus or "autoimmune" thyroid disease. Such animal models aid the study of the genetics and pathogenesis of the PGF illnesses. In partic-

ular, these animals allow investigators to test the effects of treatment with, for example, antilymphocyte globulin or bone marrow transplants (92) on the course of endocrine disease.

The obese chicken develops thyroiditis and hypothyroidism (93, 94). The genetics of the thyroiditis in these chickens has been studied in detail. Disease susceptibility appears to be under polygenic control with genes linked with histocompatibility alleles contributing to susceptibility (95–97). These chickens are frequently IgA deficient. It is noteworthy that 3% of the patients with type I diabetes are reported to be IgA deficient (98).

NZO mice exhibit an insulin resistance syndrome. These mice and related mice (NSB/NZW) develop multiple autoantibodies, particularly anti-DNA antibodies. In addition to their lupus erythematosus-like syndrome,

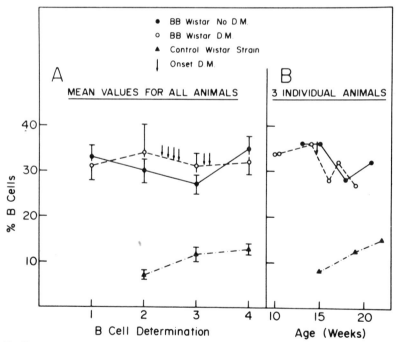

Figure 7.   Percentage of B cells of BB Wistar and control Wistar rats. (A) Mean ± SEM percentage of surface immunoglobulin-positive cells (B cells) of Ficoll-Hypaque purified lymphocytes of BB Wistar rats, which did and did not develop overt diabetes, and control Wistar rats. Determinations are grouped in 3-week intervals starting at 10 weeks of age. (B) Percentage of surface immunoglobulin-positive cells of three representative individual rats, one BB Wistar that developed diabetes, one BB Wistar that did not develop diabetes, and one animal of the control rat strain.

Table 4. Comparison of circulating white blood cells[a]

	Control Strain	BB Wistar	Difference
Experiment 1			
White blood count	12,612 ± 1677	7,422 ± 805	5190
Polymorphonuclear leukocytes	1,982 ± 419	2,600 ± 560	−618
Monocytes	418 ± 64	283 ± 68	135
Lymphocytes	10,290 ± 1220	4,549 ± 409	5741[b]
B lymphocytes	1,338 ± 171	1,581 ± 224	−243
Non-B lymphocytes	8,953 ± 1058	2.968 ± 246	5985[b]
Experiment 2			
B lymphocytes	1,569 ± 242	1,495 ± 595	74
Non-B lymphocytes	6,245 ± 765	2,412 ± 451	3833[b]
W3/13 + non-B	5,929 ± 727	2,111 ± 396	3818[b]
W3/25 + non-B	4,996 ± 612	169 ± 32	4827[b]
W3/25 − non-B	1,249 ± 153	2,243 ± 419	−994

From Jackson et al. (105).
[a] *In experiment 1, mean ± SEM of four control rats and five BB Wistar rats; experiment 2, mean ± SEM of five control rats and three BB Wistar rats.*
[b] *p < .01 by Student's t test.*

many of these mice strains develop "insulitis" and impaired glucose tolerance, though overt diabetes mellitus has not been reported (99).

An inbred strain of rats (BB) which does develop overt diabetes mellitus has been studied extensively. Approximately half of these inbred rats between 60 and 120 days of age develop overt diabetes mellitus, characterized by β cell destruction with insulitis (100, 101). A number of immunologic interventions have been used to prevent or decrease the incidence of diabetes in these animals. These interventions include therapy with antilymphocyte globulin (102), neonatal thymectomy (103), and infusion of bone marrow cells from normal rats into neonatal BB rats (92). In addition to their development of diabetes mellitus, these animals develop thyroiditis, as reported recently by E. Sternthal and co-workers (104); the prevalence of thyroiditis is increased by exposure of the BB rats to iodine (104).

We have recently discovered that the BB rat has a severe T cell lymphocytopenia (105). This T cell lymphocytopenia was first detected because of the greatly increased percentage of circulating B cells in these animals. This

elevation of the percentage of B lymphocytes precedes the development of diabetes and is independent of its occurrence (Fig. 7). As shown by the experimental results in Table 4, the increased percentage of B cells results from a severe deficiency of T cells. Several monoclonal antibody reagents are now available to aid in the quantitation of rat T cells (W3/13 "all T cells") or T cell subsets (W3/25, "help, graft versus host" T cells). The deficiency of T cells is secondary to a lack of circulating W3/25 cells. It is likely this marked aberration of immunoregulation contributes to the development of diabetes mellitus in the BB rat, but that by itself, this abnormality of circulating T cells is not sufficient to cause diabetes.

6. CONCLUSIONS

The component illnesses of the PGF syndrome, as well as the syndrome itself, cause significant morbidity and mortality. Many of the diseases, if recognized prior to an irreversible morbid event (e.g., Addison's disease, pernicious anemia, Graves' disease, atrophic hypothyroidism), can be adequately treated. Treatment in these diseases is not directed at the underlying "immunologic" abnormalities, but rather replaces the missing hormone (or vitamin) or (as is the case with Graves' disease) results in destruction of the overactive gland. Treatment of several of the component illnesses of the PGF syndrome is not adequate. In particular, studies of patients with type I diabetes mellitus treated with insulin reveals that within 30 to 40 years of the onset of diabetes, more than one-half die from the chronic complications of this disease and many are blinded or disabled (106). It is hoped, but clearly not proved, that improved insulin regimens and home glucose monitoring will help decrease this morbidity and mortality. Myasthenia gravis is another PGF illness in which for many patients, long-term therapy proves to be inadequate. Our current knowledge of the immunogenetics, disease associations, and immunologic abnormalities of these illnesses have led to initial studies of immunosuppression in these disorders (107–109). It is hoped that more precise definition of the immunopathogenesis of these illnesses and improved drugs for immunologic therapy will lead to improved therapy or prevention of this group of illnesses.

REFERENCES

1. M. B. Schmidt, *Verh. Dtsch. Pathol. Ges.* 212–221 (1926).

2. G. S. Eisenbarth and R. J. Jackson, in N. Farid, Ed., *HLA in Endocrine and Metabolic Diseases*, Academic Press, New York, 1981.

3. J. W. Irvine, *Recent Prog. Horm. Res.* **36**, 509–556 (1980).

4. F. Jens, D. Cohn, C. Kirkegaard, M. Christy, K. Siersback-Nielsen, T. Friis, and J. Nerup, *Act. Endocr.* **91**(4), 674–679 (1979).

5. W. J. Riley, N. K. Maclaren, and M. Neufeld, *J. Pediatr.* **97**, 191–195 (1980).

6. G. S. Eisenbarth, P. W. Wilson, F. Ward, C. Buckley, and H. Lebovitz, *Ann. Int. Med.* **91**, 528–533 (1979).

7. M. Neufeld, R. M. Blizzard, and N. Maclaren, *Clin. Res.* **27**, 812A (1979).

8. M. Neufeld, N. Maclaren, and R. Blizzard, *Pediatr. Ann.* **9**, 154–162 (1980).

9. D. Fritze, C. Herrmann, F. Naeim, G. S. Smith, E. Zeller, and R. L. Walford, *Ann. N.Y. Acad. Sci.* **274**, 440–450 (1976).

10. F. Naeim, J. C. Keesey, C. Herrmann, J. Lindstrom, E. Zeller, and R. L. Walford, *Tissue Antigens* **12**, 381–386 (1978).

11. J. Chanarin, S. Knight, J. O'Brien, and D. James, *Br. J. Haematol.* **33**, 539–541 (1976).

12. J. Mawhinney, J. W. M. Lawton, A. G. White, and W. J. Irvine, *Clin. Exp. Immunol.* **22**, 47–53 (1975).

13. B. Ungar, J. D. Mathews, B. D. Tait, and D. C. Cowling, *Br. Med. J.* **1**, 798–800 (1977).

14. A. H. Goldstone, D. Voak, J. C. Cawley, and W. J. Irvine, *Clin. Exp. Immunol.* **25**, 352–354 (1976).

15. P. B. Anderson, S. H. Fein, and W. G. Frey, III, *J. Am. Med. Assoc.* **244**, 2068–2070 (1980).

16. G. F. Bottazo, A. G. Cudworth, T. J. Moud, D. Doniach, and H. Festenstein, *Br. Med. J.* **2**, 1253–1255 (1978).

17. R. J. Collen, B. M. Lippe, and S. A. Kaplan, *Am. J. Dis. Child* **133**, 589–600 (1979).

18. G. S. Eisenbarth, P. Wilson, F. Ward, and H. E. Lebovitz, *N. Engl. J. Med.* **298**, 92–94 (1978).

19. N. R. Farid, B. Larsen, R. Payne, E. P. Noel, and L. Sampson, *Tissue Antigens* **16**(1), 23–29 (1980).

20. W. Riley, N. Mclaren, J. McLaughlin, M. Neufeld, J. Silverstein, and A. Rosenbloom, *Clin. Res.* **27**, 813A (1979).

21. D. H. VanThiel, W. I. Smith, B. S. Rabin, S. E. Fisher, and R. Lester, *Ann. Int. Med.* **86**, 10–19 (1977).

22. A. Kawa, Y. Nakamura, Y. Kono, Y. Maedo, and L. Kanehisa, *Experientia* **35**, 547–548 (1979).

23. M. W. Spinner, R. M. Blizzard, and B. Childs, *J. Clin. Endocrinol. Metab.* **28**, 795–804 (1968).

24. K. Arulananthem, J. M. Dwyer, and M. Genel, *N. Engl. J. Med.* **300**, 164–168 (1979).

25. M. J. Brueton, H. M. Chapel, and L. P. Mackintosh, *Tissue Antigens* **15**, 101–103 (1980).

26. L. M. Pachman, O. Jonasson, R. A. Cannon, Y. M. Friedman, *Lancet* **2**, 1238 (1977).

27. L. M. Pachman, and N. Cooke, *J. Pediatr.* **96**, 226–234 (1980).

28. I. Stephen, Z. Katz, M. Falchuk, M. V. Dahl, G. N. Rogentine, and W. Strober, *J. Clin. Invest.* **51**, 2877–2980 (1972).

29. A. G. White, R. S. C. Barnetson, J. A. G. DaCosta, and D. B. L. McClelland, *Br. J. Derm.* **89**, 133–136 (1973).

30. B. G. Solheim, Y. Ek, P. O. Thune, K. Baklien, A. Bratlie, B. Rankin, A. B. Thoresen, and E. Thorsby, *Tissue Antigens* **7**, 57–59 (1976).

31. P. P. Seah, L. Fry, J. W. Kearney, E. Campbell, J. F. Mowbray, J. S. Stewart, and A. V. Hoffbrand, *Br. J. Derm.* **94**, 131–138 (1976).

32. S. I. Katz, R. P. Hall, III, T. J. Lawley, and W. Strober, *Ann. Intern. Med.* **93**, 857–874 (1980).

33. F. C. Grumet, A. Coukell, J. G. Bodmer, W. F. Bodmer, and H. O. McDevitt, *N. Engl. J. Med.* **285**, 193–196 (1971).

34. K. M. Nies, J. C. Brown, E. L. Dubois, F. P. Quismorio, G. J. Friou, and P. J. Terasaki, *Arthritis Rheum.* **17**, 397–402 (1974).

35. F. Kissmeyer-Nielsen, K. E. Kyerbye, E. Andersen, and P. Halberg, *Transplant Rev.* **22**, 164–167 (1975).

36. M. A. Goldberg, F. C. Arnette, W. B. Bias, and L. E. Shulman, *Arthritis Rheum.* **19**, 129 132 (1976).

37. P. L. Stokes, P. Asquith, G. K. T. Holmes, P. Mackintosh, and W. T. Cooke, *Lancet* **2**, 162–164 (1972).

38. J. J. Keuning, A. S. Pena, A. Van Leeuwen, J. P. Van Hoof, J. J. Van Rood, *Lancet* **1**, 506–507 (1974).

39. M. Ambrus, E. Hernadi, and G. Bajtai, *Clin. Immunol. Immunopathol.* **7**, 311–314 (1976).

40. J. R. Mackay, and P. J. Morris, *Lancet* **2**, 793–795 (1972).

41. D. Ivanyi, J. Drizhal, E. Erbenova, J. Horejs, M. Salavec, H. Macurova, C. Dostal, J. Balik, and J. Juran, *Tissue Antigens* **7**, 45–51 (1976).

42. T. M. Chused, S. S. Kassan, G. Opelz, H. M. Moutsopoules, and P. Terasaki, *N. Engl. J. Med.* **296**, 895–897 (1977).

43. E. Hinzova, D. Ivanyi, K. Sula, J. Horejs, C. Dostal, and J. Dfizhal, *Tissue Antigens* **9**, 8–10 (1977).

44. J. D. Clough, C. J. Aponte, and W. E. Braun, *Clin. Immunol. Immunopathol.* **7**, 324–329 (1977).

45. K. H. Fye, P. Terasaki, J. P. Micholski, T. E. Daniels, G. Opelz, and N. Talal, *Arthritis Rheum.* **21**, 337–342 (1978).

46. A. Ayala, E. S. Canales, S. Karchmer, D. Alarcon, and A. Zarate, *Obstet. Gynecol. N.Y.* **53**, 985–1015 (1979).

47. E. Thorsby, A. Engeset, and S. O. Lie, *Tissue Antigens* **1**, 147–152 (1971).

48. B. B. Levine, R. H. Stember, and M. Fotino, *Science* **178**, 1201–1203 (1972).

49. F. J. Poynton, and L. B. Cole, *Br. J. Child. Dis.* **22**, 30 (1925).

50. M. W. Thompson, *Am. J. Hum. Genet.* **3**, 159–166 (1951).

51. C. Hooft, E. Devos, J. Kriekemans, and J. Van Damme, *Helv. Paediatr. Acta* **23**, 478–488 (1968).

52. J. K. Visakorpi, *Lancet* **2**, 1192 (1969).

53. E. T. Bossak, C. J. Wang, and D. Adlesbeig, *J. Mt. Sinai Hosp.* **24**, 112–129 (1957).

54. E. P. Taxay, S. Roath, and S. Mitchel, *Diabetes* **9**, 106–109 (1960).

55. J. M. Malins and N. Mayne, *Diabetes* **18**, 858–866 (1969).

56. M. J. Lancaster-Smith, J. Perrin, E. T. Swarbrick, and J. T. Wright, *Postgrad. Med. J.* **50**, 45–48 (1974).

57. C. H. Walsh, B. T. Cooper, A. D. Wright, J. M. Malins, and W. T. Cooke, *Q. J. Med. New Ser. XIVII* **185**, 89–100 (1978).

58. B. T. Cooper, G. K. T. Holmes, and W. T. Cooke, *Br. Med. J.* **1**, 537–539 (1978).

59. P. Hughes, K. Gelsthorpe, R. W. Doughty, N. R. Rowell, F. D. Rosenthal, and J. B. Aneddon, *Clin. Exp. Immunol.* **31**, 351–356 (1978).

60. M. B. Gordon, I. Klein, A. Dekker, G. P. Rodnon, and T. A. Medsger, *Ann. Intern. Med.* **95**, 431–435 (1981).

61. *Rice's Practice of Medicine*, Harper & Row, New York, 1970.

62. L. W. Freeman, *Am. J. Dis. Child.* **131**, 1252–1254 (1977).

63. S. O'Regan, *CMA J.* **121**, 1168–1169 (1979).

64. G. S. Eisenbarth and M. A. Crum P., *Diabetes* **1**, 30, Abstr. 260 (1981).

65. S. Holt and J. Blockwell, *Postgrad. Med. J.* **56**, 15–17 (1980).

66. M. Rudolf, J. Dwyer, and M. Genel, *Am. Diabetes Assoc., 40th Ann. Meet. 1980, Washington, D.C.*, Abstr. 210 (1980).

67. M. Fisher, M. Nussbaum, C. A. L. Abrams, and I. R. Shenker, *Am. J. Dis. Child* **134**, 93–94 (1980).

68. R. J. Collen, B. M. Lippe, and S. A. Kaplan, *Am. J. Dis. Child* **133**, 598–600 (1979).

69. J. S. Marshal, A. S. Weisberger, R. P. Levey, R. T. Breckenridge, *Ann. Int. Med.* **67**, 411–414 (1967).

70. G. Remuzzi, M. Livio, M. B. Donati, and G. deGaetano, *Ann. Intern. Med.* **87**, 250–251 (1977).

71. B. M. Segal and M. I. Weintraub, *Ann. Intern. Med.* **85**, 761–772 (1976).

72. W. J. Irvine, A. G. Stewart, and L. Scarth, *Clin. Exp. Immunol.* **2**, 31–69 (1967).

73. J. Nerup, *Acta Endocrinol.* **76**, 142–158 (1974).

74. T. R. Gamlen, A. Aynsley-Green, W. J. Irvine, and C. J. McCallum, *Clin. Exp. Immunol.* **28**, 192–195 (1977).

75. G. F. Bottazo, A. Florin-Christensen, and D. Doniach, *Lancet* **2**, 1279–1783 (1974).

76. A. C. MacCuish, E. W. Barnes, W. J. Irvine, and L. J. P. Duncan, *Lancet* **2**, 1529–1531 (1974).

77. W. J. Irvine, R. S. Gray, and C. J. McCallum, *Lancet* **2**, 1097–1102 (1976).

78. F. Ginsberg-Fellner, M. Dobersen, E. M. Mark, C. Nechemias, R. U. Hausknecht, P. Rubinstein, and A. L. Notkins, *Diabetes* **29**, Abstr. 212 (1980).

79. M. S. Rose, J. Chanarin, D. Doniach, J. Brostoff, and S. Ardeman, *Lancet* **2**, 9–13 (1970).

80. W. Wilson, C. E. Buckley, III, and G. Eisenbarth, *J. Clin. Endocrin. Metab.* **52**, 284–288 (1981).

81. C. Boitard, M. Debray-Sachs, A. Pouplard, and R. Assan, *Diabetes* **46**, 259, Abstr. 46 (1981).

82. G. Bersani, P. Zanco, D. Padovan, and C. Betterie, *Diabetologia* **20**, 47–50 (1981).

83. J. Nerup, V. Andersen, and G. Bendixen, *Clin. Exp. Immunol.* **4**, 355–363 (1969).

84. W. J. Irvine, A. C. MacCuish, C. J. Campbell, and L. J. P. Duncan, *Acta Endocrinol.* **83**, Suppl. 205, 65–76 (1976).

85. J. A. Simpson, P. O. Behan, M. D. Heather, *Ann. N.Y. Acad. Sci.* **274**, 382–389 (1976).

86. K. Buschard, J. Rygaard, and S. Madsbad, *Diabetologia* **19**, 262, Abstr. 61 (1980).

87. A. Galluzzo, C. Giordano, C. Sparacino, and G. D. Bompiani, *Diabetologia* **19**, 275, Abstr. 133 (1980).

88. M. W. Verghese, F. E. Ward, and G. S. Eisenbarth, *Human Immunol.* **3**, 173–179 (1981).

89. P. Pozilli, D. Andreani, M. Sensi, E. Wolf, M. Taylor, G. F. Bottazzo, and A. G. Cudworth, *Proc. Int. Cong. Endocrinol.* **VI**, 639 (1980).

90. G. S. Eisenbarth, *Anal. Biochem.* **111**, 1–16 (1981).

91. R. Jackson, M. Bowring, M. Morris, B. Haynes, and G. S. Eisenbarth, *N. Eng. J. Med.* **306**, 785 (1982).

92. A. Naji, W. K. Silvers, D. Bellgrau, and C. F. Barker, *Science* **213**, 1390–1392 (1981).

93. G. Wick, R. S. Sundick, and B. Albini, *Clin. Immunol. Immunopathol.* **3**, 272–300 (1974).

94. M. E. Gershwin, J. Montero, J. Eklund, H. Abplanalp, R. M. Ikeda, A. A. Benedict, L. Tam, and K. Erickson, *Genetic Control of Autoimmune Disease*, Elsevier, Amsterdam, 1978, pp. 271–285.

95. L. D. Bacon, J. H. Kite, Jr., and N. R. Rose, *Science* **186**, 274–275 (1974).

96. L. D. Bacon, R. K. Cole, C. R. Polley, and N. R. Rose, *Genetic Control of Autoimmune Disease*, Elsevier, Amsterdam, 1978, pp. 259–270.

97. N. R. Rose, L. D. Bacon, R. S. Sundick, *Trans. Rev.* **31**, 264–285 (1976).

98. W. J. Smith, B. S. Rabin, A. Huellmantel, D. H. VanThiel, and A. Drash, *Diabetes* **27**, 1092–1097 (1978).

99. L. C. Harrison and A. Illin, *Nature* **279**, 334–336 (1979).

100. A. F. Nakhooda, A. A. Like, C. S. Chappel, F. T. Murray, and E. B. Marliss, *Diabetes* **26**, 100–112 (1977).

101. A. F. Nakhooda, A. A. Like, C. S. Chappel, C. N. Wei, E. B. Marliss, *Diabetologia* **14**, 199–207 (1978).

102. A. A. Like, A. A. Rossini, D. L. Gubersky, M. C. Appel, and R. M. Williams, *Science* **206**, 1421–1423 (1979).

103. A. A. Like, R. M. Williams, E. Kislowskis, and A. A. Rossini, *Clin. Res.* **29**, Abstr. 542 (1981).

104. E. Sternthal, A. Like, K. Serantis, and L. Braverman, *63rd Meeting, Endocr. Soc.*, Abstr. 756 (1981).

105. R. Jackson, N. Rassi, M. A. Crump, B. Haynes, and G. S. Eisenbarth, *Diabetes* **30**, 887–889 (1981).

106. T. Deckert, J. E. Poulson, and M. Larsen, *Acta Med. Scand. Suppl.* **624**, 48–53 (1979).

107. A. D. Roses, C. W. Olanow, M. W. McAdams, and R. J. M. Lane, *Neurology* **31**, 220–224 (1981).

108. R. B. Elliot, J. R. Crossley, C. C. Berryman, and A. G. James, *Lancet* **2**, 1–4 (1981).

109. R. Jackson, R. Dolinar, S. Srikenta, M. Morris, and G. S. Eisenbarth, *Diabetes* **31**, Suppl. 2, Abstr. 192 (1982).

11

Immunology of Infertility

Gilbert G. Haas, Jr.

Department of Obstetrics and Gynecology
School of Medicine
The University of Pennsylvania
Philadelphia, Pennsylvania

Contents

1. INTRODUCTION

The mechanisms of immune tolerance that are critical for successful reproduction are among the most intriguing phenomena in biology. Fetal/maternal interactions are discussed in Chapter 12. Similarly, it is of interest to review the female's ability to suppress sensitization by the sperm/seminal plasma antigenic challenge that occurs at the time of each intercourse, and the failure of the suppressive mechanism to result in infertility.

Sensitization to sperm antigens is probably prevented by the binding of "natural" antibodies to the sperm surface (1), similar to the binding of anti-A or anti-B antibodies to erythrocytes from an AB-incompatible fetus that prevents immunization of the mother by fetal Rhesus antigens. Others (2) have suggested that the endocervix coats the majority of sperm with IgG immunoglobulins, while the small number of sperm that will achieve the upper female reproductive tract remain uncoated. Sperm coated with immunoglobulin would eventually be phagocytosed by endometrial or endocervical macrophages (3), a possible mechanism for eliminating abnormal sperm from the opportunity of achieving fertilization. In this hypothesis, women with antibody-mediated infertility would place antibodies against sperm-specific antigens on even those sperm that had successfully negotiated the cervix and uterine fundus. The probability that the uterus actively selects sperm by immunologic processes is strengthened by the observation that sperm recovered from the mouse and rabbit uterus are associated with antibodies whereas those found in the oviduct are not (4). Since in humans only

200 sperm reach the oviduct (5), it has been proposed that the inhospitable environment of the uterus to spermatozoa may have necessitated the redundant number of sperm necessary for successful reproduction (6). Theoretically, seminal plasma components might mask the immunogenicity of sperm (7); however, ejaculated sperm (which are coated with seminal plasma components) are equally as immunogenic as epididymal sperm (which are not) when inseminated under comparable conditions (8).

The clearing of senescent sperm by macrophages from the female reproductive tract is triggered by the attachment of immunoglobulin molecules to the sperm surface (see Ref. 4 for review). In vitro, the binding of immunoglobulin to sperm must be a result and not a cause of the senescent changes, and there appears to be no reason to reject the hypothesis that "natural" antibodies to sperm are involved in mediating unresponsiveness to sperm antigens (4).

It has been suggested that "naturally occurring" antibodies to sperm are a response to the (adjuvant?) effect of infection by microorganisms carrying cross-reacting antigens, since absorption with a variety of bacteria successfully removes antibody detected by immunofluorescence (9). The age-related incidence of antisperm antibodies follows the course and titer of antibodies to A or B blood group antigens in blood group O individuals, that is, peaking early (90% of prepubertal children have detectable "natural" antisperm antibody by immunofluorescence) and gradually declining thereafter (60% of young adults have similar antibodies). Antibodies to "self"-antigens, however, are usually found late in life. Tung et al. (9) hypothesized that some of the antigens identified by immunofluorescence were indeed foreign, are not protected by the development of immune tolerance, and elicit a putative antibody response when they are exposed to the immune system.

It is known that sensitization of the cell-mediated immune system by histocompatibility antigens enhances fetal survival (10). Although the fetus is generally thought to be the antigenic stimulus for this phenomena, it has been suggested that the response may be induced by spermatozoa during their passage through the uterus, preparing the mother for the ensuing implantation of the developing blastocyst (11). When the uterus is challenged by antigenically foreign epididymal sperm, it acquires the capacity to respond to subsequent inoculations by a striking hypersensitization reaction (10). Paradoxically, reproductive function is enhanced in these sensitized uteri.

Early investigations into the immunogenicity of sperm suspected that alloantigens, such as blood group or histocompatibility antigens, were responsible for antigenic sensitization that resulted in infertility (12, 13). Landsteiner and Levine (14) were the first to report the presence of ABO blood group substances on human spermatozoa, and this observation has been confirmed most recently by Kerek (15). However, it is unclear whether the antigens are inherent components of the sperm cells or are merely secreted into the seminal plasma and later become associated with sperm (16). Similar controversy exists regarding Rh, MNS, and P antigen systems. Anti-A and anti-B sera do not induce sperm agglutination (17) or complement-dependent sperm immobilization (18). Moreover, the blood type of donor sperm used in antisperm antibody assays appears to be irrelevant (19).

The presence of HLA-antigens on spermatozoa has been suggested by several investigators (20, 21) but denied by others (22). The possibility that there may be haploid expression of HLA antigens (and ABO determinants) continues to be debated in the literature. Previous supportive test results may be due to nonspecific inhibition of HLA cytotoxicity assays (22). Because immuno-electron microscopic studies indicate a much lower density of HLA antigen on sperm when compared to lymphocytes (23), this may account for some of the discrepancies. It has been suggested that if Ia antigens are present on sperm, their levels must be quite low, and that contaminating epithelial or macrophage cells in the ejaculate might be the cause of results confirming their presence (22). Regardless, antibodies to histocompatibility antigens do not result in sperm agglutination or immobilization (24).

Although several sperm-coating antigens presumably derived from the seminal plasma have been isolated (25–27), sperm-agglutinating and sperm-immobilizing antibodies in human sera do not seem to be directed against sperm-coating antigens in humans (27, 28) or in animals (29). There is evidence that some seminal plasma antigens may be modified by bacterial contaminants and subsequently provoke an immune response that may result in human subfertility (30, 31).

There appears to be cross-reactivity of sperm antigens between mammalian species (32) and between different animal phyla (33). Some mouse and human sperm differentiation antigens appear to be identical (34). Both guinea pig and human sperm can react with selected anti-human sperm sera from infertile couples; "naturally occurring" human sperm antibodies in these patients can be completely absorbed by either guinea pig sperm or spleen (35). Antisera against mouse teratocarcinoma and mouse sperm cross-react (36), as does one type of mouse sarcoma (37), mouse kidney (38), and mouse brain tissue (38, 39). Autoallergic orchitis has been induced with brain homogenate (40) and parotid gland homogenate (41). A direct proof that human sperm antibodies cross-react with human brain or parotid gland has never been given. However, some antisperm antibodies detected by immunofluorescence can be absorbed by adrenal tissue (42). Of more interest to the study of antibody-mediated infertility is the cross-reactivity of some antisera between mouse preimplantation embryos and sperm (36–39). Recently, it has been reported that human sperm and human lymphocytes share common antigens (43). Despite these observations, there does not appear to be an increased cross-reactivity between antisperm antibodies from infertile or vasectomized men and other human tissue (28). Immobilizing sperm antibodies

have been reported in the majority of a small group of female patients with systemic lupus erythematosus (44).

2. CELL-MEDIATED INFERTILITY

The identification of a cell-mediated immune response to spermatozoa antigens as a cause of infertility remains elusive (45–50). The inability to isolate specific germ surface antigens is a major hindrance to the assay techniques typically employed to detect cell-mediated immunity.

3. ANTIBODY-MEDIATED INFERTILITY

The possibility that heterologous antibodies could be produced against animal sperm was first reported at the turn of the century (51, 52). Although a vast literature has accumulated since that time, many aspects of the field remain ambiguous and confusing. Problems have frequently arisen because of inadequacies of the assay systems employed and the inherent characteristics of the fragile sperm cell itself. It is also becoming apparent that much of the clinical information regarding *circulating* antisperm antibodies may in some cases not mirror the immunologic milieu of the reproductive tract.

In early investigations it was difficult to raise homologous antibodies to sperm antigens in animals (32, 53). However, when appropriate adjuvants were employed, a temporary sterility could be produced that correlated with measurable antibodies against homologous sperm (54). Since sperm are mixed with seminal plasma at the time of ejaculation, it was possible that antibodies against semen could primarily be raised against seminal plasma "coating" antigens. However, the use of epididymal sperm (free of seminal plasma) as a sensitizing antigenic material consistently produced antibodies that would result in infertility. Antibodies against seminal plasma did not have this capability (55). In addition, epididymal or ejaculated sperm could, but seminal plasma could not, absorb the antibody activity. It thus appeared that sperm-specific antigens were involved in the sterility that subsequently resulted.

Several impairments of animal reproductive function could be correlated with the presence of antisperm antibodies. These included decreased survival of blastocytes (56), a decreased ovum fertilization rate in the tube (29, 57), impeded penetration of spermatozoa into the female genital tract (57), increased phagocytosis of spermatozoa in the uterus (55), and early embryonal mortality (58). Although animal models provide insight into the possible sequelae of spontaneously acquired immunity against human sperm antigens, the latter is associated with a weaker immune reaction than that found in the hyperimmunized animal in which adjuvants and repeated sensitizations are used to maximalize the antibody response.

3.1.   Human Antisperm Antibodies

The presence of autoantibodies against human sperm in men was predicted in 1921 by Wegelin (59). In 1922 the sera from two sterile women were reported to agglutinate and immobilize their husband's sperm (60). Wilson (61) reported that the sera from some infertile men could agglutinate and immobilize sperm. The presence of spontaneous sperm agglutination with the early loss of sperm motility were found in two men whose semen parameters were otherwise normal. Previously, an abnormal salt content or pH of the seminal plasma or bacterial contamination was considered to be the cause of spontaneous sperm agglutination in a male's ejaculate. In Wilson's patients (62), however, the agglutinating factor could also be found in the patient's serum and could agglutinate sperm from normal fertile donors. In addition, the sperm were able to absorb the agglutinating factor from the serum, implying that agglutination in the ejaculate resulted from the presence of sperm

autoantibodies. Sperm agglutinated in this manner could not penetrate cervical mucus in vivo or in vitro. The spouses of both of these men achieved a pregnancy following insemination with donor sperm.

Because of the isolating effect of the blood–testes barrier (63, 64) developing spermatozoal antigens can fail to sensitize the male's immune system during spermiogenesis. Antisperm antibodies in males have been associated with a history of testicular trauma (65), genital tract infection (66), disruption of the genital tract at the time of vasectomy (67), or for unknown reasons. The exact mechanism in which sensitization to sperm antigens occurs is unclear in this latter group of individuals. Whether the initial stimulus is an antigenically similar microorganism remains problematic.

The possible ways a female prevents sensitization to foreign sperm antigens have already been discussed. However, in some males and females the production of antisperm antibodies occurs and can interfere with any of several steps in the reproductive process (Figs. 1 and 2). These include (1) increased phagocytosis by Sertoli cells (68); (2) degeneration of spermatids (69); (3) a decrease in sperm motility (70); (4) interference with capacitation (71) or the acrosome reaction (72); (5) prevention of cervical mucus penetration (73, 74); (6) activation of macrophages and the subsequent enhancement of the phagocytic clearing of spermatozoa (75); (7) sperm cytotoxicity, if adequate levels of complement are present (18); (8) adverse peristalsis interfering with sperm migration through the uterus (76) or fallopian tubes (77); (9) inhibition of sperm enzyme activity (78, 79); (10) impairment of sperm/egg interaction (80, 81); or (11) embryonal loss or destruction (71, 82).

Men who have undergone a vasectomy provide a readily available model for circulating antisperm antibodies since they can be identified in approximately 50% of these men (83). In many animals testicular destruction occurs following sensitization to testicular spermatozoal antigens (54), but such destruc-

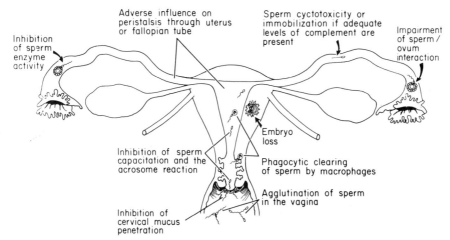

Figure 1. Possible ways that antisperm antibodies could interfere with fertility in the female.

tive changes rarely occur following vasectomy in humans (64). In fact, azoospermia following a vasovasostomy is more likely to be associated with continued vaso-occlusion rather than antisperm antibodies. Nevertheless, several reports indicate that of males who undergo a successful vas reanastomosis, only 18 to 60% will regain their fertility if antisperm antibodies are identified (85). Sperm agglutination is not the reason for their infertility, since 50% of the men who do impregnate their partners have sperm agglutination in their ejaculate (86).

Alexander (see Refs. 67 and 83 for references) has summarized five theories that may explain individual variation in the dynamics of antisperm antibody production following a vasectomy. The first hypothesis is

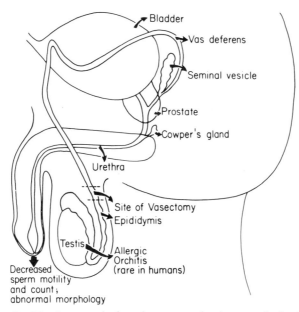

Figure 2. Possible adverse results from the presence of antisperm antibodies in the male.

that leakage of sperm from the severed vas at the time of surgery initiates an immune response, and the presence or absence of antisperm antibodies depends on the surgical technique that was employed. Since rapid, transient antibody production does not occur in man, this hypothesis appears invalid. Vasectomy in experimental animals without ligation of the vas does not effect the antibody response or result in higher titers of antibody. Therefore, the leakage of spermatozoa during the vasectomy procedure is not per se the major antigenic stimulus that initiates antibody production.

The second hypothesis is that the major site of antigen stimulation occurs around granulomas (areas of inflammation that often form near the vasectomy site). However, the presence or absence of granulomas does not always correlate with the formation of antisperm antibodies.

The third hypothesis is that spermatozoa undergo degeneration in the epididymis proximal to the site of blockage. Soluble sperm antigens might then leak from the reproductive tract at this level. Rhesus monkeys that have been vasectomized are found to have immune complexes in the basal lamina surrounding the vas efferentes, which supports this possibility.

In vasectomized Rhesus monkeys the highest levels of antisperm antibodies develop in those animals with the highest initial sperm counts. For this reason the number of sperm, and hence the amount of antigenic load, may be important.

A fifth possibility is that the response to sperm antigens is genetically determined. Antisperm antibodies never develop in some inbred strains of mice, but their presence is common in other strains.

In infertile males who have not undergone a vasectomy, self-agglutination of sperm has been associated with sterility. Both immunoglobulin and nonimmunoglobulin factors have been reported to result in agglutination (87). Wilson (61) observed that seminal plasma from men with sperm autoagglutination was capable of causing sperm agglutination in normal semen. Although antisperm antibodies have been identified in the IgG fraction of seminal plasma, some report that it is primarily a result of IgA antibodies (74). IgM does not appear to play a role, for it is rarely found in semen, probably because its high molecular weight restricts transudation into reproductive tract fluids (88). Both IgG and IgA have been found as a normal constituent of human seminal plasma; however, Sullivan and Quinlivan (89) detected IgA in the seminal plasma of infertile men, but not in samples from men who fathered a child.

Using a radioimmunobinding assay we have found that some men can have IgA or IgG associated with their sperm in increased amounts when compared to sperm from fertile donors (90). This occasionally can occur without the presence of elevated levels of similar antisperm antibodies in the circulation.

In men, the distribution of immunoglobulins in semen parallels the distribution of acid phosphatase, a product of the prostate gland. This implies that the prostate is the site of entrance of circulating immunoglobulins or the immunoglobulins are produced by the gland (91). The concentration of IgG in seminal plasma is only 1% of that found in the circulation (91). Because the concentrations of seminal IgA are greater than the concentration of seminal albumin, the local production of IgA may be occurring. We have found that frequently the amount of IgG per sperm is greater in the second portion of the ejaculate (unpublished results). Intrauterine insemination of the first portion of such ejaculates can result in pregnancies in couples with infertility secondary to antibodies on the male partner's sperm.

Although certain of the seminal plasma components may be anticomplementary (92), increased amounts of C^3 and C^4 components of complement have been identified in seminal plasma from infertile males (89). These complement components, along with IgA, could result in sperm autoagglutination. This could account for some of the abnormalities of semen parameters that may be associated with males with antisperm antibodies.

The female reproductive tract, particularly the endocervix, is well endowed with immunologically competent plasma cells that could produce local antibodies against sperm (93). These cells are increased following vaginal infection (94). These local immune mechanisms can possibly be influenced by several factors (see Ref. 95 for references): (1) large numbers of biologically redundant sperm may be immunologically different from the residual majority, presupposing a filtering process by either the endocervical canal or a higher level of the female reproductive tract; (2) sperm are phagocytosed by somatic cells of the uterine cervix, as well as by macrophages, and semen is chemotactically attracted to macrophages and neutrophils; (3) other foreign antigens gaining access to the genital tract (i.e., at the time of a vaginal infection) may produce an adjuvant effect; (4) lymphocytes and semen within the male's ejaculate may contribute to the induction of female sterility because of the foreign histocompatibility antigens on their surface; and (5) factors may be present that modify the immune response to sperm, including various immunosuppressive chemicals (i.e., seminal plasma) or precipitins directed against complement components.

It is known that bacterial toxins (96) and cell wall fragments (97) can elicit either a humoral or a local antibody response when they are introduced into the rabbit, primate, and probably the human vagina. The local response may be short-lived (1 to 7 weeks) in the face of continued elevation of circulating antibodies (at least 7 to 10 months) (98). For this reason, although humoral antisperm antibodies have been detected by a variety of techniques in infertile women (99), the clinical significance remains obscure. Although the uterine cervix appears to be the primary site of secretory IgA antibody activity in the female reproductive tract (24, p. 29), the epithelial surfaces of the uterine fundus and the fallopian tube appear to also participate to a

limited degree, but the vagina is probably inactive (see Ref. 24, pp. 24–29 for review). Usually an antigenic stimulus to any mucus membrane results in the formation of both local and circulating antibodies, but in some circumstances, antigens may not reach the circulation in sufficient quantity, and a systemic response may not occur (100, 101). From the above observations it becomes clear that in the female, both false positive and false negative inferences can be made when serum is used as an antibody source.

Although many of the complement components are not present in the secretions of the cervix or uterus (102), follicular fluid contains a respectable representation of these proteins (102). Perhaps follicular fluid, entrapped within the cumulus cells surrounding the ovum, may play an important role in complement-dependent immobilization of sperm at the site of fertilization in patients with immobilizing antisperm antibodies.

Agglutination or complement-dependent immobilization does not appear to be the mechanism by which antisperm antibodies in women perturb reproductive function, since they are rarely noticed in the female reproductive tract (103). Kramer and Jager (104) have suggested that IgA antisperm antibodies, either associated with the male's sperm or present in the female's cervical mucus, attach by their Fc component to the mucin glycoprotein. They have described a characteristic in situ shaking motion of sperm when they are involved in such a sperm/antibody/glycoprotein complex. However, F(ab)$_2$ fragments of antisperm antibodies also inhibit sperm penetration (105), which argues against Fc binding as playing an important role. Investigators have found a correlation between circulating or cervical mucus antisperm antibodies and a poor postcoital test (103, 106, 107), but interpretation of these data is difficult because of the multiple factors (e.g., infection, improper timing, abnormal semen) that can affect sperm/cervical mucus interaction. Isojima has shown that complement-dependent cervical mucus immobilizing antibodies (IgG) can inhibit sperm penetration in vivo (73), but this is not consistent with the low quality of complement (11.5% of that found in serum) present in cervical mucus (108). An increased incidence of spontaneous abortion has been found in humans (109) and animals (55) with antisperm antibodies. This association is denied by other investigators (110). It would be possible for antisperm antibodies to be a cause of early pregnancy loss since sperm isoantigenic determinants are detectable on the surface of fertilized ova, but are not present prior to fertilization (111). This implies that syngamy results in the intermingling of sperm and egg membrane components, conserving sperm membrane antigens, and allowing binding of antisperm antibodies to the fertilized egg.

3.2. Human Sperm Antigens

Although the site of antibody attachment to sperm can be suggested by immunofluorescence (42) or immunoperoxidase (112) techniques, the isolation of spermatozoal antigens has proved difficult. The apical body and perinuclear material are keratinous and contain many disulfide bonds (113) which may account for the problem. Various detergents and physical separation techniques (such as sonication) have been used to dissociate the sperm membrane; however, the antigenic determinants may be lost following these procedures, or inadequate solubilization may occur (113). The task of antigen isolation becomes especially difficult when the absorption of agglutinating and immobilizating antibody activity is used to follow antigens through the isolation process. Despite these obstacles, the isolation of several sperm antigens has been reported. However, none has been consistently capable of absorbing antisperm antibody activity from the serum of infertile patients with suspected antibody-mediated infertility. Menge and Protzman (29) isolated nine antigens from rabbit sperm that could be absorbed by testicular material and epididymal sperm but not by seminal plasma.

Katsh and Katsh (114) isolated a polypeptide–polysaccharide complex that resulted in aspermatogenesis in 100% of guinea pigs treated with milligram amounts of the substance. Kolk (115) detected an antigen on human sperm heads swollen by the addition of trypsin and dithiotretiol. The 47-amino acid protamine could not absorb sperm-agglutinating antibody and appeared to originate from the nucleus. Tung (116) described antigens in seven specific sperm regions identified by immunofluorescence assays for sperm antibodies in men following a vasectomy. He noted that immunofluorescence assays probably detect many subcellular antigens (possibly secondary to the action of alcohol fixation) (28) which would not be detected by agglutination, immobilization, or radioimmunobinding assays. Because the detected antibodies infrequently bound complement, he doubted that they had a serious pathological role in infertility. Mettler and Skrabei (117) disrupted human spermatozoa with the detergents Hyamine 2389 and Triton X-100. Four of the seven separated fractions repeatedly inhibited the sperm-immobilizing activity of human sera. None of the seven fractions was able to absorb activity from human sperm-agglutinating sera. These investigators concluded that sperm-agglutinating and sperm-immobilizing antibodies react with different sperm antigens. In a later paper (118) they separated several low molecular weight compounds following sperm disruption by autolysis. The small peptides were then attached to Cytochrome C to test their ability to form precipitates when various test sera were added. One of the 17 fractions consistently produced precipitates when added to human sperm-immobilizing sera and rabbit anti-human sperm serum. No precipitation reaction was found with human sperm-agglutinating sera.

Because spermatozoa progress through a series of complex changes during differentiation, several groups have studied the changes in surface antigens during this process (119). O'Rand and Romrell (120) hypothesized that sperm-specific molecules foreign to the male could be synthesized and inserted into the differentiating sperm membrane without eliciting an immune response because of the protection of the blood–testes barrier. In the rabbit 50% of sperm surface alloantigens detected by female rabbit anti-rabbit sperm antibodies appear after the mid-spermatid stage of spermatogenesis (121), and thus are produced after the process of self-recognition. Using a sperm immobilization technique it was substantiated that these sperm-specific macromolecules from mature rabbit sperm could function as autoantigens (120). Bechtol et al. (122) employed monoclonal antibodies against mouse testes to define two spermatozoal differentiation antigens in the mouse. Because they used viable testicular cells as an antigen source, they felt that their technique focused on the surface antigenic structure of sperm. This is not possible when cellular material is enzymatically digested and used as a sensitizing antigen. The importance of the specificity of monoclonal antibodies coupled with radioimmunobinding assays in these reports (122, 123) and another using guinea pig sperm

(124) cannot be overestimated. Identification of human seminal plasma antigens using monoclonal antibodies has only recently been reported (125). The localization and isolation of human sperm surface antigens and the discovery of their role in reproductive processes may eventually produce antigenic material for antifertility vaccines or discriminate which sperm antigens are critical to the sensitization of a particular patient with antibody-mediated infertility.

3.3. Assays for Antisperm Antibody

The most appropriate assay to use to identify men and women with antibody-mediated infertility remains controversial. The most commonly used assays are sperm agglutination (Table 1), immobilization (Table 2), and immunofluorescence. Immunofluorescence and immunoperoxidase techniques have been plagued by high levels of false positive test results in individuals not likely to have antisperm antibodies (28). In addition, they have demonstrated an unacceptable level of interpretation variation when the results from several laboratories are compared (28). The use of FITC-labeled F(ab)$_2$ fragments can reduce

Table 1. The advantages and disadvantages of agglutination assays for antisperm antibodies

Advantages	1. Simple assay procedure
	2. Rapidly performed
Disadvantages	1. Nonspecific sperm agglutination can occur
	2. Sperm agglutination rarely occurs in the female reproductive tract
	3. Agglutination cannot occur when antigen is in excess
	4. Cannot directly identify antibodies on the sperm surface
	5. Incapable of identifying antigen/antibody complexes
	6. Subjectively interpreted
	7. Cannot quantitate results
	8. Cannot monitor antigens in an isolation procedure

Table 2. The advantages and disadvantages of sperm immobilization assays for antisperm antibodies

Advantages	1. Low false positive rate
	2. Simple assay procedure
	3. Rapidly performed
Disadvantages	1. Measures only IgG$_{1-3}$ and IgM
	2. Cannot measure secretory IgA
	3. Insufficient complement in reproductive tract to support complement-dependent events
	4. Usually only positive when antibody is in excess
	5. Subjectively interpreted
	6. Range of positive and negative results are arbitrarily determined

Table 3. The advantages and
disadvantages of radioimmunobinding
assays for antisperm antibodies

Advantages	
	1. Can measure any class of immunoglobulin
	2. Can measure antibodies directly on the sperm surface
	3. Can measure sperm-associated complement
	4. Objectively interpreted
	5. Quantitative
	6. Proper controls can eliminate false positive results
	7. Capable of following sperm antigens through an isolation procedure
Disadvantages	1. Requires radiolabeled reagents
	2. Relatively lengthy procedure

nonspecific binding (126), since sperm have Fc receptors (127). Although immunocytochemical assays may not be appropriate as a screening test, they may be useful in localizing the antigen/antibody binding site in patients already shown to have antisperm antibody activity.

The use of sperm agglutination assays has also resulted in what many consider to be an unacceptably high rate of false positive test results (128, 129). Although immobilization assays have a negligible false positive rate

(18), this form of testing requires the presence of complement. It is probable that not all antibody-mediated events in the reproductive tract are complement-dependent or occur secondary to immunoglobulins of a class capable of activating complement.

Several investigators have developed radiolabeled or enzyme-linked assay systems (119, 122–124, 130, 131) (Table 3) that are capable of measuring immunoglobulins of all classes in serum, seminal plasma, cervical mucus, or directly on sperm. These assay systems appear to be highly quantitative (130, 131), have a low false positive rate (131) (Table 4), and are capable of selectively identifying each class of immunoglobulin (131). In addition, these assay systems probably can be modified to identify complement components associated with sperm, sperm-associated immunoglobulin fragments, or circulating antibody complexes.

The importance of antibodies on the male partner's sperm as opposed to in his circulation is being studied by a variety of new testing methods including a mixed agglutination reaction (132), a modification of the Coombs' assay (133), and a radioimmunobinding assay (90). From these early test results it appears that, compared to women, there is less of a dichotomy between locally produced antibodies on the male's sperm and those found in the circulation. Nonetheless, some men whose infertility is antibody-mediated could be missed if only circulating antibodies were assayed.

Table 4. Results of radiolabeled antiglobulin test for plasma IgG antisperm antibody

Group	Positive Test[a]	
	Men	Women
1314 patients with infertility	51/639 (8%)	61/675 (9%)
10 vasectomized men	6/10 (60%)	—
63 fertile controls	0/10	0/53

[a] The results are expressed as the number and percentage of patients with increased (> 2 S.D.) plasma IgG antisperm activity when compared to a group of fertile controls.

Antisperm antibodies in cervical mucus have also been studied (101, 103, 134–136). Effective assays for cervical mucus antibodies must overcome the increased viscoelasticity of the mucus sample, the ability of the high molecular weight mucin glycoprotein to entrap immunoglobulins within its matrix, and the small amount of material that is available for study. Although more mucus is present during the peri-ovulatory phase of the menstrual cycle, the immunoglobulin components are more diluted at that time, and therefore timing may not be of critical importance. Early investigations in this area simply added mucus to an appropriate buffer (103). The high molecular weight mucus components were removed by centrifugation, and any antibodies in the supernatant were identified with immobilization or agglutination assays. It became apparent, however, that this methodology retained many of the immunoglobulins in the mucin glycoprotein matrix, and an unacceptably high false negative rate resulted (137). Bromelin, a proteolytic enzyme from the pineapple, has been used to solubilize mucus more effectively (135, 137). It has been demonstrated that this technique results in an increased amount of immunoglobulins being freed for measurement (137). Although it would appear that IgG immunoglobulins might be susceptible to denaturation by the enzyme, this does not seem to occur (137). Secretory IgA molecules are known to be resistant to proteolytic digestion, but the effect of bromelin on secretory IgA has not been clearly defined. The possibility also exists that the enzyme might detrimentally affect the sperm surface (95, p. 126). We have found that bromelin can markedly diminish the number of sperm present in a radioimmunobinding assay at the conclusion of the procedure (unpublished results). The methodology that possibly has the least effect on sperm surface antigens and cervical mucus antibodies is mechanical liquefaction of the mucus sample. This involves repeated passages of the mucus through a small bore needle (95, p. 126). It has already been mentioned that some women have antisperm antibodies in their cervical mucus in spite of having negative antibody assays when their serum is tested. For this reason, the development of assays for locally produced antisperm antibodies will greatly improve the ability to monitor the response of women to therapies for antibody-mediated infertility.

3.4. Antibodies against Female Gametes

It has been noted only recently that ovarian or ovum-specific antigens can produce antibodies that interfere with fertility. The difficulties in achieving an adequate antibody response may be due to the large number of eggs necessary to sensitize animal models. Porter (138) was one of the early investigators who demonstrated that the production of isoantibodies against ovary-specific antigens was possible. It appeared that the ovary contained numerous antigens which could evoke a xenoantibody response. Many of these antigens, however, cross-react with other tissues (139) and are probably histocompatibility antigens.

Recently, attention has been specifically focused on the antigenic determinants of the zona pellucida, the envelope of acellular material surrounding the egg. Because sperm must first pass through this material prior to fertilization, the possibility that antigenic binding sites on the zona surface could be isolated and used for an antifertility vaccine or to test for the presence of anti-zona antibodies as the cause of infertility in women. Many of the ovary-specific antigens are found in the zona pellucida, theca interna, and atrophic follicles (140). Experiments have shown that not only does anti-zona antibody block fertilization in vitro (141), but it also is capable of preventing sperm penetration in vivo (141, 142). Although isoimmunization with denuded ova only reduces fertilization rates slightly, anti-zona antibody or anti-ovary antibody can completely prevent fertilization in vitro (143, 144). Trounson et al. (145) demonstrated in the human that antibodies to porcine zona pellucida could inhibit fertilization by reducing the number of sperm attaching to the zona.

Recent studies have shown that zona antigen is not species specific since antisera to porcine and bovine zona pellucida cross-react with human zona (146). This is a fortuitous finding since pig and cattle ovaries are readily available in large quantities, and pig and cattle zona antigens have been purified by a variety of methods. Anti-zona antibodies have been found in both infertile (147) and elderly women (148). Radioimmunoassays have been used to identify anti-porcine zona antibodies (149), and it seems probable that such specific assays will be valuable in screening large numbers of infertile women.

F(ab)$_2$ fragments of anti-zona antisera react equally as well with zona as do their whole serum counterparts, implying that nonspecific attachment of the Fc fragment to the zona is not occurring (150). Groups of infertile women have been found to have anti-zona antibodies, but some of these women subsequently became pregnant (151). The reversibility of the antibody response is a major consideration if induced anti-zona antibodies react with follicular ova, since an extended length of infertility or permanent sterility could follow vaccination with zona antigens.

3.5.   Therapy for Antisperm Antibody Activity

Several modes of therapy have been proposed for infertile patients with antisperm antibodies. These include condom therapy if the female partner is found to have the antibody activity (152–156), low- and high-dose corticosteroid therapy (131, 157–160), treatment of genital infections (161), the use of donor cervical mucus (162), artificial insemination with husband (163) or donor sperm (62), insemination with previously frozen sperm (164), sperm washing techniques (165), intrauterine insemination (166), inhibition of antibody response by passive immunization (167), and high-dose estrogen therapy during

the proliferative phase (168). The results of all these therapies have not been overwhelmingly remarkable, and, in the case of corticosteroids, the amount and duration of therapy remains empirical. No large controlled study to date has been established to assess the efficacy of such therapy over the effect of placebo.

3.6.   Antifertility Vaccines

The search for additional effective but safe contraceptive techniques has raised considerable interest in the possibility of developing antifertility vaccines. An early report in this area involved injection of whole semen into women (169). Although a U.S. patent was eventually awarded for this procedure, side effects limited its use. Several more defined proteins show promise as an antifertility vaccine. These include gonadotropin releasing factor (GHRF) when it is used as a hapten and administered with appropriate adjuvants (170), sperm antigens (169), zona pellucida antigens (171), human chorionic somatomammotropin (hCS) (172), luteinizing hormone (LH) (173), and the entire molecule or various subunits of human chorionic gonadotropin (hCG) (174, 175). Of these, antibodies against the beta subunit of hCG show the most promise. Although studies with many of these antigens have been limited because of inhibitions regarding human research, the beta subunit of hCG has been coupled to tetanus toxoid and tested as an antifertility vaccine in humans (174). Infertility was noted 6 weeks after the injection of the antigen, and the effect lasted from 300 to 500 days in the better responders (174). The response, however, was quite variable, and this area requires further investigation.

4.   AUTOIMMUNE OVARIAN FAILURE

Several types of ovarian failure have been associated with the presence of antisperm antibody activity, including polyglandular syndromes (176–178), gonadotropin-resistant ovary (179), Turner's syndrome (180), and premature menopause (180–182). In many of these cases the patient exhibits organ-specific autoantibodies which react against ovarian granulosa and theca interna cells, as well as other steroid-producing glandular tissue. The ovarian antigens cross-react with the adrenal and thyroid glands, and thus result in polyglandular syndromes including Addison's disease, Hashimoto's thyroiditis, and ovarian failure in association with ovarian antibodies. Chronic candidiasis was also found in these women which may be secondary to antibody cross-reactivity between ovary and the patient's T lymphocytes. It is possible that the gonadotropin-resistant ovary syndrome (Savage syndrome) might be caused by the formation of antibodies against gonadotropin receptor (179, 181, 182). Such antibodies, however, have not been found by some investigators (183).

There has also been an association between the existence of Turner's syndrome and autoimmune diseases (95, p. 134). Early follicular genesis in the developing embryo is normal in women with Turner's syndrome; however, the primordial follicles disappear at a later stage of fetal and prepubetal development.

REFERENCES

1. R. J. T. Hancock, *Arch. Androl.* **2**, 171 (1979).
2. J. Cohen and S. H. Gregson, in J. Cohen and W. F. Hendry, Eds., *Spermatozoa, Antibodies and Infertility*, Blackwell, Oxford, 1978, pp. 17–29.
3. C. R. Austin, *J. Endocrin.* **14**, 335 (1957).
4. J. Cohen and D. C. McNaughton, *J. Reprod. Fertil.* **39**, 297 (1974).
5. E. S. E. Hafez, in E. S. E. Hafez, Ed., *Human Semen and Fertility Regulation in Men*, CV Mosby, St. Louis, 1976, p. 121.
6. M. Kaye, in J. P. Hearn, Ed., *Immunological Aspects of Reproduction and Fertility Control*. University Park Press, Baltimore, 1980, p. 10.
7. C. Prakash, in N. Gleicher, Ed., *Reproductive Immunology*, Alan R. Liss, New York, 1981, pp. 405–406.
8. R. J. T. Hancock, in J. Cohen and W. F. Hendry, Eds., *Spermatozoa, Antibodies and Infertility*, Blackwell, Oxford, 1978, pp. 4–5.
9. K. S. K. Tung, W. D. Cooke, Jr., T. A. McCarty, and P. Robitaille, *Clin. Exp. Immunol.* **25**, 73 (1976).
10. A. E. Beer and R. E. Billingham, *J. Reprod. Fertil. (Suppl.)* **21**, 59 (1974).
11. B. G. Dorsman, A. E. Tumboh-Oeri, and T. K. Roberts, *J. Reprod. Fertil.* **53**, 277 (1978).
12. E. Matsunaga and S. Itoh, *Ann. Hum. Genet.* **22**, 111 (1958).
13. S. J. Behrman, J. Buettner-Janusch, R. Heglar, H. Gershowitz, and W. L. Tew, *Am. J. Obstet. Gynecol.* **79**, 847 (1960).
14. K. Landsteiner and P. Levine, *J. Immunol.* **12**, 415 (1926).
15. G. Kerék, *Int. J. Fertil.* **19**, 181 (1974).
16. S. Shulman, *Reproduction and Antibody Response*, CRC Press, Cleveland, 1975, pp. 21–22.
17. E. Fernández-Collazo and E. Thierer, *Fertil. Steril.* **23**, 376 (1972).
18. S. Isojima, K. Tsuchiya, K. Koyama, C. Tanaka, O. Naka, and H. Adachi, *Am. J. Obstet. Gynecol.* **112**, 199 (1972).
19. S. Mathur, H. O. Williamson, S. C. Landgrebe, C. L. Smith, and H. H. Fudenberg, *J. Immunol. Meth.* **30**, 381 (1979).
20. M. Fellous and J. Dausset, *Nature* **225**, 191 (1970).
21. A. Halim, K. Abbasi, and H. Festenstein, *Tissue Antigens* **4**, 1 (1974).
22. H. Y. Law and W. F. Bodmer, *Tissue Antigens* **12**, 249 (1978).
23. G. Kerek, P. Biberfeld, and B. A. Afzelius, *Int. J. Fertil.* **18**, 145 (1973).
24. H. J. Ingerslev, *Acta Obstet. Gynecol. Scand. (suppl.)* **100**, 8 (1981).
25. T. S. Li and S. J. Behrman, *Fertil. Steril.* **21**, 565 (1970).
26. A. G. Hunter, *J. Reprod. Fertil.* **20**, 413 (1969).
27. T. S. Li, M. A. Pelosi, V. V. Gowda, H. Caterini, and H. A. Kaminetzky, *Int. J. Fertil.* **23**, 38 (1978).
28. B. Boettcher, T. Hjort, P. Rumke, S. Shulman, and O. E. Vyazov, *Acta Pathol. Microbiol. Scand. Sect. C* (suppl.), 258 (1977).
29. A. C. Menge and W. P. Protzman, *J. Reprod. Fertil.* **13**, 31 (1967).
30. C. Chen and M. J. Simons, in B. Boettcher, Ed.,

Immunological Influence on Human Fertility, Academic Press, New York, 1977, pp. 255–261.

31. C. Chen and M. J. Simons, in B. Boettcher, Ed., *Immunological Influence on Human Fertility*, Academic Press, New York, 1977, pp. 263–270.

32. A. U. Smith, *Proc. R. Soc. Lond. (Biol.)* **136**, 472 (1949).

33. A. C. Lopo and V. D. Vacquier, *Nature*, **288**, 397 (1980).

34. M. Fellous, G. Gachelin, M. Buc-Caron, P. Dubois, and F. Jacob, *Dev. Biol.* **41**, 331 (1974).

35. M. D'Almeida and G. A. Voisin, *Clin. Exp. Immunol.* **28**, 163 (1977).

36. C. G. Webb, *Dev. Biol.* **76**, 203 (1980).

37. E. H. Goldberg and S. Tokuda, *Transplant. Proc.* **9**, 1363 (1977).

38. J. K. Chaffee and M. Schachner, *Dev. Biol.* **62**, 185 (1978).

39. A. Zimmermann, M. Vadeboncoeur, and J. L. Press, *Dev. Biol.* **72**, 138 (1979).

40. S. Katsh and D. W. Bishop, *J. Embryol. Exp. Morphol.* **6**, 94 (1958).

41. T. Nagano and K. Okumuru, *Virchow's Arch. (Zellpathol.)* **14**, 237 (1973).

42. J. Hjort and K. B. Hansen, *Clin. Exp. Immunol.* **8**, 9 (1971).

43. S. Mathur, J. Goust, H. O. Williamson, and H. H. Fudenberg, *Fertil. Steril.* **34**, 469 (1980).

44. Z. H. Marcus and E. V. Hess, *Arthritis Rheum.* **24**, 569 (1981).

45. B. D. Tait, J. U. Barrie, I. Johnston, and P. J. Morris, *Fertil. Steril.* **27**, 389 (1976).

46. Z. H. Marcus, L. Nebel, Y. Stahl, and G. Domingue, *Fertil. Steril.* **27**, 713 (1976).

47. Z. H. Marcus, J. H. Herman, and E. V. Hess, *Arch. Androl.* **1**, 89 (1978).

48. M. S. Nemirovsky, *Arch. Androl.* **3**, 43 (1979).

49. J. Dor, L. A. Nebel, Y. Soffer, S. Mashiach, and D. M. Serr, *Int. J. Fertil.* **24**, 94 (1979).

50. H. Tinneberg, R. Birke, and L. Mettler, *J. Reprod. Fertil.* **58**, 469 (1980).

51. K. Lansteiner, *Zantralbl. Bakteriol.* **25**, 546 (1899).

52. E. Metchnikoff, *Ann. Inst. Pasteur (Paris)* **13**, 737 (1899).

53. A. J. Weil and A. E. Finkler, *Proc. Soc. Exp. Biol. Med.* **98**, 794 (1958).

54. J. Freund, M. M. Lipton, and G. E. Thompson, *J. Exp. Med.* **97**, 711 (1953).

55. A. C. Menge, *Proc. Soc. Exp. Biol. Med.* **127**, 1271 (1968).

56. C. B. Metz and J. Anika, *Biol. Reprod.* **2**, 284 (1970).

57. D. B. A. Symons, *J. Reprod. Fertil.* **14**, 163 (1967).

58. C. B. Metz, *Fed. Proc.* **32**, 2057 (1973).

59. C. Wegelin, *Beitr. Z. Pathol. Anat. Allg. Pathol.* **69**, 281 (1921).

60. S. R. Meaker, *Boston Med. Surg. J.* **187**, 535 (1922).

61. L. Wilson, *Proc. Soc. Exp. Biol. Med.* **85**, 652 (1954).

62. L. Wilson, *Fertil. Steril.* **7**, 262 (1956).

63. W. B. Neaves, *J. Cell Biol.* **59**, 559 (1973).

64. R. C. Jones, in B. Boettcher, Ed., *Immunological Influence on Human Fertility*, Academic Press, New York, 1977, pp 67–86.

65. R. Haensch, *Arch. Gynaekol.* **208**, 91 (1969).

66. B. Fjällbrant, *Acta Obstet. Gynecol. Scand. (Suppl.)* **4**, 1 (1968).

67. N. J. Alexander and D. J. Anderson, *Fertil. Steril.* **32**, 253 (1979).

68. J. P. Hagedoorn and J. E. Davis, *Physiologist (abstr.)* **17**, 236 (1974).

69. R. Kubota, *Jap. J. Urol.* **60**, 373 (1969).

70. P. Rümke and G. Hellinga, *Am. J. Clin. Pathol.* **32**, 357 (1959).

71. A. C. Menge, *J. Reprod. Fertil. (Suppl.)* **10**, 171 (1970).

72. K. S. K. Tung, A. Okada, R. Yanagimachi, *Biol. Reprod.* **23**, 877 (1980).

73. K. Ikuma, K. Kubota, Y. Takada, T. Kamata, K. Koyama, and S. Isojima, *Jap. J. Fertil. Steril.* **25**, 1 (1980).

74. S. Jager, J. Kremer, J. Kuiken, and T. van Slochteren-Draaisma, *Int. J. Androl.* **3**, 1 (1980).

75. C. R. Austin, *J. Reprod. Fertil.* **1**, 151 (1960).

76. Y. Ashitaka, S. Isojima, and H. Ukita, *Fertil. Steril.* **15**, 213 (1964).

77. S. J. Behrman, in S. J. Behrman and R. W. Kistner, Eds., *Progress in Infertility*, Little, Brown, Boston, 1975, p. 807.

78. B. S. Dunbar, M. G. Muñoz, C. T. Cordle, and C. B. Metz, *J. Reprod. Fertil.* **47**, 381 (1976).

79. F. N. Syner, R. Kuras, and K. S. Moghissi, *Fertil. Steril.* **32**, 214 (1979).

80. A. C. Menge and C. S. Black, *Fertil. Steril.* **32**, 214 (1979).

81. G. G. Haas, Jr., J. E. Sokoloski, and D. P. Wolf, *Am. J. Reprod. Immunol.* **1**, 40 (1980).

82. W. R. Jones, *Acta Endocrinol. (Suppl.)* **194**, 76 (1974).

83. N. J. Alexander, in B. Boettcher, Ed., *Immunological Influence on Human Fertility*, Academic Press, New York, 1977, p. 25.

84. T. Hjort, in B. Boettcher, Ed., *Immunological*

Influence on Human Fertility, Academic Press, New York, 1977, p. 117.

85. *Population Report on Sterilization*, Series D, No. 3, Vasectomy reversibility—A status report, George Washington University Medical Center, St. Louis, 1976, pp. 41–59.

86. M. J. Sullivan and G. E. Howe, *J. Urol.* **117**, 189 (1977).

87. B. Boettcher, *J. Reprod. Fertil. (Suppl.)* **21**, 151 (1974).

88. P. Rümke, *Clin. Exp. Immunol.* **17**, 287 (1974).

89. H. Sullivan and W. L. G. Quinlivan, *Fertil. Steril.* **34**, 465 (1980).

90. G. G. Haas, Jr., R. Weiss-Wik, and D. P. Wolf, *Fertil. Steril.* **38**, 54 (1982).

91. A. Hekman and P. Rumke, in E. S. E. Hafez, Ed., *Human Semen and Fertility Regulation in Men*, C. V. Mosby, St. Louis, 1976, p. 252.

92. P. M. Kövary, A. Dykgers, and H. Niermann, *Arch. Androl.* **1**, 99 (1978).

93. D. P. Sinha, T. D. Anderson, E. J. Holborow, and V. C. Nandakumar, *Br. J. Obstet. Gynecol.* **84**, 948 (1977).

94. E. J. Chipperfield and B. A. Evans, *Clin. Exp. Immunol.* **11**, 219 (1972).

95. W. R. Jones, in J. P. Hearn, Ed., *Immunological Aspects of Reproduction and Fertility Control*, University Park Press, Baltimore, 1980, pp. 116–117.

96. E. B. Bell and B. Wolf, *Nature* **214**, 423 (1967).

97. S. Yang and G. F. B. Schumacher, *Fertil. Steril.* **32**, 588 (1979).

98. R. J. O'Reilly, L. Lee, and B. G. Welch, *J. Infect. Dis.* **133**, 113 (1976).

99. N. R. Rose, T. Hjort, P. Rümke, M. J. K. Harper, and O. Vyazov, *Clin. Exp. Immunol.* **23**, 175 (1976).

100. P. L. Ogra and S. S. Ogra, *J. Immunol.* **110**, 1307 (1973).

101. K. S. Moghissi, A. G. Sacco, and K. Borin, *Am. J. Obstet. Gynecol.* **136**, 941 (1980).

102. G. F. B. Schumacher, in G. F. B. Schumacher and D. S. Dhindsa, Eds., *Immunological Aspects of Infertility and Fertility Regulation*, Elsevier/North Holland, New York, 1980, p. 93.

103. N. Sudo, S. Shulman, and M. L. Stone, *Am. J. Obstet. and Gynecol.* **129**, 360 (1977).

104. J. Kramer and S. Jager, *Fertil. Steril.* **27**, 335 (1976).

105. T. Hjort, K. B. Hansen, and F. Poulsen, in J. Cohen and W. F. Hendry, Eds., *Spermatozoa, Antibodies and Infertility*, Blackwell, Oxford, 1978, pp. 101–115.

106. M. Telang, J. V. Reyniak, and S. Shulman, *Int. J. Fertil.* **23**, 200 (1978).

107. Y. Soffer, Z. H. Marcus, I. Bukovsky, and E. Caspi, *Int. J. Fertil.* **21**, 89 (1976).

108. R. J. Price and B. Boettcher, *Fertil. Steril.* **32**, 61 (1979).

109. W. R. Jones, in E. Diczfalusy, Ed., *Immunological Approaches to Fertility Control*, Karolinska Institutet, Stockholm, 1974, pp. 385–386.

110. H. J. Ingerslev and M. Ingerslev, *Fertil. Steril.* **33**, 514 (1980).

111. M. G. O'Rand, *J. Exp. Zool.* **202**, 267 (1977).

112. R. E. Mancini, O. Gutierrez, and E. F. Collazo, *Fertil. Steril.* **22**, 475 (1971).

113. L. Mettler, T. Gradl, and P. Scheidel, in E. S. E. Hafez, Ed., *Human Semen and Fertility Regulation in Men*, C. V. Mosby, St. Louis, 1976, pp. 273–274.

114. S. Katsh and G. F. Katsh, *Fertil. Steril.* **12**, 522 (1961).

115. A. H. J. Kolk, T. Samuel, and P. Rumke, *Clin. Exp. Immunol.* **16**, 63 (1974).

116. K. S. K. Tung, *Clin. Exp. Immunol.* **20**, 93 (1975).

117. L. Mettler and H. Skrabei, *Int. J. Fertil.* **24**, 44 (1979).

118. L. Mettler and H. Skrabei, *Arch. Androl.* **4**, 45 (1980).

119. K. S. K. Tung, L. B. Han, and A. P. Evan, *Dev. Biol.* **68**, 224 (1979).

120. M. G. O'Rand and L. J. Romrell, *Dev. Biol.* **75**, 431 (1980).

121. L. J. Romrell and M. G. O'Rand, *Dev. Biol.* **63**, 76 (1978).

122. K. B. Bechtol, S. C. Brown, R. H. Kennett, *Proc. Natl. Acad. Sci. USA* **76**, 363 (1979).

123. E. D. Schmell, B. J. Gulyas, and J. T. August, *Fertil. Steril. (abstr.)* **35**, 247 (1981).

124. D. G. Miles, P. Primakoff, and A. R. Bellvé, *Cell* **23**, 433 (1981).

125. M. Shigeta, T. Watanabe, S. Maruyama, K. Koyama, and S. Isojima, *Clin. Exp. Immunol.* **42**, 458 (1980).

126. T. Hjort and F. Poulsen, *Arch. Androl.* **1**, 83 (1978).

127. S. S. Witkin, S. K. Shahani, S. Gupta, R. A. Good, and N. K. Day, *Clin. Exp. Immunol.* **41**, 441 (1980).

128. A. E. Beer and W. B. Neaves, *Fertil. Steril.* **29**, 3 (1978).

129. W. F. Jones, *Fertil. Steril.* **33**, 577 (1980).

130. L. A. Hill and J. K. Hampton, Jr., *Fertil. Steril.* **33**, 302 (1980).

131. G. G. Haas, Jr., D. B. Cines, and A. D. Schreiber,

N. Engl. J. Med. **303**, 722 (1980).

132. S. Jager, J. Kremer, and T. van Slochteren-Draaisma, *Int. J. Fertil.* **23**, 12 (1978).

133. S. Mathur, H. O. Williamson, S. Landgrebe, C. L. Smith, and H. H. Fudenberg, *J. Immunol. Methods* **30**, 381 (1979).

134. S. Shulman and M. R. Friedman, *Am. J. Obstet. Gynecol.* **122**, 101 (1975).

135. S. Jager, J. Kremer, J. Kuiken, and T. van Slochteren-Draasima, in B. Boettcher, Ed. *Immunological Influence on Human Fertility*, Academic Press, New York, 1977, pp. 289–293.

136. C. Chen and W. R. Jones, *Fertil. Steril.*, **35**, 542 (1981).

137. H. J. Ingerslev and F. Poulsen, *Fertil. Steril.* **33**, 61 (1980).

138. C. W. Porter, *Int. J. Fertil.* **10**, 637 (1965).

139. C. A. Shivers, in E. Diczfalusy, Ed., *Immunological Approaches to Fertility Control*, Karolinska Institutet, Stockholm, 1974, pp. 223–242.

140. B. S. Dunbar and C. A. Shivers, *Immunol. Commun.* **5**, 375 (1976).

141. Y. Tsunoda and M. C. Change, *J. Reprod. Fertil.* **46**, 379 (1976).

142. Y. Tsunoda, T. Soma, and T. Sugie, *Gamete Res.* **4**, 133 (1981).

143. L. E. Glass and J. E. Hanson, *Fertil. Steril.* **25**, 484 (1974).

144. M. C. Chang, *Res. Reprod.* **10**, 2 (1978).

145. A. O. Trounson, C. A. Shivers, R. McMaster, and A. Lopata, *Arch. Androl.* **4**, 29 (1980).

146. A. G. Sacco, *Biol. Reprod.* **16**, 164 (1977).

147. C. A. Shivers and B. S. Dunbar, *Science* **197**, 1082 (1977).

148. T. Nishimoto, T. Mori, I. Yamada, and T. Nishimura, *Fertil. Steril.* **34**, 552 (1980).

149. M. Gerrity, E. Niu, and B. S. Dunbar, *J. Reprod. Immunol.* **3**, 59 (1981).

150. A. G. Sacco, *J. Exp. Zool.* **204**, 181 (1978).

151. World Health Organization, Special Programme of Research, Development and Research Training in Human Reproduction, Sixth Annual Report, 1977, p. 141.

152. R. R. Franklin and C. D. Dukes, *Am. J. Obstet. Gynecol.* **89**, 6 (1964).

153. R. H. Glass and R. A. Vaidya, *Fertil. Steril.* **21**, 657 (1970).

154. R. C. Kolodny, B. C. Koehler, G. Toro, and W. H. Masters, *Obstet. Gynecol.* **38**, 576 (1971).

155. M. J. Hanafiah, J. A. Epstein, and A. J. Sobrero, *Fertil. Steril.* **23**, 493 (1972).

156. R. Price and B. Boettcher, *Fertil. Steril.* **35**, 583 (1981).

157. H. G. Kupperman, *N.Y. State J. Med.* **53**, 3031 (1953).

158. A. Halim, D. Antoniou, P. W. Leedham, J. P. Blandy, G. C. Tresidder, *Proc. Roy. Soc. Med.* **66**, 373 (1973).

159. S. Shulman, B. Harlin, P. Davis, and J. V. Reyniak, *Fertil. Steril.* **29**, 309 (1978).

160. W. F. Hendry, J. Stedronska, L. Hughes, K. M. Cameron, and R. C. B. Pugh, *Lancet* **2**, 498 (1979).

161. B. Fjällbrant and S. Nilsson, *Int. J. Fertil.* **22**, 255 (1977).

162. J. H. Check and A. E. Rakoff, *Fertil. Steril.* **28**, 113 (1977).

163. M. M. Usherwood, A. Halim, and P. R. Evans, *Br. J. Urol.* **48**, 499 (1976).

164. N. J. Alexander and R. Kay, *Fertil. Steril.* **28**, 1234 (1977).

165. S. Shulman, P. Davis, P. Lade, and J. V. Reyniak, in B. Boettcher, Ed., *Immunological Influence on Human Fertility*, Academic Press, New York, 1977, pp. 281–288.

166. J. Kremer, S. Jager, J. Kuiken, and T. van Slochteren-Draaisma, in J. Cohen and W. F. Hendry, Eds., *Spermatozoa, Antibodies and Infertility*, 1978, pp. 123–127.

167. S. S. Lacy, G. L. Curtis, and W. L. Ryan, *Urology* **17**, 566 (1981).

168. H. J. Ingerslev, *Fertil. Steril.* **34**, 561 (1980).

169. M. J. Baskin, *Am. J. Obstet. Gynecol.* **24**, 892 (1932).

170. H. M. Fraser, in J. P. Hearn (Ed.), *Immunological Aspects of Reproduction and Fertility Control*, University Park Press, Baltimore, 1980, pp. 143–171.

171. R. J. Aiken and D. W. Richardson, in J. P. Hearn, (Ed.), *Immunological Aspects of Reproduction and Fertility Control*, University Park Press, Baltimore, 1980, pp. 173–201.

172. V. C. Stevens, in *Development of Vaccines for Fertility Regulation*, Scriptor, Copenhagen, 1976, p. 93.

173. E. R. González, *J. Am. Med. Assoc.* **244**, 1414 (1980).

174. H. Nash, G. P. Talwar, S. Segal, T. Luukkainen, E. D. B. Johansson, J. Vasquez, E. Coutinho, and K. Sundaram, *Fertil. Steril.* **34**, 328 (1980).

175. G. P. Talwar, in J. P. Hearn, Ed., *Immunological Aspects of Reproduction and Fertility Control*, University Park Press, Baltimore, 1980, pp. 217–227.

176. A. M. Vazquez and F. M. Kenny, *Obstet. Gynecol.* **41**, 414 (1973).

177. M. Edmonds, L. Lamki, D. W. Killinger, and R. Volpé, *Am. J. Med.* **54**, 782 (1973).

178. K. P. McNatty, R. V. Short, E. W. Barnes, and W. J. Irvine, *Clin. Exp. Immunol.* **22**, 378 (1975).

179. P. R. Koninckx and I. A. Brosens, *Fertil. Steril.* **28**, 926 (1977).

180. S. Mathur, R. S. Jerath, R. S. Mathur, H. O. Williamson, and H. H. Fudenberg, *J. Reprod. Immunol.* **2**, 247 (1980).

181. W. J. Irvine, M. M. W. Chan, L. Scarth, F. O. Kolb, M. Hartog, R. I. S. Bayliss, and M. I. Drury, *Lancet* **2**, 883 (1968).

182. M. M. Ruehsen, R. M. Blizzard, R. Garcia-Bunuel, and G. S. Jones, *Am. J. Obstet. Gynecol.* **112**, 693 (1972).

183. G. E. Austin, C. B. Coulam, and R. J. Ryan, *Mayo Clin. Proc.* **54**, 394 (1979).

12

Pregnancy and the Immune State

Norbert Gleicher
Israel Siegel

Department of Obstetrics and Gynecology
Mount Sinai Hospital Medical Center of Chicago
and Rush Medical College
Chicago, Illinois

Contents

1. INTRODUCTION

The term "immune response" or "immune state" has become a popular word in both professional as well as lay publications. Even sophisticated physicians tend to utilize these terms without recognizing that they represent a conglomerate of multiple factors, many of which have still not been either recognized or clearly defined. Nowhere does the difficulty of defining "immune response" become more apparent than in such specific clinical situations as, for example, when immunotherapy has to be monitored or in association with transplantation and pregnancy. As is explained in more detail below, the "immune response," in other words, the ability of the immune system to function, can still not be adequately evaluated. What is at our disposition is a basic knowledge of a variety of factors that are at work (e.g., cellular immunity, humoral immunity, complement system), some of the interconnections between those factors, and certain clinical situations in which some of those factors do change while others may or may not. In summary, "immune response" is a generally poorly defined term which in the clinical or laboratory practice is even more difficult to define. This chapter summarizes the human immunologic experience in association with pregnancy.

Once an attempt is made to define "immune response" in association with a very specific clinical situation, one can assume that changes in measured immune function may, or will, occur in conjunction with this very specific clinical situation. Pregnancy represents such a specific immunologic situation, not so much because clear changes in immune function have been described in association with human pregnancy, but rather because the fetus is recognized as an allograft and thus "needs protection" from rejection. Once the fetus had been recognized as an allograft, the logical consequence in the thinking process of investigators was the search for factors that protect the fetus from immunologic rejection by the mother. Investigations have consequently gone through many phases: first they seemed to suggest local mechanisms in the placenta and then cellular and/or humoral factors; most recently, some local placental factors have again been considered as the protective mechanisms. More importantly, however, the understanding of the maternal "immune response" has attained increasing importance because it may also shed light on the understanding of tolerance and transplantation biology in general (1).

The development of tolerance to antigenic tissue represents probably the most important among the many poorly understood mechanisms in human reproduction. It encompasses not only the ability of the maternal host to tolerate the fetal allograft, but also the ability of the fetus to tolerate its own as well as maternal antigens (2). The importance of understanding the mechanisms of tolerance does not rest with its reproductive repercussions, but is even greater in its application to the understanding, therapy, and cure of disease. In other words, the same mechanism that allows survival of the fetal allograft within the maternal immune system may permit malignant tissue to survive within the cancer host, to give one example (3). In that context, what is beneficial for pregnancy may be detrimental for the cancer patient. Understanding the mechanism of fetal allograft survival may thus benefit not only our understanding of pregnancy-associated phenomena, but also our understanding of cancer biology, transplantation biology, autoimmune disease, and a large number of related and still poorly understood clinical phenomena.

2. CELLULAR ASPECTS OF MATERNAL IMMUNE RESPONSE

Cellular aspects of any form of "immune response" are generally characterized by white cell function. This is also largely the topic of this review; however, most recent evidence in our own laboratory indicates a possible important function for red cells in the immune system as well (4, 5). Both these cellular aspects are therefore discussed here.

2.1. White Cells

The view of pregnancy as a state of depressed cellular immunity is supported by a number of observations, both clinically and in the laboratory, of conditions that have been considered largely or solely white cell dependent. Thus an increase in incidence and severity of infection, an enhancement of malignant tumors, and *in vivo* observations, such as prolonged persistence of human skin grafts during the third trimester of pregnancy and depressed skin reactivity to tuberculin during pregnancy, have been described (3). *In vitro* assay systems, such as maternal lymphocyte stimulation with mitogens (Fig. 1), represent by now almost classical experiments supporting the so-called cellular immune depression of pregnancy. These human observations were confirmed by investigations in a number of animal models which showed the nonspecific reduction of cell-mediated immunity, for instance, during the second half of pregnancies resulting from mating between H-2 incompatible mice (3).

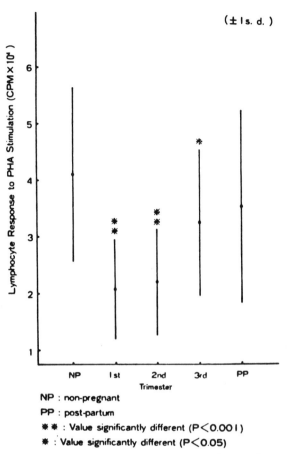

Figure 1.   Lymphocyte response to stimulation by PHA (25 μg/ml) in normal pregnant, postpartum, and nonpregnant women. PHA stimulation was found significantly decreased during pregnancy (27). (Courtesy of the authors and Alan R. Liss, Inc.)

If we assume consequently that pregnancy is associated with a decrease in cell-mediated immunity, it still remains to be determined whether the observed decline in cellular immunity does in fact occur primarily, and then allows tolerance of the fetal allograft, or whether it represents a phenomenon appearing secondarily. Whatever the immunologic mechanisms are that result in the tolerance of the fetal allograft, it always must be considered whether a factor independent of those mechanisms that we evaluate in our cellular immunity assays does, in fact, allow fetal survival. The decline in cellular immunity may then represent an immunologic situation

occurring secondarily to a still undefined primary event.

The evaluation of cellular immune capacity by any method is still difficult and rarely satisfactorily reproducible. Cell-mediated immunity depends on a number of widely varying factors that must be controlled for. Surgery, for instance, has repeatedly been shown to affect immune competence, and many of the patients involved in immunologic studies of pregnant populations have undergone surgery shortly before evaluation. Similarly, factors such as age, sex, and intercurrent disease, so frequently very dominating factors in pregnant patients, are often inadequately controlled for despite their clearly established significance.

Counts

Even the simplest aspects of maternal cellular immune function in pregnancy have remained controversial. Thus the composition of the white cells of peripheral blood, which may provide valuable information about the state of the host's immune system, has remained, despite the ease and availability of manual or automated methods for the determination of cell differentials, relatively unknown and statistically inconclusive.

Changes in the number of peripheral white cells in pregnancy were first demonstrated in 1835 by Nasse (cited in Ref. 6). This phenomenon was subsequently shown to be due to an increased number of peripheral neutro-

phils. In 1924, Heyns (cited in Ref. 6) described a lymphocytopenia and eosinopenia that occur during labor. Despite the fact that peripheral white cell changes in pregnancy have been known to occur for close to a century and a half, a normal range for blood counts during various stages of pregnancy has not yet been established. Studies of maternal peripheral blood cell counts during pregnancy have remained too limited in number for any given stage of pregnancy. This fact partly accounts for the widely conflicting results obtained by different investigators.

Total Number Of Lymphocytes.   The total number of peripheral blood lymphocytes was shown to decrease (6–10), increase (6), or remain unaltered (7, 11–16) during pregnancy. Recent studies by Pitkin and Witte (8) reported

Table 1.   Absolute numbers of white cells (10^6/ml)

	Pregnant Subjects	Nonpregnant Controls	p Value[a]
	Total White Cells		
Range	5.1–21.4	4.0–11.4	
Mean ± S.D.	11.44 ± 3.72	6.89 ± 1.91	$p < .0005$
N	86	37	
	Segmented Neutrophils		
Range	1.8–17.7	1.60–9.35	
Mean ± S.D.	7.96 ± 2.90	3.76 ± 1.54	$p < .0005$
N	101	35	
	Band Neutrophils		
Range	0.015–7.2	0.044–0.615	
Mean ± S.D.	1.05 ± 1.35	0.238 ± 0.189	$p < .0025$
N	96	27	
	Lymphocytes		
Range	0.4–5.0[b]	1.4–4.0	
Mean ± S.D.	0.9 ± 0.98	2.20 ± 0.30	$p < .05$
N	90	38	
	Monocytes		
Range	0.07–2.0	0.09–0.830	
Mean ± S.D.	0.618 ± 0.421	0.347 ± 0.235	$p < .0005$
N	92	36	

From Siegel and Gleicher (9), with the permission of the authors and Masson Publishing, Inc.
[a] *By Student's* t *test.*
[b] *14 out of 90 pregnancy bloods showed less than 10^6 lymphocytes per milliliter as compared to 0 out of 38 in the nonpregnant control group (p < .0005 by chi square).*

Table 2.   Percentages of white cells

	Pregnancy Blood	Nonpregnant Control Bloods	p Value[a]
	Segmented Neutrophils		
Range	18–88	38–70	
Mean ± S.D.	67.78 ± 12.28	54.37 ± 9.67	p < .0005
N	84	38	
	Band Neutrophils		
Range	1–70	1–11	
Mean ± S.D.	8.85 ± 11.66	3.33 ± 2.54	p < .0005
N	84	27	
	Lymphocytes		
Range	3–38	17–50	
Mean ± S.D.	18.03 ± 9.79	34.15 ± 9.07	p < .0005
N	90	41	
	Monocytes		
Range	1–16	1–11	
Mean ± S.D.	5.72 ± 3.69	5.71 ± 3.41	N.S.
N	92	36	

From Siegel and Gleicher (9), with the permission of the authors and Masson Publishing, Inc.
[a] By Student's t test.

a decreased number of lymphocytes in pregnancy, but the results were not statistically significant. In a very recent study of our own (9), we found a significant decrease in the number of lymphocytes in early labor ($p <$ .05). In addition, we noted that a significant percentage of pregnant women in early labor had lymphocyte counts of less than 1 million per milliliter ($p <$ .0005) (Tables 1 and 2).

Total Number Of Monocytes.   Efrati et al. (13) and Baines et al. (17) reported that the total number of monocytes did not change during pregnancy. Pitkin and Witte (8) reported an increase in the number of monocytes in pregnancy, but the result fell short of statistical significance ($p = $ .07). Plum et al. (7) showed an increase in the proportion of monocytes in Ficoll-Hypaque-isolated peripheral mononuclear cells. The total numbers of the monocytes were not reported, however. We have utilized standard automated hospital techniques

to study the total number of monocytes in late pregnancy (9) (Tables 1 and 2) and were able to demonstrate for the first time a highly significant rise in the total number of peripheral monocytes in late pregnancy ($p <$ .0005). As a consequence of these findings, we postulated (9) that the increase in the total number of monocytes may affect immune responses through an increase in the monocyte/lymphocyte ratio (Table 3), which can suppress certain immune responses (18) during monocyte-lymphocyte interactions (19, 20).

Percentage of T Cells.   Attempts to demonstrate changes in the percentage of peripheral T cells resulted in reports describing a decrease in (15, 16, 21, 22) or no (6, 7, 12, 14, 22–26) significant pregnancy-associated changes. Sumiyoshi et al. (27) recently reported the first use of multiple T cell markers in a study of T cell subpopulations in human pregnancy. The results are intriguing because

Table 3.   Ratio of absolute cell numbers

	Pregnancy Bloods	Nonpregnant Control Bloods	p Value[a]
Lymphocyte-Monocyte			
Range	0.55–31.65	1.53–47.06	
Mean ± S.D.	5.09 ± 5.47	9.47 ± 8.90	$p < .0005$
N	95	35	
Segment Neutrophils-Band Neutrophils			
Range	0.71–140.78	4.50–62.97	
Mean ± S.D.	23.76 ± 25.36	29.78 ± 20.96	$p < .15$(N.S.)
N	95	25	

From Siegel and Gleicher (9), with the permission of the authors and Masson Publishing, Inc.
[a] *By Student's t test.*

they indicate an increase in a maternal suppressor T cell population. Further studies of T cell subpopulations are required and are likely to demonstrate more pregnancy-associated T cell changes.

Percentage Of B Cells. The results on B cell counts conflict, showing both an increase (14, 16, 21, 22) or no change (7, 12, 15, 21, 23) in pregnancy. Most investigators who have demonstrated a decrease in percentages of T cells have also demonstrated an increase in the percentages of the B cell population (14, 16, 21, 22). Standard complement and fluorescent markers used in the past to identify B cells also interact with monocytes. The possibility therefore exists that many of the B cells that were identified as such were in fact monocytes. This is suggested by the studies of Plum et al. (7), who have shown that apparent increases in complement receptor (EAC) and surface membrane immunoglobulin (SMIg) B cells in pregnancy have been abolished by prior removal of monocytes. Relatively few studies of B cell subpopulations have been conducted to date. Those that were performed did not solve the controversy but seemed rather to add additional conflicting results. For example, SMIgG and SMIgM B lymphocyte subpopulations were reported to increase (22, 26) or to show no changes (24, 26) in pregnancy.

In conclusion, it can thus be stated, despite largely conflicting results, that quantitative changes in both polymorphonuclear and mononuclear peripheral white cells in pregnancy seem to occur. A decrease in the total number of lymphocytes reduces the total number of T cells despite an unchanged T cell percentage. Increases in the number of monocytes are likely to affect lymphocytes through monocyte-lymphocyte interactions. Changes in proportions of suppressor and helper T cell subpopulations may affect immune responses regardless of total numbers of lymphocytes. It is apparent that additional studies to establish ranges of white cell differentials in all stages of pregnancy are urgently required. The most recent developments in the identification of cellular subsets with monoclonal markers should allow better definition of maternal (and fetal) cellular adaptations to pregnancy. Table 4 summarizes the published experience with peripheral mononuclear cell counts in pregnancy.

Function

A variety of in vitro assay systems have been utilized in association with pregnancy (29) (Table 5). These include assays that measure the secretion of lymphokines, response to mitogens (27) (Fig. 1), lymphocyte transformation, mixed leukocyte reaction, and an assay system developed in our laboratory,

Table 4.   Peripheral mononuclear cell counts in pregnancy

Mononuclear Cells[a]	Range of Counts within[b]		
	Normal	Increased	Decreased
Total lymphocyte number	7, 11–61	6	6–10
% T lymphocytes E-RFc	6, 17, 12 14, 22, 26		15, 16, 21, 22
% T lymphocytes E-RFc ("active")	12		14
% T lymphocytes IgG-FcR[c]		27	
% T lymphocytes IgM-FcR[c]			27
% B lymphocytes EAC-RFc	7, 12, 15 21, 23		
% B lymphocytes SMIg	15	14, 16 21, 22	
% B lymphocytes SMIgG	26	22	
% B lymphocytes SMIgA	22		
% B lymphocytes SMIgM	24	26	
% B lymphocytes Fc-IgG	27		
Total monocyte number	13, 17	7–9	

From Siegel and Gleicher (28), with the permission of the authors and Alan R. Liss, Inc.
[a] E-RFc: T lymphocytes adhering to sheep red cells. E-RFc ("active"): a subpopulation of T lymphocytes adhering to sheep red cells. IgG-FcR: T lymphocytes with surface IgG and Fc receptors. IgM-FcR: T lymphocytes with surface IgM and Fc receptors. EAC-RFc: B lymphocytes adhering to red cells coated with antibody and complement. SMIg: B lymphocytes having surface membrane immunoglobulins. Fc-IgG: B lymphocytes having both Fc receptors and surface IgG.
[b] Numbers indicate the reference number of published report within the respective range.
[c] Indicates concentration of cells.

the leukocyte migration enhancement factor determination (30–33). Most of these assay systems, as noted before, gave in the majority of reports an indication of depressed immunocyte function. The leukocyte migration enhancement assay was characterized by showing leukocyte migration enhancement in association with two very specific immunologic situations, namely, pregnancy (Figs. 2 and 3) and malignant neoplasia (Fig. 4). This assay depended on two factors: a humoral

factor, probably an IgG, and a factor inherent to the pregnancy white cells.

In summary, it can be stated that white cell function in pregnancies seems to undergo a change. However, it still remains to be determined if this represents a primary or secondary event.

2.2.   Red Cells

Table 6 represents a summary of Fc and complement (C) receptors on human blood

Table 5. Substances that have been implicated in suppressing (blocking) the immune tesponse and the assay systems applied (during pregnancy)

Substances	Assay Systems
Serum[a]	Colong inhibition test (mouse)
Plasma[a]	Mixed lymphocyte reaction (human)
Serum[a]	PHA stimulation test (human)
Plasma[a]	Macrophage migration inhibition test (human)
Serum[a]	Polymorphonuclear leukocyte phagocytosis (human)
Plasma (IgG)	Macrophage migration inhibition test (human)
Serum (IgG)	Microcytotoxicity assay (mouse)
Immune complexes	Various (see Ref. 24)
Placental glycoprotein	Lymphocyte transformation (human)
-Globulin	PHA stimulation test (human)
Pregnancy zone protein	PHA stimulation test (human)
Hormones	Nonpregnant experience[b]
Estrogen	Various assay systems
Progesterone	Mixed lymphocyte reaction (human)
HCG	Various assay systems

From Gleicher and Jiegel (29), with the permission of the authors and the Mount Sinai Journal of Medicine.
[a] Undefined component.
[b] In vitro *experience that may be extrapolated to pregnancy because of high circulating hormone levels.*

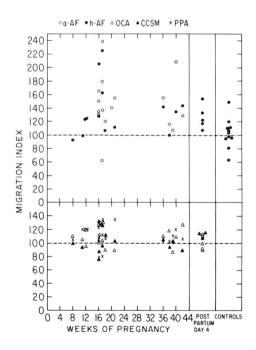

Figure 2. Leukocyte migration in pregnant and control patients. Significant leukocyte migration enhancement (LME) can be observed with autologous (a-AF) and homologous (h-AF) amniotic fluid in pregnancy, but not in nonpregnant controls. In contrast, control substances in the chambers, such as ovarian carcinoma homogenate (OCA), choriocarcinoma spent medium (CCSM), and placental pool homogenate (PPA), did not cause LME in either pregnant or control patients (30). (Courtesy of the authors and Williams & Williams.)

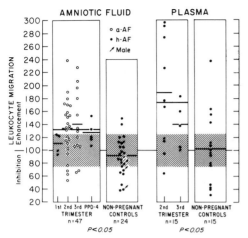

Figure 3. Leukocyte migration enhancement (LME) in pregnancy. Clearly significant LME can be seen in pregnant patients both with amniotic fluid and pregnancy plasma. The horizontal bars represent mean values, ± 2 S.D. The shaded areas represent 25% LME and LMI, generally considered significant. For numerical delineation see Table 2 (31). (Courtesy of the authors and Williams & Williams.)

cells. As may be seen from the table, erythrocytes possess a C3b-C4b receptor. In recent studies in our laboratory, we were able to demonstrate changes in what may represent this receptor's activity in association with different immunologic states. Thus we were able to show that certain malignancies are associated with a significantly decreased receptor potential, whereas certain autoimmune diseases do have a significantly increased receptor potential (35). In utilizing a red cell immunoadherence (RCIA) receptor assay, we were able to show significant changes in RCIA receptor activity in association with pregnancy (5).

In short, the addition of autologous serum to mixtures containing human red cells from pregnant and nonpregnant females and sheep red cells results in the formation of mixed aggregates containing both human and sheep red cells. The sheep red cells then act in our system as indicator cells for antigen-antibody-complement complexes. In contrast, no ag-

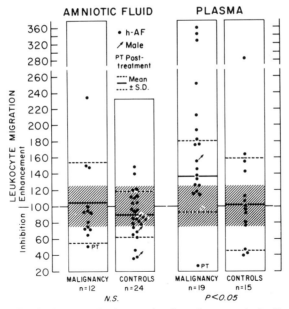

Figure 4. Leukocyte migration in cancer. Leukocyte migration enhancement is significant in cancer patients using autologous cancer plasma, but no amniotic fluid. The horizontal bars represent mean values ± 2 S.D. The shaded areas represent 25% LMI and LME, generally considered significant (32). (Courtesy of the authors and Williams & Williams.)

Table 6. Receptors for Fc and C on human blood cells

Cell Type	Fc Receptors				C Receptors						
	IgG	IgM	IgA	IgE	C1q	C3a	C3b-C4b	C3bi	C3d	C5a	C5b
Erythrocytes	−	−	−	−	−	−	+	−	−	−	−
Platelets	+	−	−	−	+	−	−	−	−	−	−
Neutrophils	+	−	+	−	−	+	+	+	+[a]	+	?[d]
Macrophages	+	−	−	?	−	?	+	+	+[a]	?	−
Eosinophils	+	−	−	?	−	+	+	−	+	+	−
Basophils-mast cells	+	−	−	+	−	+	?	−	+	+	−
B lymphocytes	+	+	−	+	+	−	+	−	+	−	+[e]
T lymphocytes	+	+	+	+	−[b]	−	−[c]	−	−[c]	−	−

From Gleicher and Theofilopoulos (34), with the permission of the authors and Masson Publishing, Inc.

[a] Recent findings suggest that neutrophils and macrophages do not have C3d (CR₂) receptors.

[b] It was originally suggested that both B and T cells have C1q receptors. However, recent studies indicate that C1q receptors are present only on B cells.

[c] C3 receptors have occasionally been described on T-type lymphoblasts.

[d] Not formally shown.

[e] Receptors for C5b are present on certain hormone lymphoblastoid (Raji) cells. The receptors for C5b have been found to be identical to C3b receptors.

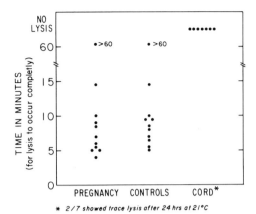

Figure 5. The presence of anti-sheep red cell antibody as indicated by time required for lysis. The absence of lysis in cord bloods indicates the absence of anti-sheep red cell antibody (5). (Courtesy of the authors and Alan R. Liss, Inc.)

gregate formation occurs when autologous cord serum is added to mixtures containing cord red cells and sheep red cells. Heat inactivation of the adult serum or the presence of 0.15 M EDTA prevents the formation of these mixed aggregates. These observations indicate that the mixed aggregates occur through complement-dependent RCIA phenomena. The addition of untreated cord serum to mixtures containing inactivated adult serum

restored the formation of mixed aggregates, indicating that the cord serum contains sufficient complement for RCIA. Natural antibodies against sheep red cells present in adult sera are absent in cord sera (Fig. 5).

Utilizing the RCIA-receptor assay (Fig. 6), RCIA-receptor activity of cord red cells was found to significantly exceed RCIA-receptor activity of the adult pregnant red cell ($p < .0025$). It is postulated that this may represent yet another aspect of immune adaption between mother and fetus.

3. HUMORAL ASPECTS OF MATERNAL IMMUNE RESPONSE

3.1. Immunoglobulins and Complement

Since immunoglobulin and complement (C) determinations were technically feasible much earlier than more sophisticated procedures such as the determination of lymphocyte populations, a large number of investigators attempted to correlate pregnancy with immunoglobulin and/or complement levels. They reported

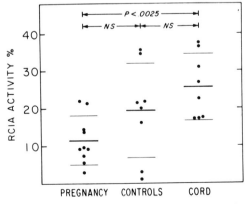

Figure 6. Red cell immune adherence activity in pregnant adults, controls, and cord blood. The horizontal bars indicate the mean ± S.D. (5). (Courtesy of the authors and Alan R. Liss, Inc.)

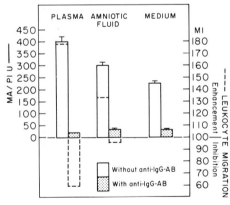

Figure 7. The influence of IG on leukocyte migration enhancement. Leukocyte migration with PL and AF before and after neutralization of IgG with gamma-chain specific anti-IgG antibody. The area of leukocyte migration is unspecifically inhibited by the addition of antibody as is witnessed by the decrease in migration area in the medium control, which does not contain IgG. But leukocyte migration with PL and AF is even more inhibited, resulting in a migration index of 100 (33). (Courtesy of the authors and Williams & Williams.)

Table 7. Immunoglobulin and complement levels in association with EPH gestosis

Ref.	Immunoglobulins[a]				Complement[a]			Comments
	IgG	IgM	IgA	IgD	Total	C3	C4	
36					S			
37	L							Patients without proteinuria; the diagnosis must be questionable
38	L	S	S					
39	L	S	S	L				
40		S						
41					S	S		
42					S			
43					L	H		Only the change in C3 reached significance
44	L	L			L	S	L	Attributes lower Ig levels to loss in urine

From Gleicher and Siegel (45), with the permission of the authors and the Mount Sinai Journal of Medicine.
[a] *L = lower; S = same; H = higher than controls.*

highly variable results in the literature. Variable results are reported not only for normal pregnancy but also for abnormal situations such as *e*dema *p*roteinuria *h*ypertension (EPH) gestosis (36–44), another name for preeclampsia/eclampsia. A number of investigators have demonstrated that a certain immunoglobulin fraction within IgG does seem to play an important role in pregnancy. A group in Boston was the first to demonstrate that certain patients with habitual abortions were lacking a very specific IgG fraction. Other investigators later confirmed this work. In our laboratory, we were able to demonstrate that the in vitro reaction, leukocyte migration enhancement, partly depends on an IgG immunoglobulin (33) (Fig. 7). The detailed function of this IgG still remains to be determined. Consequent to the above outlined work, however, it seems reasonable at the present time to suggest an immunologic workup in patients with habitual abortions. Table

7 demonstrates the large variations in published results with EPH gestosis.

3.2. Immune Complexes

Immune complexes (IC) may influence the immune response in a variety of ways. Table 8 summarizes presently recognized immune functions of ICs. Their discussion within the context of maternal immune function in pregnancy is therefore of utmost importance.

The first evidence for the presence of ICs in normal pregnancy came from histological investigations of kidney and placenta through deposits of immunoglobulins and certain complement components. Similar studies were later performed in patients with EPH gestosis (46–50). These early studies led to conflicting results, and it was thus not surprising that once assay systems for the detection of circulating ICs became available, they were applied to pregnancy (51–58). Table 9 lists the

Table 8.   Possible effects of immune complexes on immune response

Humoral Responses

Suppression
1. Antigen-specific suppression through interaction with antigen, as well as Fc-receptors on B cells
2. Nonantigen-specific suppression through interaction with Fc-receptors on B cells
   Release of suppressor factor(s) from B cells
   Effector cell blockade
   Activation of suppressor T cells
   Blockade of antigen receptors on T cells
   Blockade of T and B cell interaction
   Effect on macrophages
Enhancement
1. Increased DNA synthesis of B cells
2. Rapid localization of antigen in lymphoid follicles
3. Enhanced binding of antigen to antigen-bearing cells
4. Enhanced processing of antigen by macrophages
5. Stimulation of helper T cells
6. Close approximation of collaborating cells via Fc and C3 receptors

Cellular Responses

Inhibition of enhancement of antibody-dependent cellular cytotoxicity
Blockade of cell-mediated lymphocyte reactions
Blockade of delayed hypersensitivity
Altered traffic of lymphocytes

From Gleicher and Theofilopoulos (34), with the permission of the authors and Masson Publishing, Inc.

Table 9. Immune complexes in normal and abnormal (preeclamptic) pregnancy

Authors	Year of Publication	Method of Detection	Sample	Pregnancy		Comments
				Normal	Preeclamptic (EPH gestosis)	
Masson et al. (51)	1977	AI[a]	Serum	+		IC titers decrease to nonpregnant levels 3–4 weeks before delivery
Stirrat et al. (52)	1978	LA[b]	Serum	+	++	11/20 preeclamptic and 4/16 pregnant controls showed ICs
Knox et al. (53)	1978	Raji Cell	Serum	−	−	All sera with Raji assay negative 2/34
		C1q	Serum	−	−	Preeclamptic patients had C1q-binding 2SD above normal
Gleicher and Thefilopoulos (54)	1978	Raji cell	Plasma	−		1/20 low borderline plasma titers
			Amniotic Fluid	−		All amniotic fluids negative
Schena et al. (55)	1978–1979	^{125}I-C1q	Serum	+	++	Normal pregnancy positives 27% 1st, 8.7% 2nd, 11% 3rd trimester; puerperium 15%, preeclampsia 72%
McLaughlin et al. (56)	1979	C1q	Serum	−	−	9/12 normal, 10/12 preeclamptic sera positive
		LA	Serum	+	+	
D'Amelio et al. (57)	1979	PEGP[c]	Serum	−	−	0/30 normal pregnancies of all trimesters
		C1q	Serum			2/10 preeclamptic pregnancies, 2/11 diabetic pregnancies, 2/18 habitual aborters
Woodroffe et al. (58)	1979	C1q	Serum		−	0/14 preeclamptic pregnancies

Gleicher and Theofilopoulos (34), with the permission of the authors and Masson Publishing, Inc.
a Agglutination inhibition test.
b Latex agglutination test.
c Polyethylene glycol precipitation.

presently available experience with the detection of ICs during pregnancy. As may be noted, most of these data are rather new and still controversial. Some of the investigators were able to detect ICs in normal pregnancies; others were able to detect them only in abnormal pregnancies. No consensus could be reached at present if pregnancy does represent an IC state and, if EPH gestosis represents an IC disease, as suggested by some investigators. The best available consensus is summarized in the following fashion: if pregnancy does in fact represent an IC state, in other words, if ICs are physiologically present during normal pregnancy, then these ICs are most likely noncomplement-fixing. This statement is borne out by the fact that most of the investigators who utilized noncomplement-dependent assay systems for the detection of ICs were able to detect ICs in normal pregnancy. On the other hand, those who utilized complement-dependent assay systems usually had negative results in normal pregnancy. The picture in toxemia is even more complicated. As may be seen from Table 9, the number of investigated sera has remained extremely small. Some investigators, again, mainly those utilizing noncomplement-dependent assay systems, report an increase in ICs in association with preeclampsia. Again, it is the general consensus at present that this observation needs further confirmation. Most importantly, however, even if these observations are confirmed, it remains to be seen if noncomplement-fixing ICs do in fact have phlogogenic potential. As is presently believed, such ICs are usually small and do not have the capability to incur injury to tissue.

The discussion of pregnancy as an IC state, indicating the physiological presence of ICs during gestation, brings up the question of the influence of such physiological ICs on maternal as well as fetal organs. On the other hand, the consideration of pregnancy as an IC disease may have to be entertained in association with the EPH gestosis syndrome. In the latter, ICs may have the same, increased phlogogenic, or a totally different pathological potential. Again, the effect may be maternal as well as fetal. Last, the effect of associated IC diseases on the pregnant female and/or fetus deserves discussion. It seems feasible to assume that one IC condition superimposed upon the other may result in an additive effect. ICs do not necessarily have to be maternal in origin. Theoretically, ICs may be formed in the fetal circulation as well. Such a concept is presently supported by experimental evidence in some animal models (34). If one assumes the passage of maternal ICs transplacentally into the fetus, the fetomaternal passage may be possible as well.

Pregnancy as an IC State

Such a concept would indicate that the presence of ICs in normal pregnancy represents a normal physiological event. It could be assumed that the appearance of previously absent ICs was related to those immunologic processes which are responsible for the immunologic tolerance of the fetal allograft. We noted earlier that ICs may have influence on a large variety of immune responses (Table 8). If present in pregnancy, ICs would have to be small and noncomplement-fixing. Otherwise, it should be possible to detect such ICs with complement-dependent assay systems. A number of questions arise: what is the significance of such ICs, if present? If small, do they have the capability to cross the placental barrier into the fetus? If so, what is their significance in the fetus?

Very small ICs are usually formed with large antigen excess, typically contain a single antibody molecule divalently attached to antigen molecules ($AG_2 AB_1$), do not fix complement, and by and large cannot initiate inflammatory processes (34). Pregnancy could represent the state of significant antigen excess, although evidence in our laboratory indicates the opposite (33). Such ICs may evade entrapment by filtering organs because of the small size and eventually cross into the fetus. No obvious damage occurs in normal pregnancy to either mother or fetus. Therefore, it may be concluded that even if ICs are present in normal pregnancy, they do not have any pathological (phlogogenic) potential. It remains to be seen if such ICs are capable of exerting influence on the immune response of either mother or fetus. It has been suggested that the activation of fetal suppressor cells may occur transplacentally by ICs (3). The absence of phlogogenic potential in normal pregnancy may therefore be seen as indirect evidence that either no ICs or ICs with no phlogogenicity are present during normal pregnancy.

Pregnancy as an IC Disease

Although the presence of such small ICs with no phlogogenic potential seems feasible in normal pregnancy, it becomes difficult to construct a theoretical concept for the presence of such ICs in association with the EPH gestosis syndrome. Again, it must be presumed that if ICs are present with preeclampsia, they are of the small, noncomplement-fixing and therefore nonphlogogenic type. Larger and/or complement-dependent ICs should be detectable by a variety of assay systems, including the frequently applied Raji cell assay and the C1q binding assay. Those assays showed negative results in most reported in-

stances. One wonders if small ICs may in fact have the potential to cause "disease" as observed with the preeclampsia syndrome. Some questions do arise in conjunction with EPH gestosis: if ICs have a part in the etiology of preeclampsia, are they identical to those appearing in normal pregnancy? If so, does preeclampsia thus represent only a quantitative difference from normal pregnancy? Obviously additional studies are of utmost importance in order to clarify those questions.

The wide acceptance of the immunologic concept of EPH gestosis over the most recent years (45) will unquestionably provide additional answers within the near future. Some considerations concerning clinical applications of such an approach seem indicated. If the fetus is seen as an allograft, it can, on the basis of transplantation experience, be assumed that IC disease may develop. Such a process has been recognized in association with rejection mechanisms of kidney, bone marrow, and other transplants (59). The importance of such a concept lies in the therapeutic approach to the preeclampsia syndrome. If it in fact represents an immunologic rejection mechanism, it should be treated as such.

ICs have been reported to decrease platelets

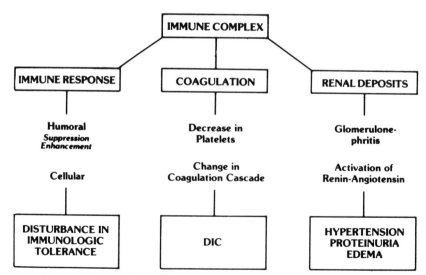

Figure 8.   Concepts of the induction of EPH gestosis by the presence of immune complexes (45). (Courtesy of the authors and *Mount Sinai Journal of Medicine.*)

and have been implicated in changes of the coagulation cascade. ICs may therefore be implicated in the frequent association of disseminated intravascular coagulation (DIC) with preeclampsia. The mechanism of IC-induced DIC is still poorly understood, but the association has been reported in a number of IC diseases. Figure 8 represents a graphic demonstration of how ICs could induce most if not all of the major signs and symptoms of EPH gestosis (preeclampsia).

3.3. Other Substances

Table 5 demonstrates a large variety of substances that have been implicated in suppressing (blocking) the "immune response" in a number of *in vitro* assay systems during pregnancy. As may be seen from this table, in earlier studies, serum and/or plasma without more detailed definition was implicated in suppressing the *in vitro* response (60–67). Later on, a number of more specific substances were implicated, including certain placental glycoproteins (68) and α-globulins (69).

Almost all steroid hormones have been implicated at one time or another to be immunodepressants (70–76). Although most of those probably are immunodepressants in very specific *in vitro* situations, it seems reasonable to state at present that systemic immunosuppressive action of any of the pregnancy hormones does not seem to play an important role in pregnancy. Estrogens, also used as immunodepressants in some clinical situations such as corneal transplants (70), do not seem to influence the pregnancy situation. The progesterones are even less likely to play any significant part. The most intensively investigated and best documented hormone in its immunologic influence upon pregnancy is human chorionic gonadotropin (hCG) (77–79). Even in very early investigations of pregnancy immunology hCG was thought to represent an immunosuppresive factor. Earlier studies, clearly demonstrating such immunosuppressive action by a number of *in vitro* assays, were later refuted by many investi-

gators, with some reporting that not hCG but rather contaminants of utilized reagents were responsible for the immunosuppressive action that had been demonstrated in association with hCG. Most recent investigations, however, indicate that hCG may have immunosuppressive capability, dependent on concentration. Nevertheless, the real immunologic activity of hCG in normal and abnormal pregnancy has not been determined as of yet. However, hCG represents the ideal link to the oncofetal antigens. Similar to other oncofetal antigens, hCG has been recently demonstrated to reappear in association with almost all malignancies (80–87). It has therefore been suggested by a number of investigators that hCG and/or oncofetal antigens may be closely involved in the induction of immunologic tolerance (3, 88). Because pregnancy and malignancy do represent the only biological systems in which clearly antigenic tissue is being tolerated by a seemingly intact immune system, oncofetal antigens and hCG may represent a common link. It would exceed the present discussion to go into further detail. It should be noted, however, that some oncofetal antigens such as alpha fetoprotein (AFP) have also been indicated in immunosuppressive activities (89).

4. THE FETAL FACTOR IN MATERNAL IMMUNE RESPONSE

The immunologic maternal/fetal interaction not only represents tolerance of the fetal allograft by the maternal immune system, but also requires a very delicate balance in the tolerance of the maternal immunogenic function by the fetal immune system (2). This aspect is not reviewed here. What is relevant to the present review, however, is the recognition that fetal immunologic parameters may affect the maternal immune system. Long before suppressor cell activity had been recognized in the maternal compartment, such suppressor cell activity had been recognized in fetal cord blood (90, 91). It was then suggested that those fetal suppressor cells may be activated by transplacental passage of an activating factor from the mother and then in turn suppress maternal as well as fetal activity (91). Interestingly, it was shown early during those studies that fetal suppressor cells are capable of suppressing not only fetal lymphocytes but also maternal lymphocytes. Unpublished studies by F. Siegal of The Mount Sinai School of Medicine in collaboration with us indicate that at term, suppressor and helper cell function in cord blood is equal to that of the adult. It seems, therefore, very attractive to speculate that a delicate balance between maternal as well as fetal activity is necessary for the normal immunologic homeostasis of pregnancy (2).

5. MATERNAL IMMUNE RESPONSE IN ABNORMAL PREGNANCIES

If pregnancy is seen as a delicate balance of different forces within the immune system, a defect in any of those forces, and thus a defect in the overall balance, may very well result in an abnormal pregnancy. Such a concept underlies the immunologic theory of EPH gestosis, and has also attracted increasing attention in certain cases of abortion as well as trophoblastic disease. It would exceed the framework of this review to describe abnormalities in association with EPH gestosis, abortion, and trophoblastic disease in detail. Figure 9, however, gives a short summary of a concept suggested by Takeuchi (92). The

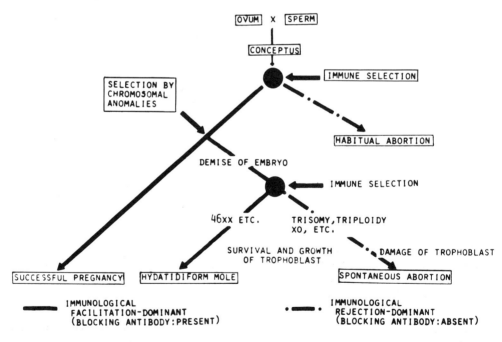

Figure 9. Scheme of the hypothesis on "immune selection" of the conceptus into hydatidiform mole or spontaneous abortion after demise of the embryo: if the conceptus does not develop the blocking antibody (BA), it results in spontaneous abortion. The woman in such a situation is prone to be an habitual aborter. If the conceptus develops the BA, it continues to grow successfully to a "feto-placental unit." If the early demise of the embryo occurs due to a chromosomal anomaly, in most cases BA begins to decrease, resulting in spontaneous abortion; however, in a few cases, BA does not decrease, and the conceptus develops into hydatidiform mole (92). (Courtesy of the authors and Alan R. Liss, Inc.)

influence of abnormalities of the immune response on congenital abnormalities of the fetus represents one of the most fascinating aspects of developmental biology and is under increasing investigation.

6. CONCLUSIONS

Pregnancy as a very specific immunologic state has not yet been clearly defined. It has become apparent recently that immunologic changes do occur in association with pregnancy. It still remains to be determined if changes in immunologic parameters that we are presently able to detect with still rather primitive methodology represent a primary or only a secondary change following a primary impulse that is still unknown. This review is not presented to take sides between the two major schools of thought in reproductive immunology, those who believe in a systemic maternal immune adaption and those who believe in a local placental immune adaption to pregnancy. Rather, it is presented to allow an understanding of what is presently known about the maternal immune response in pregnancy. With increasing sophistication and increasing knowledge, clinical application of our newly derived knowledge will follow. EPH gestosis, habitual abortion, and trophoblastic disease may represent the most obvious examples for an early application to clinical practice. It should not be forgotten, however, that immunologic disease of pregnancy, transplantation biology and medicine, oncology, and many fields in internal medicine and basic biology also have to learn and gain from a better understanding of the maternal immune response in pregnancy.

REFERENCES

1. R. E. Billingham, *Mt. Sinai J. Med.* **47**, 550 (1980).
2. I. Siegel and N. Gleicher, *Mt. Sinai J. Med.* **47**, 474 (1980).
3. N. Gleicher, G. Deppe, and C. J. Cohen, *Obstet. Gynecol.* **54**, 335 (1979).
4. I. Siegel, T. L. Liu, and N. Gleicher, *Lancet*, **2**, 556–559 (1981).
5. I. Siegel and N. Gleicher, *Am. J. Reprod. Immunol.* **1**, 88 (1981).
6. W. C. Andrews and R. W. Bonsnes, *Am. J. Obstet. Gynecol.* **61**, 1129 (1951).
7. J. Plum, M. Thiery, and L. Sabbe, *Clin. Exp. Immunol.* **31**, 45 (1978).
8. R. M. Pitkin and D. L. Witte, *J. Am. Med. Assoc.* **242**, 2696 (1979).
9. I. Siegel and N. Gleicher, *Diagnost. Gynecol. Obstet.*, **3**, 123–126 (1981).
10. F. W. Tysol and L. Lowenstein, *Am. J. Obstet. Gynecol.* **60**, 1187 (1950).
11. P. Brain, R. H. Marston, and J. Gordon, *Br. Med. J.* **4**, 488 (1972).
12. M. G. Dodson, R. H. Kerma, C. F. Lange, S. S. Stefani, and J. A. O'Leary, *Obstet. Gynecol.* **49**, 299 (1977).
13. P. Erfati, B. Presentey, M. Margalith, and L. Rozenszajn, *Obstet. Gynecol.* **23**, 429 (1964).
14. P. Gergely, J. Dzvonyar, G. Szegedi, B. Fekete, G. Szabo, and G. Petranyi, *Klin. Wochenschr.* **52**, 601 (1974).
15. J. R. Scott and T. L. Feldbush, *J. Am. Med. Assoc.* **239**, 2769 (1978).
16. A. J. Strelkauskas, I. J. Davies, and S. Dray, *Clin. Exp. Immunol.* **32**, 531 (1978).
17. M. G. Baines, H. F. Pross, and K. G. Millar, *Clin. Exp. Immunol.* **28**, 453 (1977).
18. A. Novogrodsky, K. H. Stenzel, and A. L. Rubin, *J. Immunol.* **118**, 852 (1977).
19. I. Siegel, *J. Immunol.* **105**, 879 (1970).
20. V. Persson, L. Hammarstrom, E. Moller, G. Moller, and C. I. E. Smith, *Immunol. Rev.* **40**, 78 (1978).
21. R. Bulmer and K. W. Hancock, *Clin. Exp. Immunol.* **28**, 302 (1977).
22. D. B. Cornfield, J. Jencks, R. A. Binder, and C. E. Rath, *Obstet. Gynecol.* **53**, 203 (1979).
23. S. A. Birkeland and K. Kristoffersen, *Scand. J. Immunol.* **10**, 415 (1979).
24. P. D. Campion and H. L. F. Currey, *Lancet* **2**, 830 (1972).
25. G. Garewal, S. Sehgal, and B. K. Aikat, *Br. J. Obstet. Gynecol.* **875**, 221 (1978).
26. Y. W. Loke, S. S. Brook, and G. E. Allen, *Am. J. Obstet. Gynecol.* **122**, 561 (1975).
27. Y. Sumiyoshi, I. Gorai, F. Hirahara, K. Tanaka, and H. Minapuchi, *Am. J. Reprod. Immunol.*, **1**, 145–149 (1981).

28. I. Siegel and N. Gleicher, *Am. J. Reprod. Immunol.*, **1**, 154–155 (1981).

29. N. Gleicher and I. Siegel, *Mt. Sinai J. Mea.* **47**, 511 (1980).

30. N. Gleicher, C. J. Cohen, T. D. Kerenyi, and S. B. Gusberg, *Am. J. Obstet. Gynecol.* **133**, 386 (1979).

31. N. Gleicher, P. C. Beers, T. D. Kerenyi, C. J. Cohen, and S. B. Gusberg, *Am. J. Obstet. Gynecol.* **136**, 1 (1980).

32. N. Gleicher, P. C. Beers, T. D. Kerenyi, C. J. Cohen, and S. B. Gusberg, *Am. J. Obstet. Gynecol.* **136**, 126 (1980).

33. N. Gleicher, P. C. Beers, T. D. Kerenyi, C. J. Cohen, and S. B. Gusberg, *Am. J. Obstet. Gynecol.* **136**, 5 (1980).

34. N. Gleicher and A. N. Theofilopoulos, *Diagnost. Gynecol. Obstet.* **2**, 7 (1980).

35. I. Siegel and N. Gleicher, *Immunol. Commun.*, **10**, 433–449 (1981).

36. S. Thomson, W. M. Arnott, and G. D. Matthew, *Lancet* **1**, 734 (1939).

37. C. H. W. Horne, P. W. Howie, and R. B. Goudie, *J. Clin. Pathol.* **23**, 514 (1970).

38. B. Benster and E. J. Wood, *J. Obstet. Gynaecol. Br. Commonw.* **77**, 518 (1970).

39. J. W. W. Studd, *J. Obstet. Gynaecol. Br. Commonw.* **78**, 786 (1971).

40. N. M. Burdash, J. M. Blake, Jr., and L. L. Hester, *Am. J. Obstet. Gynecol.* **116**, 827 (1973).

41. J. L. Kitzmiller, L. Stoneburner, and P. F. Yelonsky, *Am. J. Obstet. Gynecol.* **117**, 312 (1973).

42. H. E. Fadel, M. D. E. Soliman, and M. M. El-Mehairy, *Int. J. Gynecol. Obstet.* **12**, 6 (1974).

43. R. S. Tedder, M. Nelson, and V. Eisen, *Br. J. Exp. Pathol.* **56**, 389 (1975).

44. S. L. Yang, A. M. Kleinman, and P. Y. Wei, *Am. J. Obstet. Gynecol.* **122**, 727 (1975).

45. N. Gleicher and I. Siegel, *Mt. Sinai J. Med.* **47**, 442 (1980).

46. R. H. Morris, P. Vassalli, and R. T. McClusky, *Clin. Obstet. Gynecol.* **11**, 522 (1968).

47. O. M. Petrucco, N. M. Thomson, J. R. Laurence et al., *Br. Med. J.* **1**, 473 (1974).

48. K. S. K. Tung, *Fed. Proc.* **32**, 4292 (1973).

48. K. S. K. Tung, *Fed. Proc.* **32**, 4292 (1973).

49. K. S. K. Tung, *J. Immunol.* **112**, 185 (1974).

50. K. S. K. Tung, *Am. J. Pathol.* **70**, 4a (1973).

51. P. L. Masson, M. Delire, and C. L. Cambiaso, *Nature* **266**, 542 (1977).

52. G. M. Stirrat, C. W. G. Redman, and R. J. Levinsky, *Clin. Obstet. Gynecol.* **11**, 522 (1968).

53. G. E. Knox, S. Stagno, J. E. Volanakis et al., *Am. J. Obstet. Gynecol.* **132**, 87 (1978).

54. N. Gleicher and A. N. Theofilopoulos, *Diagnost. Gynecol. Obstet.* **2**, 7 (1980).

55. F. P. Schena, C. Manno, L. Selvaggi, et al., *Lancet* **1**, 216 (1979).

56. P. J. McLaughlin, G. M. Stirrat, C. W. G. Redman et al., *Lancet* **1**, 934 (1979).

57. R. D'Amelio, P. Bilotta, A. Pachi et al., *Clin. Exp. Immunol.* **37**, 33 (1979).

58. A. J. Woodroffe, M. Foldes, P. E. McKenzie et al., *Aust. N.Z. J. Med.* **9**, 129 (1979).

59. A. N. Theofilopoulos and F. J. Dixon, *Adv. Immunol.* **28**, 89 (1979).

60. K. E. Hellström, I. Hellström, and J. Brawn, *Nature* **224**, 914 (1969).

61. P. Curzen, E. Jones, and J. Gaugas, *Br. Med. J.* **2**, 49 (1972).

62. S. Kasakura, *J. Immunol.* **107**, 1296 (1971).

63. J. A. McIntyre and W. P. Faulk, *Lancet* **2**, 821 (1979).

64. C. A. St. Hill, R. Finn, and V. Denye, *Br. Med. J.* **2**, 513 (1973).

65. V. Youtananukorn and P. Matangkasombut, *Nat. New Biol.* **242**, 110 (1973).

66. R. H. Persellin and J. K. Leibfarth, *Arthritis Rheum.* **21**, 316 (1978).

67. H. Pence, W. M. Petty, and R. E. Rocklin, *J. Immunol.* **114**, 525 (1975).

68. R. R. Riggio, J. E. Parrillo, Jr., F. G. Bull, G. H. Schwartz, K. H. Stenzel et al., *Transplantation* **12**, 400 (1971).

69. S. R. Cooperbrand, R. C. Davis, K. Schmid, and J. A. Mannick, *Transplant. Proc.* **1**, 516 (1969).

70. S. R. Waltman, R. M. Burde, and J. Berrios, *Transplantation* **11**, 194 (1971).

71. R. J. Ablin, G. R. Bruns, P. Guinan, and I. M. Bush, *J. Immunol.* **113**, 705 (1974).

72. R. J. Ablin, G. R. Bruns, P. Guinan, N. Sadoughi, and I. M. Bush, *Urol. Res.* **2**, 69 (1974).

73. R. J. Ablin, G. R. Bruns, P. D. Guinan, H. A. Sheik, and I. M. Bush, *J. Lab. Clin. Med.* **87**, 227 (1976).

74. R. J. Ablin, G. R. Bruns, P. D. Guinan, H. A. Sheik, and I. M. Bush, *Eur. Urol.* **5**, 359 (1979).

75. R. J. Ablin, R. A. Bhatti, P. D. Guinan, and W. Khin, *Clin. Exp. Immunol.* **38**, 83 (1979).

76. H. Kobayashi, T. Mori, A. Suzuki, T. Nishimoto, H. Nishimoto et al., *Am. J. Obstet. Gynecol.* **134**, 255 (1979).

77. M. D. Kaye and W. R. Jones, *Am. J. Obstet. Gynecol.* **109**, 1029 (1971).

78. D. M. Jenkins, M. G. Acres, J. Peters, and J. Riley, *Am. J. Obstet. Gynecol.* **114**, 13 (1972).

79. T. Han, *Clin. Exp. Immunol.* **18**, 529 (1974).

80. M. A. Naughton, D. A. Merrill, L. M. McManus, L. M. Fink, E. Berman, et al., *Cancer Res.* **35**, 1887 (1975).

81. G. D. Braunstein, J. L. Vaitukaitis, P. P. Carbone, et al., *Ann. Intern. Med.* **78**, 39 (1973).

82. L. H. Rees and J. C. Ratcliffe, *Clin. Endocrin.* **3**, 263 (1973).

83. S. W. Rosen, B. D. Weintraub, J. L. Vaitukaitis, H. H. Sussman, J. M. Hershman et al., *Ann. Intern. Med.* **82**, 71 (1975).

84. C. R. Kahn, S. W. Rosen, B. D. Weintraub, S. S. Fajans, and P. Gordon, *N. Engl. J. Med.* **297**, 565 (1977).

85. Y. Yoshimoto, A. R. Wolfsen, F. Hirose, and W. D. Odell, *Am. J. Obstet. Gynecol.* **134**, 729 (1979).

86. A. Borkowski and C. Muquardt, *N. Engl. J. Med.* **301**, 298 (1979).

87. C. J. M. Lips, J. van der Sluys Veer, J. A. van der Donk, R. H. van Dam, and W. H. L. Hackeng, *Lancet* **1**, 16 (1978).

88. P. Alexander, *Nature* **235**, 137 (1972).

89. R. Masseyeff, *Pathol. Biol.* **20**, 703 (1972).

90. N. Moriya, T. Nagaoki, N. Okuda, and N. Taniguchi, *J. Immunol.* **123**, 1795 (1979).

91. M. B. A. Oldstone, A. Thesin, and L. Moretta, *Nature* **269**, 333 (1977).

92. S. Takeuchi, *Am. J. Reprod. Immunol.* **1**, 23 (1980).

13

Postpartum Autoimmune Endocrine Syndromes

Nobuyuki Amino
Kiyoshi Miyai

The Central Laboratory for Clinical Investigation
Osaka University Hospital
Fukushima-ku
Osaka, Japan

Contents

1. INTRODUCTION

Pregnancy has been described as a successful allograft of foreign tissue, and gestational physiological changes in immune reactions are receiving increasing attention (1, 2). On the other hand, autoimmune diseases are considered to be induced by a disturbance of immunologic surveillance. Therefore pregnancy is of special interest to the clinical immunologist because many autoimmune diseases occur more commonly in women, often during the childbearing age.

Hashimoto's disease and Graves' disease are now recognized as autoimmune disorders (3), and pregnancy markedly influences the clinical course of these diseases (4, 5). Especially after delivery, disease is aggravated and transient thyrotoxicosis and/or hypothyroidism are frequently observed (4, 6). Postpartum hypothyroidism has long been known to occur as a result of hypopituitarism since the report by Sheehan in 1937 (7). In 1948, however, Roberton reported the frequent occurrence of hypothyroidism after delivery in association with endemic goiter and suggested that iodine deficiency in the postpartum period might be one factor inducing these changes (8). In 1955 Fraser and Garrod (9) reported four cases of primary myxedema dating from "postpartum shock or hemorrhage." They did not discuss its possible relation to autoimmune abnormalities since the concept of autoimmune thyroiditis was unknown at that time.

This chapter deals with recent progress in the effect of pregnancy on autoimmune thyroid diseases and describes the various types of postpartum thyroid dysfunction which are tentatively called "postpartum autoimmune endocrine syndromes."

2. HASHIMOTO'S DISEASE AND PREGNANCY

Many studies have been reported on the complication of hypothyroidism with pregnancy (10) but few data are available on the effect of pregnancy on the clinical course of Hashimoto's disease. In 1975 Nelson and Palmer (11) observed a remission of goitrous hypothyroidism during pregnancy in a patient with Hashimoto's thyroiditis. They suggested that Hashimoto's thyroiditis might undergo spontaneous remission during pregnancy.

Figure 1 shows the spontaneous changes of goiter size, serum TSH, and free T_4 index in pregnancy in 15 patients with Hashimoto's disease. Goiter size and serum TSH decreased significantly in late pregnancy when compared with values in early pregnancy. In two patients the serum free T_4 index in early pregnancy was slightly low but returned spontaneously to normal in late pregnancy. These data indicate that Hashimoto's disease is ameliorated during pregnancy (12).

After delivery, however, various changes in the free T_4 index were observed, as shown in Figure 2. Patients were divided into the following three groups according to the severity of hypothyroidism 2 to 6 months postpartum: in group a, the maximal level of serum TSH was more than 50 microunits per milliliter; in group b, the serum TSH was 10 to 50 microunits per milliliter; and in group c, the serum TSH was less than 10 microunits per milliliter. In group a, four of six patients showed marked thyrotoxicosis 1 to 3 months postpartum. After thyrotoxicosis, these patients all developed hypothyroidism 3 to 4 months postpartum and then their TSH levels returned to the normal range 6 to 8 months postpartum. Two other patients developed overt hypothyroidism without preceding thyrotoxicosis. In group b, four of five patients showed mild thyrotoxicosis at 2 to 4 months postpartum and then developed mild hypo-

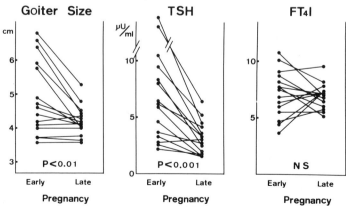

Figure 1. Comparison of goiter size (transverse width), serum TSH, and free T_4 index (FT$_4$I) between early and late pregnancy in untreated patients with Hashimoto's disease. NS = No significant difference.

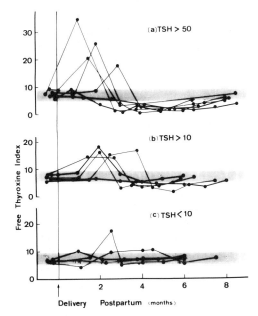

Figure 2. Change of free T$_4$ index after delivery in 15 patients with Hashimoto's disease. (*a*) The maximal level of serum TSH was more than 50 microunits per milliliter in the postpartum hypothyroid state; (*b*) the serum TSH was 10 to 50 microunits per milliliter at the time of postpartum hypothyroidism; (*c*) the serum TSH was less than 10 microunits per milliliter at 2 to 6 months postpartum. Shaded areas indicate normal ranges of the free T$_4$ index.

thyroidism with a serum TSH of less than 50 microunits per milliliter at 3 to 5 months postpartum. None of the four patients in group *c* developed hypothyroidism, although two showed very mild transient thyrotoxicosis 3 to 4 months postpartum. All cases of thyrotoxicosis were induced by thyroid destruction, because of the later development of hypothyroidism, a low T$_3$/T$_4$ ratio (13), and/or low radioactive iodine uptake. In the early

Figure 3. Serial changes of goiter size, titer of antithyroid microsomal antibody (MCHA), and peripheral lymphocyte count during and after pregnancy in 15 patients with Hashimoto's disease. In the upper panel, open circles indicate goiter sizes with serum TSH levels of more than 10 microunits per milliliter, and closed circles indicate those with serum TSH levels of less than 10 microunits per milliliter.

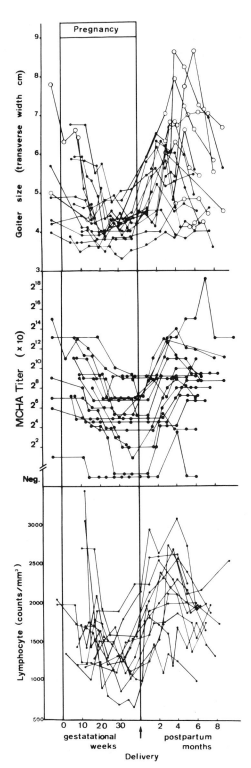

phase of transient hypothyroidism, no increase of serum TSH was observed in six patients, although both the free T_4 index and the free T_3 index were clearly lower than normal. No relation was found between the occurrence of postpartum hypothyroidism and breast feeding or iodine ingestion. These data indicate that postpartum hypothyroidism is the consequence of postpartum transient thyrotoxicosis, and marked thyroid destruction in the early postpartum period leads to more obvious hypothyroidism.

The sequential changes of goiter size, the antithyroid microsomal antibody (MCHA) titer, and the peripheral lymphocyte count in these 15 patients are shown in Figure 3. The goiter increased 1 month postpartum, before increase of serum TSH. The goiter enlarged further in the period of increased TSH 4 to 6 months postpartum in nine patients who developed hypothyroidism. In all patients, the titer of MCHA decreased gradually as pregnancy progressed and increased after delivery to a peak at about 2 to 5 months postpartum. The extent of increase in the MCHA titer after delivery varied in each patient, but the ratio of the maximum titer to that in late pregnancy was 2^4 or more in all patients who developed postpartum hypothyroidism. Peripheral lymphocyte counts also decreased in pregnancy and increased after delivery to a peak at about 2 to 4 months postpartum. All these data indicate that amelioration of Hashimoto's disease during pregnancy and aggravation after delivery are related to immunologic changes associated with gestation.

3.   TRANSIENT POSTPARTUM HYPOTHYROIDISM

For establishing a method for prediction of postpartum development of hypothyroidism, various parameters were measured in 32 patients with Hashimoto's disease, who could be observed in early pregnancy and the postpartum period. As shown in Table 1, age, goiter size, thyroid function tests, the titers of antithyroid antibodies, and the peripheral lymphocyte counts in early pregnancy in patients who developed postpartum hypothyroidism (group A) were compared with those who did not develop hypothyroidism (group B). Only the titer of MCHA was found to be significantly different in the two groups. Individual values of the MCHA titer are shown in Figure 4. An interesting finding was that 11 of 21 patients (52%) in group A but only 1 of 11 patients (9%) in group B delivered a female baby (Fig. 4). The difference between these incidences was significant ($p < .05$). Eleven of 12 patients (92%) with female babies developed postpartum hypothyroidism, whereas 10 of 20 patients (50%) with male babies developed postpartum hypothyroidism. The difference between these incidences was also significant. Considering these data, it is suggested that the development of postpartum hypothyroidism may be predicted in patients with a female baby and a high titer of microsomal antibody (more than 10×2^7) in

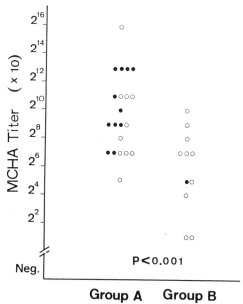

Figure 4. Comparison of titers of antithyroid microsomal antibody in early pregnancy in Hashimoto's patients who developed postpartum hypothyroidism (Group A) and those did not develop hypothyroidism (Group B). Open circles: patients who delivered a male baby. Closed circles: patients who delivered a female baby.

Table 1. Comparison of age and goiter size, thyroid function, antithyroid antibody, and peripheral lymphocyte count in early pregnancy in patients with Hashimoto's disease who did and did not develop postpartum hypothyroidism[a]

	No. Examined	Age	Goiter Size[b] (cm)	Free T$_4$ Index	TSH (μU/ml)	TGHA[c] (10×2^n)	MCHA[c] (10×2^n)	Peripheral Lymphocytes (Counts/mm^3)
Group A	21	27.9 ± 2.8	4.7 ± 1.0	7.1 ± 2.0	11.9 ± 16.7	2.0 ± 3.0	9.8 ± 2.7	1587 ± 416
Group B	11	26.6 ± 2.8	4.3 ± 0.8	8.0 ± 1.6	4.7 ± 2.6	1.3 ± 2.0	5.8 ± 2.8	1688 ± 753
Significance of difference		NS	NS	NS	NS	NS	$p < .001$	NS

[a] Values are means $\pm$ SD. Group A = Patients who developed postpartum hypothyroidism. Group B = Patients who did not develop postpartum hypothyroidism.
[b] Goiter size is expressed as transverse width of the thyroid gland.
[c] Titers of antithyroglobulin (TGHA) and antithyroid microsomal hemagglutination antibody (MCHA) are expressed as 10×2^n. Values are means $\pm$ SD. Negative reactions for antibodies are treated as n = 0.

Table 2. Recurrence of transient postpartum hypothyroidism

Case No.	Episode	Sex of Baby	Months Post-partum	Serum Values at Hypothyroidism[a]		
				T_4 (μg/dl)	T_3 (ng/dl)	TSH (μU/ml)
1	1	Female	4	1.4	73	363
	2	Female	4	2.1	121	250
2	1	Female	4.5	5.0	ND	30
	2	Male	5.5	2.4	100	44
	3	Male	5.5	2.3	108	58
3	1	Male	3	3.2	ND	ND
	2	Female	3	3.4	99	15
4	1	Male	5	2.2	92	31
	2	Male	5	2.7	150	56
5	1	Male	4	4.9	120	18
	2	Male	4	6.4	137	13

[a] ND = not done.

early pregnancy. Furthermore, postpartum hypothyroidism can also be predicted in the patients who had previous postpartum hypothyroidism. Table 2 shows the recurrence of postpartum hypothyroidism in five patients with Hashimoto's disease. The time when hypothyroidism occurred after delivery and the severity of hypothyroidism are almost the same in the two consecutive episodes in each patient.

As described above, transient thyrotoxicosis usually precedes postpartum hypothyroidism. However, patients often attend hospital with a complaint of thyroid enlargement at the time of hypothyroidism and thyrotoxicosis is frequently missed (14). Table 3 summarizes the characteristics of transient postpartum hypothyroidism.

4. GRAVES' DISEASE AND PREGNANCY

Because of the prevalence of Graves' disease in women of childbearing age, this disease is often complicated by pregnancy (10). During

Table 3. Transient postpartum hypothyroidism

Goiter	1. A high incidence of previous goiter
	2. Thyroid enlargement at 1–3 months postpartum
	3. Goiter decreases in size spontaneously at 6–12 months postpartum, but does not disappear
Thyroid function	1. Increase of T_4 and T_3 at 1–2 months postpartum, but low radioactive iodine uptake
	2. Decrease of T_4 and T_3, and increase of TSH at 3–5 months postpartum, but high radioactive iodine uptake
	3. Spontaneous recovery to euthyroidism at 6–12 months postpartum
Antithyroid antibody	1. Transient increase of antithyroid microsomal hemagglutination antibody (MCHA) at 3–5 months postpartum
	2. Titers of MCHA decrease thereafter, but do not disappear.

pregnancy the symptoms of Graves' disease have been reported to remain unchanged or often to become ameliorated (10, 15, 16), but rarely to be aggravated (17). It is difficult, however, to evaluate the effect of pregnancy on Graves' disease when the patients are receiving antithyroid drugs. To clarify this point, spontaneous changes of serum thyroid hormones were examined in patients with Graves' disease who were considered to be in a state of clinical remission or near remission, during and after pregnancy without antithyroid drugs. Figure 5 shows serial changes of the serum free T_4 index in 41 pregnancies in 35 patients with Graves' disease. Eighteen patients (44%) showed a transient increase of the free T_4 index at 10 to 15 weeks of pregnancy but a normal free T_4 index in the second and third trimesters (18). After delivery 32 cases (78%) developed various degrees of thyrotoxicosis, mostly at 2 to 4 months postpartum (18). The serum free T_3 index also showed a similar

elevation at 10 to 15 weeks of pregnancy and after delivery.

These patients with Graves' disease were divided into the following four groups according to postpartum changes of thyroid function: (1) persistent thyrotoxicosis—free T_4 index more than 20 with high radioactive iodine uptake and thyrotoxicosis persisting for more than 2 months; (2) transient thyrotoxicosis—a high free T_4 index with normal or high radioactive iodine uptake and transient thyrotoxicosis; (3) no change—free T_4 index within the normal range after delivery; (4) destruction-induced thyrotoxicosis—a high free T_4 index with low radioactive iodine uptake and/or subsequent development of transient hypothyroidism. The serum free T_4 index and free T_3 index were significantly higher in the first two groups but not in the latter two groups. Individual values of the free T_4 index in weeks 10 to 15 of pregnancy are shown in Figure 6. Sixteen of 18 patients

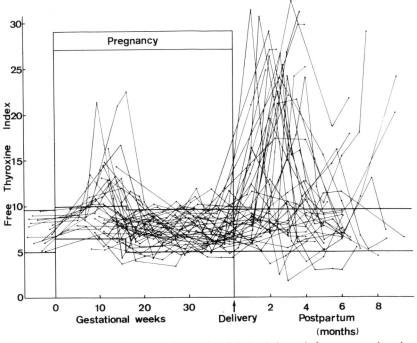

Figure 5. Spontaneous sequential changes of serum free T_4 index during and after pregnancy in patients with Graves' disease who were considered to be in a state of remission or near remission. Horizontal lines indicate normal range of free T_4 index. (Data from Ref. 18.)

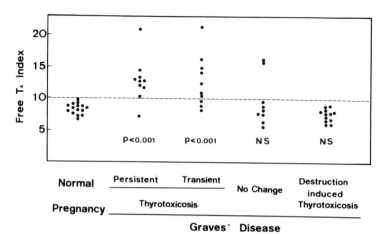

Figure 6. Free T$_4$ index at 10 to 15 weeks of pregnancy in normal women and patients with Graves' disease. Patients with Graves' disease were divided into four groups according to postpartum changes of thyroid function. (Data from Ref. 18.)

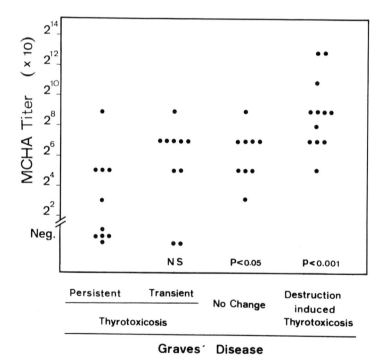

Figure 7. Antithyroid microsomal antibodies at 10 to 15 weeks of pregnancy in patients with Graves' disease who were considered to be in a state of remission or near remission. Patients were divided into four groups according to postpartum changes of thyroid function.

(89%) who had a high free T$_4$ index of more than 10 showed recurrence of stimulation-induced thyrotoxicosis of either the persistent or transient type. On the contrary, only 4 of 23 patients (17%) whose free T$_4$ index in early pregnancy was less than 10 showed recurrence of stimulation-induced thyrotoxicosis, whereas the others remained euthyroid or developed postpartum destructive thyrotoxicosis, similar to that in Hashimoto's disease.

The titers of antithyroid microsomal antibodies (MCHA) in early pregnancy were higher in the latter two groups. Individual data are shown in Figure 7. These data indicate that Graves' disease was aggravated in early pregnancy and after delivery, and ameliorated in the latter half of pregnancy. Postpartum relapse of persistent hyperthyroidism could be predicted by the early increase in the free T$_4$ index in pregnancy. It is also suggested that Graves' disease may progress toward a pathological state compatible with Hashimoto's disease after complete remission, as suggested by Wood and Ingbar (19). An earlier study suggested the possible effect of increased

thyroxine-binding globulin on amelioration of Graves' disease during pregnancy (20). However, as described above, Hashimoto's disease was also ameliorated during pregnancy. Amelioration of Graves' disease in later pregnancy may be induced by physiological suppression of immune reactions, which is discussed below.

5. TRANSIENT POSTPARTUM THYROTOXICOSIS

Transient thyrotoxicosis induced by thyroid destruction is often observed after delivery in patients with Hashimoto's disease (12, 21). Moreover, various types of postpartum thyrotoxicosis are also observed in patients with Graves' disease (5, 18), as described above. Collecting these cases together, postpartum thyrotoxicosis can be devided into the following four groups: (1) persistent thyrotoxicosis-increased thyroid hormones with high radioactive iodine uptake (RAIU) and thyrotoxicosis persisting for more than 2 months; (2) transient thyrotoxicosis with normal or

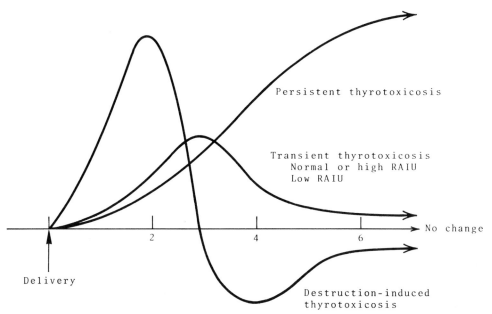

Figure 8. Changes of free thyroxine index in various types of postpartum thyrotoxicosis. Numbers indicate months postpartum.

high RAIU; (3) transient thyrotoxicosis with low RAIU; and (4) transient thyrotoxicosis with low RAIU followed by transient hypothyroidism. Typical patterns of these thyrotoxicoses are illustrated in Figure 8. The first two groups of thyrotoxicosis are stimulation-induced thyrotoxicosis, and antithyroid therapy is necessary only in the first group. Persistent thyrotoxicosis usually develops 3 to 4 months postpartum. Most of destruction-induced thyrotoxicosis in the last group develops 1 to 3 months postpartum.

Measurement of RAIU is the best way to differentiate these types of thyrotoxicosis at present. However, the RAIU test is contraindicated in women who are breast-feeding. Furthermore, lactation markedly influences the RAIU of the thyroid gland, since a significant amount of radioiodine is secreted into milk. Recently it was found that the serum ratio of T_3 to T_4 was useful in the differentiation of stimulation-induced thyrotoxicosis from destruction-induced thyrotoxicosis. A T_3/T_4 ratio less than 20 (nanograms/micrograms) in thyrotoxic patients is a laboratory signal of destruction-induced thyrotoxicosis (13), although this usefulness is not accepted by all workers (22). Patients with postpartum thyrotoxicosis, in whom the serum T_3/T_4 ratio is low, may be followed with a mild tran-

quilizer or β-blocker when they report moderate or severe symptoms of thyrotoxicosis.

6. INCIDENCE OF POSTPARTUM THYROID DYSFUNCTION

Transient thyrotoxicosis or hypothyroidism or transient thyrotoxicosis followed by hypothyroidism was frequently observed after delivery in patients with autoimmune thyroid diseases in Japan (4, 5, 14). Similar postpartum syndromes have been observed in Canada (6), England (23), and the United States (24, 25). The physiological and immunologic changes associated with gestation may induce postpartum aggravation of autoimmune thyroid disease, as described below. In has been suggested that the subclinical forms of the disease might develop into overt disease after delivery (14, 21). Subclinical autoimmune thyroiditis has been found in 8.5% of women in the general population of Japan (26). Therefore a population survey of postpartum thyroid dysfunction was performed (27).

Table 4 shows the abnormalities of thyroid function present 3 to 8 months after delivery. Two of the 507 subjects were diagnosed as having "simple goiter" before pregnancy, but the other 505 had no previous history of

Table 4.   Summary of patients with abnormal thyroid function at 3–8 months postpartum among 507 subjects

Type of Thyroid Abnormality	No. of Patients (%)	Number of Cases		
		Goiter	TGHA[a]	MCHA[a]
Transient thyrotoxicosis alone	13 (2.6)	6	5	11
Transient thyrotoxicosis followed by transient hypothyroidism	7 (1.4)	4	3	6
Persistent thyrotoxicosis	0 (0)	0	0	0
Transient hypothyroidism alone	7 (1.4)	7	3	7
Persistent hypothyroidism	1 (0.2)	1	1	1
Total	28 (5.5)	18	12	25

[a] Number of patients who had positive antithyroglobulin (TGHA) and antithyroid microsomal hemagglutination antibodies (MCHA). (Data from Ref. 27).

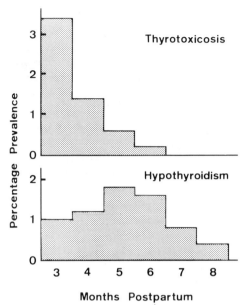

Figure 9. Percentage prevalence of postpartum thyrotoxicosis and hypothyroidism in various periods postpartum.

a thyroid abnormality. In all, 28 of the 507 subjects (5.5%) had thyrotoxicosis or hypothyroidism. Pituitary hypothyroidism was not observed in this screening study. Figure 9 shows the percentage prevalence of postpartum thyrotoxicosis and hypothyroidism in various postpartum periods.

The high prevalence of postpartum thyroid dysfunction associated with antithyroid antibodies in this study strongly supports the hypothesis that these postpartum abnormalities are induced by aggravation of subclinical autoimmune thyroid disease (14, 21).

It is known that postpartum hypothyroidism occurs as a result of hypopituitarism (28). The incidence of postpartum hypopituitarism has been estimated to be 0.003% (4 of 124,752 deliveries) (29). This study, however, revealed a higher rate (3.0%) of primary hypothyroidism in the postpartum period, although in most cases the disorder was transient. The prevalence of persistent primary hypothyroidism was only 0.2% but this figure was still far higher than that for postpartum pituitary hypothyroidism ($p < .001$).

The thyrotoxic state usually persisted for 1 to 2 months, but in three cases it persisted for nearly 3 months. None of the patients with postpartum thyrotoxicosis had neck pain or fever. All cases of thyrotoxicosis except one were considered to have been induced by thyroid destruction, because of the later development of hypothyroidism, a low T_3/T_4 (nanograms/micrograms) ratio (<20), or low radioactive iodine uptake. Table 5 compares the symptoms of patients with post-

Table 5.   Frequency of symptoms observed in 20 patients with postpartum thyrotoxicosis and 254 postpartum controls

Symptom	Thyrotoxicosis No. (%)	Controls No. (%)
Shoulder stiffness	13 (65)	119 (47)
Fatigue	11 (55)[a]	75 (30)
Increased appetite	8 (40)	72 (28)
Increased sweating	4 (20)	23 (9)
Palpitation	4 (20)[b]	13 (5)
Nervousness	3 (15)	39 (15)
Hypersensitivity to heat	2 (10)	22 (9)
Weight loss	1 (5)	8 (3)
Total no. examined	20	254

[a] *Significantly different from controls at* $p < .02$ *by chi-square test.*
[b] *Significantly different from controls at* $p < .05$ *by chi-square test.*
(Data from Ref. 27.)

partum thyrotoxicosis with those of postpartum controls. Control subjects had many symptoms. Therefore, only fatigue and palpitation were significantly different in prevalence when the patients were compared with the controls. However, the severity of these symptoms was more marked in the patients in whom thyrotoxicosis continued for more than 2 months.

At 3 months postpartum, antithyroid antibodies were found in 62 subjects (12.2%). This prevalence was significantly higher than that in the nonpregnant controls of similar age (7.8%) ($p < .002$). The development of postpartum thyroid dysfunction was not related to age, parity, breast feeding, or the economic situation of the mother. Interestingly, 22 of 28 patients (79%) with postpartum thyroid dysfunction gave birth to girls, in contrast to 208 of 442 controls (47%) ($p < .01$). In all, 30 subjects had antithyroid-antibody titers of 10×2^7 or higher 3 months postpartum, and of these, 18 had girls and 12 had boys. In 13 of the former 18 subjects (72%) and in three of the latter 12 subjects (25%) postpartum thyroid dysfunction occurred ($p < .05$). It is possible that the gestational and postpartum state of immunologic surveillance in women who conceive females differs from that in women who conceive males.

Interestingly, the condition of three of these patients mimicked so-called postpartum psychosis (30, 31): one with postpartum depression and two with postpartum acute transitory excitement. It is interesting to speculate that an acute, dramatic change in serum levels of thyroid hormones may induce overt psychosis in subjects with a predisposition to psychosis.

7.   POSTPARTUM AUTOIMMUNE HYPOPHYSITIS

Hypopituitarism occurring after delivery has long been known as a Sheehan's syndrome (7) and a spasm involving the arteries which supply the anterior lobe was suggested as a pathogenic factor (32), although underlying pathophysiology was not completely understood.

Recently there have been reports that such pituitary dysfunction might also be induced by lymphoid hypophysitis of autoimmune nature (33–41). Reported cases are summarized in Table 6. Lymphoid hypophysitis was diagnosed postmortem in cases 1 to 7 and antemortem in cases 8 and 9. All patients were females and five of nine cases have occurred within 14 months postpartum. Very interestingly, cases 1 and 7 seemed to be complicated with postpartum thyroiditis. Case 1 had developed tiredness and listlessness associated with thyroid enlargment after delivery (33), suggesting the complication with postpartum primary hypothyroidism. Case 7 had increased free thyroxine index with low radioactive iodine uptake (39), suggesting destructive thyrotoxicosis at 3 months after delivery. In case 8 a low titer of antibodies apparently reacting with all cell types of the anterior pituitary was demonstrated (40). Cases 1 to 8 had signs and symptoms of pituitary insufficiency but case 9 had hyperprolactinemia and mimicked postpartum amenorrhea–galactorrhea syndrome (42).

Levine (43) had induced an experimental allergic adenohypophysitis in rats, similar to human lymphoid hypophysitis, by injecting autologous pituitary homogenate with adjuvant. He found that the severity of hypophysitis was greater in postpartum rats. Engelberth and Jezkova (44) reported that 18% of women at the fifth to seventh postpartum day had pituitary autoantibodies. Twenty-five percent of women with positive pituitary antibodies, but 4% of women without antibodies, developed some signs of hypopituitarism at 6 to 12 months after delivery. They also found a high titer of antibodies in a woman with Sheehan's syndrome (44). The frequent occurrence of lymphoid hypophysitis in the postpartum period in association with postpartum thyroiditis strongly suggests that the pituitary may also be the subject of autoimmune damage during the postpartum period. It is necessary to reevaluate the pathogenesis of pituitary dysfunction in patients with so-called Sheehan's syndrome, since 79% of patients with postpartum hypopituitarism

Table 6. Reported cases of lymphoid hypophysitis

Case No.	Authors	Reported Year	Ref.	Age/ Sex	Onset	Pathology in Pituitary Gland[a]	Clinical Manifestations	Other Findings
1	Goudie and Pinkerton	1962	33	22/F	14 months postpartum	Atrophic pituitary with lymphocytic infiltration in anterior lobe	Amenorrhea, vascular collapse following surgery	Hashimoto's disease (postpartum thyroiditis), adrenal atrophy
2	Hume and Roberts	1967	34	74/F	Insidious	Atrophic anterior lobe with severe lymphocytic infiltration	Unconsciousness, scanty body hair, pallor, waxy skin	Pernicious anemia, focal chronic thyroiditis, adrenal atrophy
3	Egloff et al.	1969	35	29/F	12 months postpartum	Marked destruction of anterior lobe with lymphocytic infiltration	Recurrent hypoglycemic coma, amenorrhea	Atrophy of adrenal cortex
4	Kliaer and Norgaard	1969	36	74/F	Insidious	Pronounced lymphocytic infiltration in anterior lobe	Myxedema, shock after institution of thyroid medication	Hashimoto's disease, lymphoid adrenalitis
5	Lack	1975	37	42/F	Insidious	Lymphocytic infiltration with germinal center in adenohypophysis	Anemia, hypothyroidism, body hair, possible sepsis	Schizophrenia, adrenal atrophy
6	Gleason et al.	1978	38	60/F	Insidious	Enlarged pituitary with destructive lymphoid cell infiltrate and fibrosis	Fatigue, anorexia, recurrent hypoglycemic coma, arthralgia	

(continued on p. 260)

Table 6. (continued)

Case No.	Authors	Reported Year	Ref.	Age/Sex	Onset	Pathology in Pituitary Gland[a]	Clinical Manifestations	Other Findings
7	Richts-meier et al.	1980	39	31/F	2–3 months post-partum	Atrophic anterior lobe with heavy lymphocytic infiltration	Lethargy, ano-rexia, weakness, hypercalcemia, hypoglycemia, cardiac arrest	Postpartum thyroiditis, lymphoid adrenalitis
8	Mayfield et al.	1980	40	23/F	7 months post-partum	Lymphoid cell infiltra-tion in anterior lobe	Headache, visual disturbance fatigue anorexia	
9	Porto-carrero et al.	1981	41	25/F	5 months post-partum	Lymphocytic infiltra-tion and focal germinal center formation asso-ciated with extensive stromal fibrosis	Headache, galac-torrhea, amenorrhea	Hyperpro-lactinemia

[a] Lymphoid hypophysitis was diagnosed at autopsy in cases 1–7. Histological findings were obtained at transsphenoidal exploration in cases 8 and 9.

might have associated autoimmune thyroiditis (27, 28). Awareness of postpartum autoimmune hypophysitis may result in earlier recognition and successful treatment of what otherwise can be a potentially fatal condition (39).

8. MECHANISMS IN POSTPARTUM THYROID DYSFUNCTION

8.1. Other Autoimmune Diseases and Pregnancy

During pregnancy maternal immune reactions are regulated to prevent rejection of the fetal allograft (1, 2). Cell-mediated immunity (45, 46), as well as humoral immunity (47), is depressed during pregnancy. These physiological immunologic changes may influence the clinical course of autoimmune diseases.

An ameliorating effect of pregnancy on rheumatoid arthritis was described as early as the mid-nineteenth century (48), and this fact led Hench to discover steroid hormone therapy in 1949 (49). It is now well recognized that rheumatoid arthritis is ameliorated during pregnancy but aggravated after delivery (49, 50). Oka observed frequent onsets of rheumatoid arthritis at 0 to 6 months after delivery (50). As for systemic lupus erythematosus (SLE), it is not clear whether pregnancy affects SLE patients adversely or has a beneficial effect. Friedman and Rutherford reported the exacerbation of disease during the first trimester of pregnancy (51), but it seemed to be ameliorated in the latter half of pregnancy (51, 52). However, consistent results were obtained that disease activity exacerbated during the first 8 weeks postpartum (51, 52). The simultaneous onset of postpartum thyroiditis and SLE has also been reported (14). In patients with scleroderma, pregnancy seemed to have no effect on the course of disease (53). The course of myasthenia gravis during pregnancy is variable but the great danger is a relapse in the postpartum period,

especially during the first 3 weeks (54, 55). Some patients may develop fatal crises. The effect of pregnancy on idiopathic thrombocytopenic purpura is poorly understood, since treatment greatly modifies the spontaneous course of the disease (56), although Lorz and Frumin (57) reported a spontaneous remission of disease during pregnancy. Ulcerative colitis is often aggravated in the first 3 months of pregnancy and in the puerperium, but attacks of colitis are relatively infrequent between the fourth month and term (58). Alopecia areata, some cases of which are considered to be an autoimmune disorder, were also reported to be ameliorated during pregnancy (59). Considering all these data, it seems probable that autoimmune disease, in general, is ameliorated during pregnancy and aggravated after delivery.

8.2. Postpartum Aggravation of Hashimoto's Disease

In Hashimoto's disease, cytotoxic immune reactions, such as complement-dependent cytotoxic antibody (60), antibody-dependent cell-mediated cytotoxicity (61), direct lymphocyte cytotoxicity (62, 63), and lymphotoxin (64), have been demonstrated in vitro. These reactions are illustrated in Figure 10. However, it is unknown which is the most important destructive factor in vivo.

Titers of antithyroid microsomal antibodies and peripheral lymphocyte counts decrease

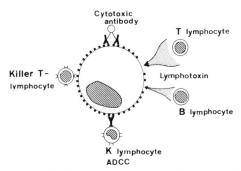

Figure 10. Cytotoxic immune reactions in Hashimoto's disease.

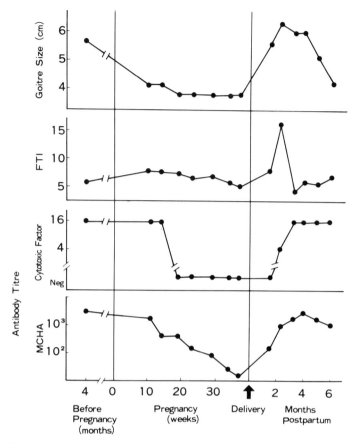

Figure 11. Changes of goiter size, free thyroxine index (FTI), cyutotoxic factor (antibody), and microsomal antibody (MCHA) during and after pregnancy in patients with Hashimoto's disease.

as pregnancy progresses, but increase after delivery in patients with Hashimoto's disease (Fig. 3). As shown in Figure 11, activities of cytotoxic antibody also decrease during pregnancy and increase at the time of postpartum aggravation. To examine changes in lymphocyte subpopulations, peripheral T, B, and K lymphocytes were enumerated in Hashimoto's disease (Table 7). During pregnancy a significant decrease in K lymphocytes was observed but not in T or B lymphocytes. At the time of postpartum aggravation, a significant increase was found in total lymphocyte counts, and B and K lymphocytes. Figure 12 shows the serial changes in peripheral T and B lymphocytes during and after delivery in

a patient with Hashimoto's disease. Immediately after delivery, the T cell percentage began to decrease and that of B cells increased. At the time of postpartum hypothyroidism, populations of T and B cells were inverted but returned to normal in association with spontaneous recovery of thyroid destruction. Figure 13 shows individual values of peripheral K lymphocyte counts in Hashimoto's disease. These data on postpartum increases in antithyroid antibodies and K and B lymphocytes suggest that antibody-dependent cell-mediated cytotoxicity (ADCC) may be important in postpartum autoimmune thyroid destruction. The role of direct lymphocyte cytotoxicity and lymphotoxin needs to be studied further.

Table 7. Peripheral T, B, and K lymphocytes in healthy subjects and patients with Hashimoto's disease[a]

	No. Examined	Total Lymphocyte (Count/mm³)	Percentage			Absolute Count/mm³		
			T Cells	B Cells	K Cells	T Cells	B Cells	K Cells
Nonpregnant healthy females	20	1768 ± 465	75.9 ± 5.5	21.8 ± 5.1	4.6 ± 1.6	1331 ± 329	393 ± 157	81 ± 39
Hashimoto's disease								
Nonpregnant	25	1899 ± 468	76.5 ± 7.8	19.0 ± 7.5	5.4 ± 2.4	1452 ± 402	368 ± 184	103 ± 67
Pregnant	16	1555 ± 297	73.8 ± 11.6	25.3 ± 12.9	3.1 ± 1.2[d]	1160 ± 263	403 ± 255	49 ± 23[d]
Postpartum[b]	36	2339 ± 429[e]	68.9 ± 9.1[d]	27.6 ± 8.9†	6.2 ± 2.4[c]	1625 ± 421[d]	635 ± 206[e]	147 ± 64[e]

[a] Values are means ± SD.
[b] Values at the time of postpartum aggravation of Hashimoto's disease.
[c-e] Difference from healthy controls at p < .05 ([c]), p < .01 ([d]), and p < .001 ([e]).

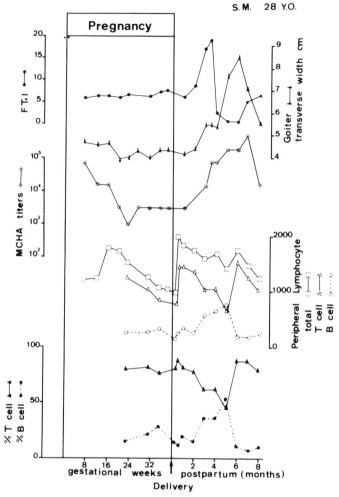

Figure 12.   Serial changes of T and B lymphocytes during and after delivery in a patient with Hashimoto's disease.

8.3.   Postpartum Aggravation of Graves' Disease

It is generally accepted that Graves' disease is an autoimmune disorder, and several reports have appeared indicating that circulating immunoglobulin plays an essential role in the development of the hyperthyroidism (see Chapter 6) (3, 65, 66). However, thyroid-stimulating antibody (TSAb) was not found in every patient with Graves' disease (66, 67) and did not always correlate with the severity of thyrotoxicosis (68). In some cases,

recurrence of hyperthyroidism was not associated with detectable activity of TSAb (69). Thus the hypothesis that humoral antibodies are entirely responsible for thyroid stimulation in Graves' disease is dependent upon the validity of the bioassay techniques available. Figure 14 shows the relation of TSAb activity and postpartum relapse of Graves' thyrotoxicosis (67). The titer of MCHA increased in association with the recurrence of hyperthyroidism. However, no TSAb activity was detectable during pregnancy or at the time of development of hyperthyroidism, but it was

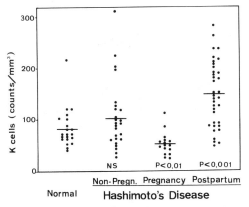

Figure 13. Peripheral K lymphocyte counts at various conditions of Hashimoto's disease. Postpartum values were obtained at the time of postpartum aggravation of disease.

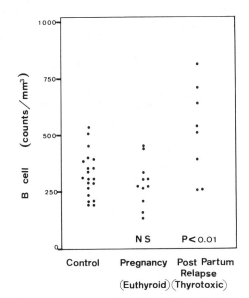

Figure 15. Increase of peripheral B lymphocyte at postpartum relapse of stimulative thyrotoxicosis in Graves' disease.

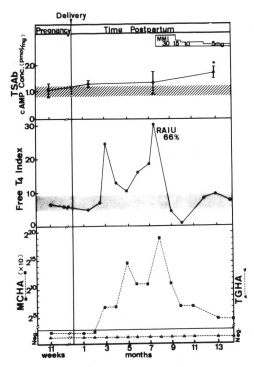

Figure 14. Changes in TSAb, FT$_4$ index, and antithyroid antibodies during pregnancy and after delivery in Graves' disease. TSAb values are shown as the mean (± SE) cAMP concentrations (picomoles per milligram tissue). The asterisk indicates positive TSAb activity. Range (mean ± SD) of cAMP concentration accumulated by thyroid slices in pooled normal Ig, normal range of FT$_4$ index. (Data from Ref. 67.)

detectable in the euthyroid state after therapy. No correlation between postpartum relapse of hyperthyroidism and TSAb activity was found in the other patients. These prospective studies suggest that circulating TSAb may not be detectable in patients with recurrent hyperthyroidism after delivery in Graves' disease.

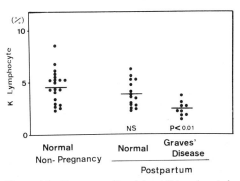

Figure 16. Percentage of peripheral K lymphocyte in normal female subjects, either at nonpregnant or postpartum period, and in patients with Graves' disease at the time of postpartum relapse of hyperthyroidism.

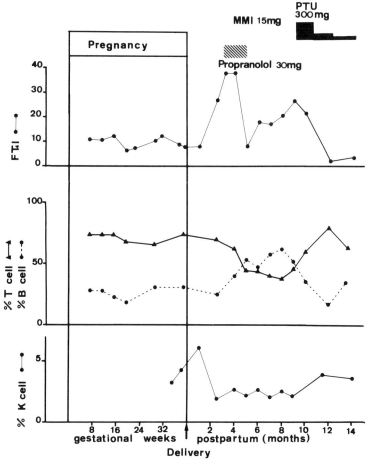

Figure 17. Serial changes of peripheral T, B, and K lymphocytes during and after delivery in the patients with Graves' disease. Hyperthyroidism relapsed 2 months postpartum.

As for lymphocyte subpopulations, a significant increase in peripheral B lymphocytes was observed at the time of relapse of Graves' thyrotoxicosis after delivery (Fig. 15). This result is compatible with the report of B lymphocyte increase in untreated patients with Graves' disease (70). Increases in B lymphocytes may be the characteristic of the "active state" in both Graves' and Hashimoto's diseases. Contrary to Hashimoto's disease, the percentage of peripheral K lymphocytes was lower at the time of postpartum recurrence of stimulative thyrotoxicosis than that of nonpregnant or postpartum normal females (Fig. 16). Figure 17 shows the serial changes of T, B, and K lymphocytes in a patient with Graves' disease in whom stimulative thyrotoxicosis relapsed after delivery. It is suggested that the higher number of K lymphocytes, which have ADCC, leads to reduced thyroid function in autoimmune thyroid disease (71). A decrease in K lymphocytes may be related to decreased activity of ADCC, and a small amount of stimulating factors may easily induce marked hyperthyroidism in Graves' disease. Further studies, including cellular immune reactions within the thyroid gland, are necessary to elucidate the precise mechanisms involved in postpartum relapse of hyperthyroidism.

8.4.   Immune Rebound Hypothesis

Autoimmune diseases often ameliorate during pregnancy and are aggravated more frequently after delivery, as described above. Many factors related to gestation have been reported to have immunosuppressive activities (see Chapter 12). These factors are summarized in Table 8. Possibly all these factors may work for protection of the fetal allograft, although it is unknown which is the most important factor during pregnancy. Immu-

Table 8.   Immunoregulatory substances in pregnancy

Pregnancy Serum Proteins

α-Fetoprotein (AFP)

Pregnancy-associated proteins

  α_2-Globulins

   Pregnancy zone protein (PZ)

   Pregnancy-associated macroglobulin (PAM)

   Pregnancy-associated globulin (PAG)

   Pregnancy-associated plasma proteins (PAPP)

  β_1-Globulins

   "Schwangerschafts-proteine"-1,2,3 (SP-1,2,3)

   Pregnancy-specific β-globulin (PSBG)

   β_1-Glycoprotein (β_1-GP)

Soluble Substance Produced by Fetal Lymphocytes

Placental Proteins

Human chorionic gonadotrophin (HCG)

Human placental lactogen (HPL)

Placental proteins 1–6 (PP1–6)

Placental transcortin

Other relatively minor proteins

Antibodies

Antibodies to paternal HLA antigens

Antibodies to placental antigens

Hormones

Glucocorticoids

Estrogens

  Estrone (E_1)

  Estradiol (E_2)

  Estriol (E_3)

Progesterone

Androgens

Aldosterone

Human chorionic gonadotrophin (HCG)

Human placental lactogen (HPL)

  = Human placental somatomammotropin (HCS)

Prolactin

Prostagrandins

  PGE_1 and E_2

  $PGF_1\alpha$ and $F_2\alpha$

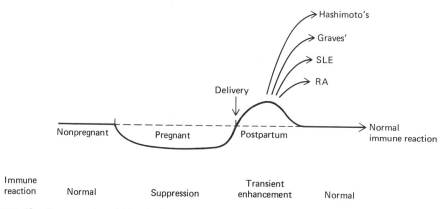

Figure 18. Immune rebound hypothesis regarding the postpartum onset of autoimmune diseases. Possible immunosuppression in pregnancy may disappear at delivery. "Transient enhancement" of the immune reactions may occur after delivery.

nosuppression induced by these factors in pregnancy may disappear rapidly at delivery and "transient enhancement" of immune reaction may occur after delivery by a somewhat similar mechanism to the "rebound phenomenon" observed after withdrawal of immunosuppressive glucocorticoid therapy. This immune rebound hypothesis is illustrated in Figure 18. Postpartum enhancement of immune reaction may protect the mother from puerperal infection. However, overt disease may develop if she has a subclinical form of autoimmune disease. Diseases occurring after delivery should, therefore, be examined from the standpoint of an autoimmune abnormality.

9. NEONATAL THYROID DISEASE DUE TO ANTIBODY TRANSFER

It is well known that maternal IgG passes easily across the placenta to the fetus, although IgA, IgM, and IgE are impermeable. Therefore IgG autoantibodies in the mother reach the fetus, may produce pathological effects, and may induce neonatal transient autoimmune diseases, such as neonatal systemic lupus erythematosus (72), neonatal myasthenia gravis (73), neonatal Graves' disease (74), neonatal transient hypothyroidism (75), and neonatal thrombocytopenia (76). These phe-

nomena are ideal experimental systems from which to elucidate the mechanisms involved in the occurrence of autoimmune disease.

9.1. Neonatal Graves' Disease

Neonatal Graves' disease or thyrotoxicosis is an uncommon disorder occurring in about 1% of babies born from mothers with present or past history of Graves' disease (77). Symptoms are tachycardia, irritability, diarrhea, goiter, staring eyes, and voracious appetites with poor weight gain. Patients frequently have heart failure which is related to a high mortality rate in this disease. Most of the mothers were hyperthyroid at the time of pregnancy but some of them were on thyroid replacement therapy for hypothyroidism due to Hashimoto's disease (78, 79). Rosenberg et al. (80) first reported the activity of long-acting thyroid stimulator (LATS) in the blood of infants and suggested that LATS tranferred from mother might induce neonatal thyrotoxicosis. The biological half-life of circulating LATS in the infant was calculated to be 6 days (81), and this was consistent with the self-resolving nature of thyrotoxicosis. Munro et al. (77) suggested that measurement of LATS or LATS-protector activities in the maternal blood might enable the prediction of neonatal thyrotoxicosis. Very recently, however, Hoffman et al. (79) reported a case of neonatal Graves' disease without detectable LATS or LATS-protector, but they found TSAb activity, measured by the method of cyclic AMP accumulation, in the blood of the infant as well as in maternal blood. Thus the measurement of TSAb in maternal blood may be essential for prediction of neonatal thyrotoxicosis.

Robinson et al. (82) suggested that fetal thyrotoxicosis should be considered when a fetal heart rate was persistently above 160 beats per minute in a mother with present or past history of Graves' disease. Prevention of neonatal thyrotoxicosis was attempted with prenatal antithyroid drug therapy (82, 83) and seemed to be successful. Figure 19 shows the relation of fetal heart rate and serum levels of free thyroxine index in the second and third trimesters in the mothers with Graves'

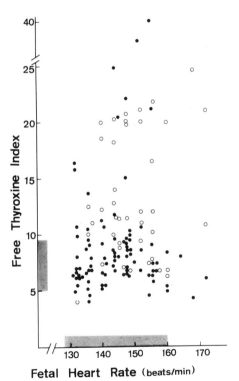

Figure 19. Relation of fetal heart rate and serum levels of free thyroxine index in mothers with Graves' disease. Shaded areas indicate the normal ranges. Patients with antithyroid drugs (○) and without drugs (●).

disease (84). No relation was found between the two, even though the possible effect of antithyroid drugs was considered. Data suggest that fetal heart rate may not always reflect the condition of fetal thyrotoxicosis or circulating TSAb activity may not correlate to the severity of maternal thyrotoxicosis.

Thyrotoxic symptoms are recognized usually in the first few hours of life, but when the mother is receiving antithyroid drugs up to the time of delivery, clinical and biochemical manifestations of thyrotoxicosis may be delayed from several days to several weeks of life. Delayed onset of neonatal thyrotoxicosis is explained by the rapid disappearance of antithyroid drugs from the neonatal blood contrary to persistence of thyroid stimulating IgG which may have a longer half-life. This disease is self-limiting. However, Levitsky et al. (85) reported a case of infantile persistent thyrotoxicosis which developed 3 months postpartum. Furthermore, Hollingsworth et al. (86) reported four familial cases with "congenital" Graves' disease in whom hyperthyroidism persisted for months or years. This congenital thyrotoxicosis occurred in infants from families with a high incidence of Graves' disease and is believed to be transmitted as an autosomal dominant trait with the predilection of the female infant (86). This type of congenital thyrotoxicosis cannot be explained by a simplistic maternal-to-fetal humoral theory. Similar types of congenital, persistent autoimmune disease were also found in myasthenia gravis (87). Fisher (88) speculated that neonatal Graves' disease could be due to (1) direct stimulation of circulating transplacentally acquired human thyroid stimulating antibodies (TSAb); (2) stimulation by circulating autonomously produced TSAb; (3) stimulation by TSAb produced by sensitized lymphocytes within the newborn's thyroid gland; (4) an inherent thyroidal hypersensitivity to TSAb; or (5) inherent thyroidal hyperactivity unrelated to TSAb.

Therapy should be started as soon as the diagnosis is established. Antithyroid drugs, iodine, β-blockers, sedatives, and glucocorticoids are used in proper combination. Propylthiouracil should be administered in doses of 5 to 10 milligrams per kilogram a day in divided doses at 8 hour intervals (88). The recommended dose of propranolol is 2 milligrams per kilogram a day divided into two or three portions (88). If patients present with severe thyrotoxic symptoms, prednisone (2 mg/kg/day) may be useful to acutely inhibit thyroid hormone secretion and block the peripheral conversion of thyroxine to triiodothyronine. Complicated congestive heart failure must be treated with digitalis (digoxin 75 μg/kg/day) and β-blockers should not be used.

9.2. Transient Neonatal Hypothyroidism

Regarding the relation of maternal thyroid antibodies to neonatal thyroid dysfunction, Blizzard et al. (89) first described the significant association between the two, although Parker et al. (90) could not confirm this association. In 1960, Sutherland et al. (91) reported on children with familial nongoitrous cretinism born of a hypothyroid mother with Hashimoto's disease. Their hypothyroidism was partially reversible. In 1973 Goldsmith et al. (92) further studied this family and suggested that the transplacental transfer of some unknown thyrosuppressive factor(s) might induce congenital, nongoitrous hypothyroidism. These studies suggested that some congenital hypothyroidism may be induced by transplacental maternal antibodies, although the exact mechanism or nature of pertinent antibodies is unclarified.

Recently Endo et al. (93) found that TSH-binding inhibitor immunoglobulins (TBII) blocked the cyclic AMP stimulation induced by TSH or TSAb. Matsuura et al. (75) reported a familial neonatal transient hypothyroidism induced by transplacental transfer of maternal TBII. This TBII did not stimulate the thyroid gland but inhibited the thyroid stimulation induced by TSH. Two siblings had congenital hypothyroidism and were treated with thyroid hormones. Replacement therapy was discon-

tinued at 12 and 17 months of life, respectively, but recurrence of hypothyroidism was not observed. Their mother had juvenile onset hypothyroidism due to Hashimoto's disease. Babies born of hypothyroid mothers with Hashimoto's disease should, therefore, be carefully examined for the possibility of transient neonatal hypothyroidism. Measurement of TBII in maternal blood may be useful for prediction of this disease.

Recent progress in mass screening for congenital hypothyroidism has found many cases of neonatal hypothyroidism. Most cases are due to thyroid dysgenesis (94, 95) and thyroid autoimmunity is an infrequent cause of congenital hypothyroidism (96). Neonatal screening has revealed different types of transient neonatal hypothyroidism (97, 98) and transient infantile hyperthyrotropinemia (99). These cases had no abnormality in thyroid autoimmunity and their underlying pathophysiology is still unknown. Autoimmune neonatal hypothyroidism should carefully be differentiated from these conditions by measurement of circulating thyroid antibodies.

REFERENCES

1. A. E. Beer and R. E. Billingham, *Adv. Immunol.* **14**, 1 (1971).

2. N. Gleicher, G. Deppe, and C. J. Cohen, *Obstet. Gynecol.* **54**, 335 (1979).

3. A. Kidd, N. Okita, V. V. Row, and R. Volpé, *Metabolism* **29**, 80 (1980).

4. N. Amino, K. Miyai, T. Onishi, T. Hashimoto, K. Arai, K. Ishibashi, and Y. Kumahara, *J. Clin. Endocrinol. Metab.* **42**, 296 (1976).

5. N. Amino, K. Miyai, T. Yamamoto, R. Kuro, F. Tanaka, O. Tanizawa, and Y. Kumahara, *J. Clin. Endocrinol. Metab.* **44**, 130 (1977).

6. J. Ginsberg and P. Walfish, *Lancet* **1**, 1125 (1977).

7. H. L. Sheehan, *J. Pathol. Bacteriol.* **45**, 189 (1937).

8. H. E. W. Roberton, *Br. Med. J. Suppl.* **2**, 2275 (1948).

9. R. Fraser and O. Garrod, *Br. Med. J.* **2**, 1484 (1955).

10. G. N. Burrow, in G. N. Burrow and T. F. Ferris, Eds., *Medical Complications During Pregnancy*, Saunders, Philadelphia, 1975, p. 196.

11. J. C. Nelson and F. J. Palmer, *J. Clin. Endocrinol. Metab.* **40**, 383 (1975).

12. N. Amino, H. Mori, Y. Yabu, T. Yamada, Y. Iwatani, R. Kuro, Y. Hisa, O. Tanizawa, and K. Miyai, in J. R. Stockigt and S. Nagataki, Eds., *Thyroid Research VIII*, The Australian Academy of Science, Sydney, 1980, p. 551.

13. N. Amino, Y. Yabu, T. Miki, S. Morimoto, Y. Kumahara, H. Mori, Y. Iwatani, K. Nishi, K. Nakatani, and K. Miyai, *J. Clin. Endocrinol. Metab.* **53**, 113 (1981).

14. N. Amino, K. Miyai, R. Kuro, O. Tanizawa, M. Azukizawa, S. Takai, F. Tanaka, K. Nishi, M. Kawashima, and Y. Kumahara, *Ann. Intern. Med.* **87**, 155 (1977).

15. H. Gardiner-Hill, *Lancet* **1**, 120 (1929).

16. E. B. Astwood, *J. Clin. Endocrinol. Metab.* **11**, 1045 (1951).

17. H. M. Clute and D. H. Daniels, *Am. J. Med. Sci.* **179**, 477 (1930).

18. N. Amino, O. Tanizawa, H. Mori, Y. Iwatani, T. Yamada, K. Kurachi, Y. Kumahara, and K. Miyai, *J. Clin. Endocrinol. Metab.* 55, 108 (1982).

19. L. C. Wood and S. H. Ingbar, *J. Clin. Invest.* **64**, 1429 (1979).

20. J. T. Dowling, N. Frienkel, and S. H. Ingbar, *J. Clin. Invest.* **35**, 1263 (1956).

21. N. Amino, R. Kuro, O. Tanizawa, F. Tanaka, C. Hayashi, K. Kotani, M. Kawashima, K. Miyai, and Y. Kumahara, *Clin. Exp. Immunol.* **31**, 30 (1978).

22. T. F. Nikolai, J. Brosseau, M. A. Kettrick, R. Roberts, and E. Beltaos, *Arch. Intern. Med.* **140**, 478 (1980).

23. B. I. Hoffbrand and S. C. Webb, *Postgrad. Med. J.* **54**, 793 (1978).

24. H. G. Fein, J. M. Goldman, and B. D. Weintraub, *Am. J. Obstet. Gynecol.* **138**, 504 (1980).

25. E. J. Shahady and G. M. Meckler, *J. Family Practice* **11**, 1049 (1980).

26. N. Amino and K. Miyai, *Lancet* **2**, 585 (1978).

27. N. Amino, H. Mori, Y. Iwatani, O. Tanizawa, M. Kawashima, I. Tsuge, K. Ibaragi, Y. Kumahara, and K. Miyai, *N. Engl. J. Med.* **306**, 849 (1982).

28. H. L. Sheehan, *Q. J. Med.* **8**, 277 (1939).

29. H. L. Sheehan, *J. Obstet. Gynaecol. Br. Commonw.* **72**, 103 (1965).

30. D. A. Boyd, *Am. J. Obstet. Gynecol.* **43**, 148 (1942).

31. C. L. Thomas and J. E. Gordon, *Am. J. Med. Sci.* **238**, 363 (1959).

32. H. L. Sheehan and J. P. Stanfield, *Acta Endocrinol.* **37**, 479 (1961).

33. R. B. Goudie and P. H. Pinkerton, *J. Pathol. Bacteriol.* **83**, 584 (1962).

34. R. Hume and G. H. Roberts, *Br. Med. J.* **2**, 548 (1967).

35. B. Egloff, W. Fischbacher, and E. von Goumoëns, *Schweiz. Med. Wochenschr.* **99**, 1499 (1969).

36. W. Kliaer and J. O. R. Norgaard, *Acta Path. Microbiol.* **76**, 229 (1969).

37. E. E. Lack, *Arch. Pathol.* **99**, 215 (1975).

38. T. H. Gleason, P. L. Stebbins, and M. F. Shanahan, *Arch. Pathol. Lab. Med.* **102**, 46 (1978).

39. A. J. Richtsmeier, R. A. Henry, J. M. E. Bloodworth, and E. N. Ehrlich, *Arch. Intern. Med.* **140**, 1243 (1980).

40. R. K. Mayfield, J. H. Levine, L. Gordon, J. Powers, R. M. Galbraith, and S. E. Rawe, *Am. J. Med.* **69**, 619 (1980).

41. C. J. Portocarrero, A. G. Robinson, A. T. Taylor, and I. Klein, *J. Am. Med. Assoc.* **246**, 1811 (1981).

42. R. A. H. Kinch, E. R. Plunkett, and M. C. Devlin, *Am. J. Obstet. Gynecol.* **105**, 766 (1969).

43. S. Levine, *Science* **158**, 1190 (1967).

44. O. Engelberth and Z. Jezkova, *Lancet* **1**, 1075 (1965).

45. R. Finn, C. A. St. Hill, A. J. Govan, I. G. Ralfs, F. J. Gurney, and V. Denye, *Br. Med. J.* **3**, 150 (1972).

46. Y. H. Thong, R. W. Steele, M. M. Vincent, S. A. Hensen, and J. A. Bellanti, *N. Engl. J. Med.* **289**, 604 (1973).

47. N. Amino, O. Tanizawa, K. Miyai, F. Tanaka, C. Hayashi, M. Kawashima, and K. Ichihara, *Obstet. Gynecol.* **52**, 415 (1978).

48. P. S. Hench, *Proc. Staff Meet. Mayo Clin.* **24**, 167 (1949).

49. P. S. Hench, E. C. Kendall, C. H. Slocumb, and H. F. Polley, *Ann. Rheum. Dis.* **8**, 97 (1949).

50. M. Oka, *Ann. Rheum. Dis.* **12**, 227 (1953).

51. E. A. Friedman and J. W. Rutherford, *Obstet. Gynecol.* **8**, 601 (1956).

52. M. Garsenstein, V. E. Pollak, and R. M. Kark, *N. Engl. J. Med.* **267**, 165 (1962).

53. W. M. Spellacy, *Obstet. Gynecol.* **23**, 297 (1964).

54. D. Fraser and J. W. A. Turner, *Lancet* **2**, 417 (1953).

55. W. C. Plauche, *Am. J. Obstet. Gynecol.* **135**, 691 (1979).

56. R. F. Heys, *Obstet. Gynecol.* **28**, 532 (1966).

57. H. M. Lorz and A. M. Frumin, *Obstet. Gynecol.* **17**, 362 (1961).

58. F. C. Walker, in *The Surgical Management of Ulcerative Colitis*, F. C. Walker, Ed., Butterworth, London, 1969, p. 39.

59. J. C. Seelen, L. A. M. Stolte, J. H. J. Bakker, and E. Verboom, *Acta Endocrinol.* **23**, 60 (1956).

60. R. J. V. Pulvertaft, D. Doniach, and I. M. Roitt, *Br. J. Exp. Pathol.* **42**, 496 (1961).

61. E. A. Calder, W. J. Penhale, D. McLeman, E. W. Barnes, and W. J. Irvine, *Clin. Exp. Immunol.* **14**, 153 (1973).

62. W. K. Podleski, *Clin. Exp. Immunol.* **11**, 543 (1972).

63. Y. Iwatani, N. Amino, H. Mori, S. Asari, F. Matsuzuka, K. Kuma, and K. Miyai, *J. Immunol. Methods* **48**, 241 (1982).

64. N. Amino and L. J. DeGroot, *Cell. Immunol.* **11**, 188 (1974).

65. T. F. Davies, P. P. B. Yeo, D. C. Evered, F. Clark, B. R. Smith, and R. Hall, *Lancet* **2**, 1181 (1977).

66. J. M. Mckenzie and M. Zakarija, in E. Klein, F. A. Horster, and D. Beysel, Eds., *Autoimmunity in Thyroid Disease*, Schattauer Verlag, Stuttgart, 1979, p. 107.

67. Y. Yabu, N. Amino, H. Mori, K. Miyai, O. Tanizawa, S. Takai, Y. Kumahara, F. Matsuzuka, and K. Kuma, *J. Clin. Endocrinol. Metab.* **51**, 1454 (1980).

68. N. Kuzuya, S. C. Chin, H. Ikeda, H. Uchimura, K. Ito, and S. Nagataki, *J. Clin. Endocrinol. Metab.* **48**, 706 (1979).

69. D. F. Gardner and R. D. Utiger, *J. Clin. Endocrinol. Metab.* **49**, 417 (1979).

70. H. Mori, N. Amino, Y. Iwatani, O. Kabutomori, S. Asari, S. Motoi, K. Miyai, and Y. Kumahara, *Clin. Exp. Immunol.* **42**, 33 (1980).

71. N. Amino, H. Mori, Y. Iwatani, S. Asari, Y. Izumiguchi, and K. Miyai, *J. Clin. Endocrinol. Metab.* **54**, 587 (1982).

72. J. D. Hardy, S. Solomon, G. S. Banwall, R. Beach, V. Wright, and F. M. Howard, *Arch. Dis. Child.* **54**, 7 (1979).

73. T. Namba, S. B. Brown, and D. Grob, *Pediatrics* **45**, 488 (1970).

74. J. M. McKenzie and M. Zakarija, *J. Endocrinol. Invest.* **2**, 183 (1978).

75. N. Matsuura, Y. Yamada, Y. Nohara, J. Konishi, K. Kasagi, K. Endo, H. Kojima, and K. Wataya, *N. Engl. J. Med.* **303**, 738 (1980).

76. L. M. Kernoff, E. Malan, and K. Gunston, *Ann. Intern. Med.* **90**, 55 (1979).

77. D. S. Munro, S. M. Dirmikis, H. Humphries, T. Smith, and G. D. Broadhead, *Br. J. Obstet. Gynaecol.* **85**, 838 (1978).

78. J. A. Thomson and I. D. Riley, *Lancet* **1**, 635 (1966).

79. W. H. Hoffman, P. Sahasrananan, S. S. Ferandos, C. L. Burk, and N. R. Roge, *J. Clin. Endocrinol. Metab.* **54**, 354 (1982).

80. D. Rosenberg, M. J. H. Grand, and D. Silbert, *N. Engl. J. Med.* **268**, 292 (1963).

81. P. Sunshine, H. Kusumoto, and J. P. Kriss, *Pediatrics* **36**, 869 (1965).

82. P. L. Robinson, N. M. O'Mullane, and B. Alderman, *Br. Med. J.* **1**, 384 (1979).

83. I. Ramsay, *Brit. Med. J.* **2**, 1110 (1976).

84. N. Amino, T. Yamada, O. Tanizawa, and K. Miyai (submitted for publication).

85. L. L. Levitsky, E. Trias, and M. S. Grossman, *Pediatrics* **46**, 627 (1970).

86. D. R. Hollingsworth and C. C. Mabry, *Am. J. Dis. Child.* **130**, 148 (1976).

87. W. T. Mclean and R. C. McKone, *Arch. Neurol.* **29**, 223 (1973).

88. D. A. Fisher, *Am. J. Dis. Child.* **130**, 133 (1976).

89. R. M. Blizzard, R. W. Chandler, B. H. Landing, M. D. Pettit, and C. D. West, *N. Engl. J. Med.* **263**, 327 (1960).

90. R. H. Parker and W. H. Beierwaltes, *J. Clin. Endocrinol. Metab.* **21**, 792 (1961).

91. J. M. Sutherland, V. M. Esselborn, R. L. Burket, T. B. Skillman, J. T. Benson, *N. Engl. J. Med.* **263**, 336 (1960).

92. R. E. Goldsmith, A. J. McAdams, P. R. Larsen, M. Mackenzie, and E. V. Hess, *J. Clin. Endocrinol. Metab.* **37**, 265 (1973).

93. K. Endo, K. Kasagi, J. Konishi, K. Ikekubo, T. Okuno, Y. Takeda, T. Mori, and K. Torizuka, *J. Clin. Endocrinol. Metab.* **46**, 734 (1978).

94. P. G. Walfish, J. Ginsberg, R. A. Rosenberg, and N. J. Howard, *Arch. Dis. Child.* **54**, 171 (1979).

95. S. H. LaFranchi, W. H. Murphey, T. P. Foley, P. R. Larsen, and N. R. M. Buist, *Pediatrics* **63**, 180 (1979).

96. J. H. Dussault, J. Letarte, H. Guyda, and C. Laberge, *J. Pediatr.* **96**, 385 (1980).

97. S. H. LaFranchi, N. R. M. Buist, W. H. Murphey, P. R. Larsen, and T. P. Foley, *Pediatrics* **60**, 538 (1977).

98. F. Delange, J. Dodion, R. Wolter, P. Bourdoux, A. Dalhem, D. Glinoer, and A. M. Ermans, *J. Pediatr.* **92**, 974 (1978).

99. K. Miyai, N. Amino, K. Nishi, T. Fujie, K. Nakatani, O. Nose, T. Harada, H. Yabuuchi, K. Doi, T. Yamamoto, R. Satake, T. Tsuruhara, and T. Oura, *Arch. Dis. Child.* **54**, 965 (1979).

Index

Acetylcholine (ACh) receptor antibodies:
  measurement of, 107-108
  and myasthenia gravis, 104-109
  properties of, 106-107
Addison's disease, 195
  and adrenocortical autoantibodies,
    182-189
  in autoimmune polyglandular syndromes (APS),
    182
  cell-mediated autoimmunity and, 187-189
  clinical disorders associated with, 194
  HLA association of, 86
  idiopathic, 196, 199
  polyglandular failure and, 193-194
  prevalence of, 97-98
Adrenal antibodies, 186
β-Adrenergic receptor antibodies:
  and atopy, 117-120
  and autonomic sensitivity, 119
  significance of, 119-120
Adrenocortical autoantibodies, 182-189
Allotope, 7
Alopecia areata, and pregnancy, 261
Alpha fetoprotein (AFP), 241
"Altered self" concept, 14
Alternative pathway, 9
Anemia, pernicious, 32, 196
Antibodies, 6-8. *See also specific antibody*
Antibody-dependent cell-mediated cytotoxicity
  (ADCC), 262
Antibody molecules:
  regions of, 8
  structural genes for, 8
Antibody synthesis, and antigenic stimulus,
  13
Antisperm antibodies, human, 210-214
  agglutination assays for, 215-217
  immobilization assays for, 215-217
  radioimmunobinding assays for, 215-216
  therapy for, activity, 218
Antithyroid microsomal antibody (MCHA),
  250, 261-262
Asthma, 198
Atopy:
  β-adrenergic receptor antibodies and,
    117-120

and autonomic function, 117-119
Autoantigens, nature of, 23. *See also specific*
  autoantigen
Autoimmune disease:
  adjuvant-induced, 21-22
  features of, 20
  genetic predisposition to, 23-27
    H gene theory, 25-26
    linkage disequilibrium theory, 23-24
    and multiple dominant genes, 23
    V gene theory, 24-25
  histocompatibility antigens and, 25-26
  and lymphoid malignancies, 53-55
  sex and, 26
  therapy and prophylaxis of, 35
Autoimmune mechanisms, 1-39

Balanced genetic polymorphism, 6
B cell(s), 10, 72-73
  alloantigens, 11
Beta (β) cell function, 172-173
  adenylate cyclase-cyclic AMP system,
    172
  and cell surface antigens, 173
  effects of antibodies on, 173
  and glucose-stimulated insulin release,
    173
  glycolytic pathway, 172
  and insulin release, 172
  and insulin synthesis, 173
  and islet cell antibodies, 172-173
Burnet's forbidden clone theory, 20-22

Candidiasis, chronic, 219
Celiac disease, 198
Cell cooperation, and infection, 13-14
Cell-mediated immune responses, 142-144
  and lymphocytes sensitized to specific antigen,
    assessment of, 142
Cells, 9-10
C genes, 8
Chromosome, 8, 14
Classical pathway, 9
Clones:
  and antigenic stimulus, 12-13
  concept of, 3-4